Who Decides Who Decides?

T0144690

By the same author

The Re-Discovery of George Gissing. London: National Book League; 1971.
[with Pierre Coustillas]

'Things to Fix': An initiative using the best ideas of Brighton Health Care staff to help patients, staff and the organisation. Brighton: Brighton Health Care NHS Trust; 1994
[with Pauline Sinkins].

The Invisible Hospital and the Secret Garden: an insider's commentary on the NHS reforms. Oxford: Radcliffe Medical Press/London: Institute of Health Services Management; 1995.

An Innocent Elopement: patients and empowerment. [Lecture], London: The Patients Association; 1996.

Sense and Sensibility in Health Care. [co-author], edited by Marshall Marinker. London: British Medical Journal Publishing; 1996.

Who Owns Our Bodies? making moral choices in health care. Oxford: Radcliffe Medical Press/Southampton: Institute for Health Policy Studies; 1997.

User Involvement in Health Care: what next? London: Association of Charitable Foundations 4th Annual Lecture on Philanthropy; 1997.

Dilemmas in Modern Health Care. [editor] London: Social Market Foundation/ Profile Books; 1997.

'If this is a question, is this an answer? Patients and empowerment: first principles, moral problems, and patient benefit'. In: Ling, Tom, editor. *Reforming Healthcare by Consent.* Oxford: Radcliffe Medical Press; 1999.

The Realities of Rationing: 'priority setting' in the NHS. London: Institute of Economic Affairs; 1999.

Socialised Medicine in Great Britain: lessons for the Oregon Plan. Address to the Cascade Policy Institute, Portland, Oregon; 1999.

'Safe in whose hands? Effective consumer power in health care'. In: Vaizey, Edward, editor. *The Blue Book On Health.* London: Politicos; 2002.

Patients, Power, and Responsibility: the first principles of consumer-driven reform. Oxford: Radcliffe Medical Press in association with the Institute of Economic Affairs; 2003.

Gissing and the City: cultural crisis and the making of books in late Victorian England. [editor], Houndsmills: Palgrave Macmillan; 2006.

Serious about Series: American cheap libraries, British railway libraries, and some literary series of the 1890s. London: Institute of English Studies; 2007.

'Coming, Ready or Not!' The realities, the politics, and the future of the NHS: nine studies in change. Brighton: Edward Everett Root Publishers; 2008.

Who Decides Who Decides?

Enabling choice, equity, access, improved performance and patient guaranteed care

Professor JOHN SPIERS
School of Humanities and Social Studies,
University of Glamorgan
Visiting Fellow at the Institute of Economic Affairs,
and at Progressive Vision
Member, Advisory Council, Reform

Formerly, member of the Board of the National Care
Standards Commission; Chairman, Brighton Health
Authority, Brighton Health Care NHS Trust, the South East
Thames NHS Management College at David Salomons House
and The Patients Association

Foreword by

Professor PHILIP BOOTH
Editorial and Programme Director at the IEA,
and Professor of Insurance and Risk Management
at the Cass Business School, London

In association with the Institute of Economic Affairs

iea
www.iea.org.uk

Radcliffe Publishing
Oxford • New York

Radcliffe Publishing Ltd
18 Marcham Road
Abingdon
Oxon OX14 1AA
United Kingdom

www.radcliffe-oxford.com

Electronic catalogue and worldwide online ordering facility.

British Library Cataloguing in Publication Data

A catalogue record for this book is available from the British Library.

ISBN-13: 978 184619 276 0

Typeset by Pindar New Zealand (Egan Reid), Auckland, New Zealand
Printed and bound by Cadmus Communications, USA

Contents

This book is dedicated with gratitude to my dear grandmother, Kate Root (née Warren) born 20 May 1888, died 10 October 1973, and my dear mother, Kate Spiers (née Root) born 27 December 1907, died 13 September 1976.

'That's who we're here for, the folks with a quarter in their pocket.'
– TOBEY MAGUIRE AS 'SEABISCUIT'S' JOCKEY JOHNNY 'RED' POLLARD

'People are different.'
– VIRGINIA POSTREL

'Our job is improving the meaning of life, not just delaying death.'
– ROBIN WILLIAMS, AS DR HUNTER 'PATCH' ADAMS

'A free system can adapt itself to almost any set of data, almost any general prohibition or regulation, so long as the adjusting mechanism itself is kept functioning. And it is mainly changes in prices that bring about the necessary adjustments.'
– FRIEDRICH VON HAYEK

'Imagination and poetry, the only things which are ever permanent.'
– WB YEATS

'Business, like love, laughs at locksmiths.'
– DAVID S. LANDES

'None who have always been free can understand the terrible fascinating power of the hope of freedom on those who are not free.'
– PEARL S BUCK

'Freedom does not always win. This is one of the bitterest lessons of history.'
– AJP TAYLOR

'Freedom exists only where people take care of the government.'
– WOODROW WILSON

'A competitive price system selects that allocation that minimizes the total production cost. . . . This assertion is true, but not obvious. Individual producers care about their individual profits, not about economy wide costs. It is something of a miracle that individual selfish decisions must lead to a collectively efficient outcome [but] economists know that this miracle occurs.'
– STEVEN E LANDSBURG

'It is striking how timid the "free world" has become since the end of the Cold War. Everyone is for democracy, but no one trusts its institutions.'
– SUSAN BUCK-MORSS

'There are many who give up, and many who procrastinate, but there are some who go on.'
– CS FORESTER

About the author

Professor John Spiers has had an unusual career. He took a First Class Honours degree in History at the University of Sussex. While a graduate student there he founded The Harvester Press, the scholarly book publishing firm. He has been innovative entrepreneur, company executive, author and an adviser to government. He built his firm from scratch, founding it at age 28. The firm won the Queen's Award for Export Achievement in 1986, being only the third publishing firm to have done so then. He has since held national appointments in healthcare, education and the arts, and he has played a leading part in healthcare studies in several national 'think-tanks'.

John is a well-known independent speaker and writer on healthcare, on which he has lectured in Britain, America, Asia, Australia, and in Europe. He is not a member of a political party. He has been for a number of years a Visiting Fellow at the Institute of Economic Affairs, specialising in healthcare policy. He was also a member of Prime Minister John Major's Citizen's Charter Advisory Panel concerned with exploring measures of specific standards of service to consumers. He served as Chairman of Brighton Health Authority, Brighton Health Care Trust, the NHS South East Region David Salomons Management Centre, and The Patients Association, whose relaunch he led in 1995. He is a Fellow of the Royal Society of Arts. He was joint Chairman of Arts for Health.

In 2001 he was a founder member of the Advisory Council of Reform, the think-tank on whose advisory council he serves. He was Health Policy Adviser to The Social Market Foundation, and Chairman of The Health Policy Committee of The Centre for Policy Studies. He was an executive member of the National Association of Health Authorities and Trusts, and in 1999 an Adjunct Scholar at The Cascade Policy Institute, Portland, Oregon studying American healthcare policy. He was also the founding Chairman of the think-tank Civitas (to which he gave its name) in 2000. In November 2007 he was one of the first four Fellows appointed by Progressive Vision in London.

John holds three academic appointments. He has been since 1998 a Visiting Professor at the University of Glamorgan, initially in the Business School and now in Humanities and Social Studies. He is a Senior Research Fellow in the Institute of English Studies, University of London, where has published books on English Literature and publishing history. He is also a Visiting Fellow in the Ruskin Programme at the University of Lancaster, and a Trustee of the Ruskin Foundation.

He was appointed in 2001 to the Board of the new National Care Standards Commission, on which he served until 2004. He once toured The Royal Sussex County Hospital at Brighton in a wheelchair (and with a wheelchair-bound woman patient and her virtually blind husband) to dramatise what he called 'the invisible hospital'. This is the one which managers too often overlook but which is often the awkward and unwelcoming reality for patients. This tour promoted user-friendly access, although it made him unpopular with local consultants. He appointed the first-ever Patient's Advocate (Ms Bec Hanley) in an NHS Hospital, in 1991. He gave the Patient's Advocate direct access to himself and to other executives. She successfully provided information as well as listening, acting as a messenger within the system, mediating in disputes and trying to solve problems – as well as seeking to prevent their recurrence. This became a model for the NHS. However, it also underlined the need for financial empowerment of the individual. He also established the first Clinical Performance Improvement Unit in an NHS Hospital, in 1993.His chief hobbies include supporting The Arsenal, whom he first saw play as a young boy in the late 1940s.

Acknowledgements

I am indebted to my dear wife Leigh for the title of the book, and for much else – for her encouragement, perceptive suggestions, forbearance, and her computer skills at every stage in the research and the writing of this book. She first used the phrase 'who decides who decides?' in her MBA project work at Ashridge Management College when she was a senior NHS manager, and before she became an art historian. This phrase best captures the essence of all the issues concerning choice.

My thanks are also due to my colleagues at the Institute of Economic Affairs: to the Director General and Ralph Harris Fellow, John Blundell and to Editorial and Programme Director Professor Philip Booth. Philip has been particularly helpful to me on long-term elderly care funding but I have also much benefited from his detailed comments on other chapters. My thanks are also due to the late Arthur Seldon. All three have been inspirational leaders. Philip has also very generously provided the Foreword. Shane Frith, founder of Progressive Vision, has been supportive too, particularly on health savings accounts.

I am grateful to my friends and colleagues Professor Rod Dubrow-Marshall and Professor Michael Connolly of the University of Glamorgan for our conversations, especially concerning public sector management.

I am indebted to one of my several medical friends – Dr William Pickering – for our discussions over some 15 years, especially concerning the regulation of medical practice and of individual clinical performance. I much value his unfailing good humour and political incorrectness. If Dr Pickering's proposal for an independent medical inspectorate were adopted we would save many lives. His work can be read in David Gladstone (ed.), *Regulating Doctors* (London: Institute for the Study of Civil Society; 2000), and in regular contributions to the *British Medical Journal*.

Everyone who considers the prospects of consumer-driven reform is indebted to the pioneering work of Professor Regina E Herzlinger, of Harvard Business School, including the essential volume which she so expertly brought together, *Consumer-Driven Health Care* (San Francisco, Calif.: Jossey-Bass/John Wiley; 2004). *Sto magnis nominis umbra.*

I am grateful, too, to my friend Lucianne Sawyer CBE – a leader in sensitive and achievable service development – for much wise advice and information concerning social care, during our several years as members of the board of the National Care Standards Commission and since.

My publisher, Gillian Nineham, has been supportive over a lengthy period, this being the fourth of my healthcare books which she has published. I am grateful to her and to her colleagues – especially to Gregory Moxon, Ollie Judkins and Jamie Etherington – for all their professional expertise, guidance, encouragement and commitment. So, too, my thanks to the production and design staff. I owe much to the professionalism (and patience!) of Jane Gadd and the team at Pindar New Zealand and especially to Brian O'Flaherty for his skilled copy-editing, and John Moriarty for indexing.

We all stand on the shoulders of others. Pliny said in his *Natural History* that 'I have prefaced these volumes with the names of my authorities. I have done so because it is, in my opinion, a pleasant thing and one that shows an honourable modesty, to own up to those who were the means of one's achievements . . .' I am indebted to a number of writers, of course, whose works I credit. Virginia Postrel's two invaluable recent works are of the highest quality and importance: *The Future and its Enemies: the growing conflict over creativity, enterprise, and progress* (New York: The Free Press; 1998), and *The Substance of Style: how the rise of aesthetic value is remaking commerce, culture, and consciousness* (New York: HarperCollins; 2003; Harper Perennial edition; 2004). I have also much valued the remarkable work by Geoff Mulgan, *Good and Bad Power: the ideals and betrayals of government* (London: Allen Lane; 2006; Penguin Books edition, 2007).

The guidance in the works of James Buchanan and Gordon Tullock on 'public choice theory' (or the economics of politics) and in particular their insights into how producer interests behave in capturing monopoly and unpriced bureaucratic 'services' for their own benefit has been important. Professor Colin Robinson has served freedom and democracy superbly with his work editing and introducing *The Collected Works of Arthur Seldon*, published by the Liberty Fund in seven volumes in 2004–05. I am, too, grateful to the staff of the library at the King's Fund in London and at the British Library for their unfailing good humour and professional expertise.

It is conventional to say that the opinions expressed are, of course, my own and not necessarily of those organisations with which I am associated and to apologise for overlooked errors. My 'errors', as ever, are my own responsibility, and, indeed, my deliberate pleasure. I used to be wrong on policy initiatives for at least five years. But reform is catching me up, it seems. I appear to have got my errors down now to a matter of months. I hope to live long enough to see change pass me in the fast lane, and to stand in its warm light.

Finally, Eduardo, come back fit as soon as possible – well, strong, confident and scoring beautiful goals again!

JS
Twyford, Sussex

Foreword

The National Health Service is approaching its 60th birthday as I write this foreword. It is clear that it is not fit for purpose. Every day patients die or live in discomfort because they are victims of a giant experiment in central planning that we would not put up with in any other area of our lives.

Why do we suffer such central planning in health provision? The answer given by many is that health is so important that it cannot be left to the market. Furthermore it is argued that, in the provision of healthcare, the virtue of equality is more important than the pursuit of quality.

But, other goods and services are vital for a comfortable and dignified life too. And we know what the result would be if we submitted the provision and distribution of food, for example, to the vagaries of central planning. Grim uniformity and malnourishment were obvious symptoms of central planning of agriculture and food distribution in the former Soviet bloc. Grim uniformity and poor health are the obvious symptoms of the central planning of healthcare. Indeed, is it not ironic that those same central planners who tell us that healthcare is so important that it must be provided by the state are sitting in their offices trying to develop strategies to deal with the health implications of obesity caused by the superabundance of food that our free market system provides?

Furthermore, modern research now shows very clearly that the NHS does not lead to equality of provision. In a system where resources are distributed as a result of the decisions of bureaucrats and politicians it is the noisy and articulate who get the better treatment. Indeed, the pursuit of an unachievable equality is inhuman. We see this in the recent decision (hopefully to be reversed) that prevented patients from purchasing their own drugs to supplement NHS care. Ultimately, as that controversy shows, it is impossible to have equality without banning individuals from spending their own money on healthcare and to do that is iniquitous.

Without price signals, resources cannot be allocated efficiently, innovation will not take place and consumer preferences can never be satisfied – after all, without price signals, consumer preferences cannot even be discovered. Nevertheless, the concerns that motivate many of the supporters of centrally planned healthcare are shared by much of the population. Good economic analysis, though, can lead to policy proposals that harness some of the benefits of markets whilst enabling the pursuit of other aims based on equity. As John Spiers, in this excellent analysis of the current conjuncture and potential policy solutions, shows current and proposed reforms do not go far enough. Patients need to be in charge of real, hard cash. If at least part of that cash – indeed much or all of it in the case of many citizens – comes from the government, then at least a minimum standard of care for all can be achieved.

Admittedly, there will not be equality. The levelling down approach of central planning is no part of the Spiers' agenda. But equality does not exist now.

By proposing a more modest objective, that of ensuring a particular standard of care for all as a minimum, John Spiers shows how market mechanisms can be unleashed that will allow all members of society to have a much higher standard of care than central planning makes possible.

But what would the great army of conscientious people who work in the NHS make of Spiers' proposals? A market structure that uses financially-empowered individual choice (with the poor receiving tax transfers so that they are on the same footing as the middle-class) will in fact offer a genuine rapprochement with clinicians. Indeed, of the three ways to manage clinicians the market is the most favourable. The other two ways – central government targets, highly prescriptive procedures and artificial cost-containment or self-management – are each less attractive.

The challenge, too, is to find solutions which can lift professional morale by encouraging more autonomous, adaptive behaviour locally. Here, the author suggests that free markets populated by mutual purchasing bodies and a pluralism of providers will have some unexpected effects. One is that they will be conciliatory to professional interests, insofar as this is legitimate in a free society: for the changes will promote the rewards and status of those professionals who continue to attract willing custom. The purchasing bodies will remunerate professional competence. Professional work itself will be a key locale of adaptive, creative development where the good is rewarded and the less good discouraged.

The mission of the IEA is to analyse and expound market solutions to economic and social problems. The central planning of healthcare has not worked. The economic and social problems it leaves in its wake are immense. John Spiers' detailed yet fluent book, co-published by the IEA, demonstrates how we can achieve better healthcare for all by harnessing the one economic system that we know is effective in allocating resources efficiently and delivering individuals and families the goods and services they need and want. As well as being of obvious value to those involved in the policy process, this book will be very useful in the world of medical and management education (particularly on MBA courses for those involved in hospital management, and on MA and MSc courses in public sector management) and also for students and teachers of economics-related courses. As such, the IEA is delighted to team up with Radcliffe Publising.

Professor Philip Booth
Editorial and Programme Director, Institute of Economic Affairs
Professor of Insurance and Risk Management, Cass Business School
July 2008

The views expressed in this book are, as in all IEA publications, those of the author and not those of the Institute (which has no corporate view), its managing trustees, Academic Advisory Council Members or Senior Staff.

Introduction: sources for courses

'If we can prevent the government from wasting the labour of the people, under the pretence of caring for them, they will be happy.'

– THOMAS JEFFERSON

'[Those] thousands of immortal creatures condemned without alternative or choice, to tread, not what our great poet calls "the primrose path to the everlasting bonfire", but one of jagged flints and stones, laid down by brutal ignorance . . .'

– CHARLES DICKENS

'Most of economics can be summarized in four words: "People respond to incentives." The rest is commentary.'

– STEVEN E LANDSBURG

This book offers messages from the inside, looking out – and from the outside, looking in.

It concerns how we can put the consumers of care in control. And how to enable the medical professionals who deliver our care to be able to do all they can for us in the best possible ways.

I focus in particular on who decides who decides. On how consumer choice can be made real. And on the positive rapprochement between consumers and clinicians, in a market of empowered customers.

The challenge of making choice in health and social care real for the isolated individual poses fundamental philosophical and cultural questions, as well as genuine operational problems.

The key cultural alternatives concern how we look at the world, at one another, at ourselves, and at government. Whether we are 'dynamist' or 'statist' in outlook. That is, whether we trust ourselves more than we trust 'the state'. Whether we believe that 'experts' can know our interests best – indeed, better than we can know them for ourselves, and in advance. Or whether we believe in market-based, adaptive, evolutionary change guided by the incremental choices of many and the self-responsibility of the individual. Whether we believe that economics or politics should rule. Whether we believe that direct incentives and rewards make an enormous difference in our lives.

If we take the view that choice is democratic and essential to a good life for the individual we must seek major structural and thus cultural changes in care. Notably on who controls the money. We do, too, need to carry healthcare professionals with us – and to free them to deliver best care in an open market where all consumers have the power of financially empowered choice. This concerns enabling change to be reconciliatory, and giving staff permission to change. It requires tax transfers to the poor, too, to enable them to be in the position now enjoyed by the middle classes. Both are very considerable challenges. Here, the evidence of social care pilots is especially important.

Today, however, there remain fundamental deficits which are in the way of making choice real in health and social care. The most striking deficits include the following.

First, the great majority of the users of public services do not control the money, and so services are not responsive to effective, subjective and priced individual demand.

Second (and consequently) there is very little data to inform choices and to make comparisons, since this would increase demand.

Third, there is no contestability in purchasing and so no competition for the willing revenues that all consumers could control as customers but do not.

Fourth, as a consequence, much care is poorly coordinated, to the great detriment of many care outcomes, notably for cancer-sufferers.

Fifth, the language of choice remains confused and confusing. Often, deliberately so.

There are two crucial distinctions which define this debate. This is the contrast between subjectivity and activism. Or between private life and political life.

The distinctions are, first, that being able to command a necessarily personal, intimate, individual, timely, effective and acceptable treatment with an outcome that you prefer as an individual — and for which you will make your own trade-offs about preferred outcomes – is very different from the diffuse, infrequent, and elusive possibilities of being able occasionally to try to discipline a system by voting once in a while. There is no way by voting that every potential service-user can express their preferences about a specific service or treatment or outcome and be sure of tangible and specific preferred results. And, second, politics only empowers the noisy, the vocal, the organised, the pressure group, and the vested interest whereas markets empower the silent, the dispersed, the unorganised and those without 'cultural clout'.[1] As Tim Harford reminds us, 'The economist Steve Landsburg goes so far as to suggest that if you want to change politics, you would be better advised to buy a lottery ticket with the intention of spending the proceeds on lobbying.'[2]

I address a series of interlinked questions which illuminate these issues. My analysis suggests there is significant potential to improve quality, increase productivity, and reduce costs while enabling better access and equity, too. On all these issues I say more, shortly. In brief summary:

First: what is the case for choice?

'Choice' is both moral and instrumental. It is moral because to take choice away from individuals in this most sensitive area of life – the provision of healthcare – undermines an individual's dignity as a free, human person. Allowing choice is also central to 'the power of change' as well as signalling an understanding of the unique nature of all people.

'Choice' is democratic. It interposes the individual – their personality, history, experience and wishes – as the essence of a clinical decision. It offers this as a counter to the decisions of external authority. Choice suggests that for many questions there is no 'right answer'. Instead, it signals individual identity and mobilises personal ideas of authenticity. It privileges necessarily changeable subjectivity about the most personal things in the world. This idea has many symbolic, practical and cultural consequences. It concerns the individual fulfilment of each of us, and the personal trade-offs about treatments, outcomes and costs which each of us must inevitably make. The issues include the notion that the more choice we have the greater our self-responsibility. This concerns *real* individual responses, too, and not just a general notion of 'self-responsibility'. Choice is integral to an economic and a social structure which can encourage self-care. This cannot be achieved by attempts to impose it centrally. We know, too, that choice has a positive impact on outcomes.

Choice is thus not only about 'efficiency' and 'value for money', although in a genuine market it can assist both of these imperatives materially. It is about authenticity. Choice is about making a service individual and special. It also has a much wider value for a free society. It involves us all, too, in the creative trial and error processes where societies evolve successfully by experimentation and adaptive responses. There is a constant ratchet effect. Choice generates unequivocal wider improvements, which cannot be predetermined by planners. These gains arise from experiment, and from the impact of previously unexpressed tacit knowledge. They are contingent, and incremental. They recognise the uncertainty of the world, and welcome trial and error as the means to reveal new possibilities. The expression of values, the negotiation of trade-offs, the ideal balance varies from person to person. The essence of 'choice' in markets is who *decides* who *decides*. Who do we *assume* has the right to be in control?

Second: how can we know what people want and are prepared to fund?

This is the elusive 'problem of knowledge'. There are two chief approaches to trying to know what people prefer, and will pay for. We can work with the aggregated knowledge of individual market decisions, or we can to try to consult and plan with service development in view. The attempt to substitute 'consultation' for individual empowerment bears directly on possible sources of the necessary knowledge on which to base decisions about what services to offer. In markets there is a daily, incremental referendum. But in public services officials try to guess preferences in advance. Thus the many complicated and often frustrating local debates, in which people feel they are told that after extensive consultation officials will now act just as they always intended in the first place.

Third: how can choice be made real for the individual?

Here, two changes are necessary in Britain. First, there should be individual financial empowerment. Here I propose the introduction of a lifelong individual health savings account (HSA), funded initially by tax reductions and with tax transfers to the poor to enable them to stand in the same position as the middle classes. The New Labour government of Mr Gordon Brown is investing £520 million in a three-year initial programme to transform social services for older and disabled people.[3] Personal budgets – already held by the disabled – now enable many in social care to define their wants, and negotiate these. This is tax-based money. This book argues that what we now need is for personal budgets to reach into every nook and cranny of all health and social care services. Thus, a health savings account would bring together all funding for all such services. I welcome the new pilot by the West Midlands Strategic Health Authority to test the viability of individual health budgets for patients.[4] This will further open up the possibilities for more radical change. The evolutionary requirement means enabling incentives, signals and risk-adjusted information to work to equip choices and reveal preferences. And also to specify the costs of our actions.

Second, there must be competitive purchasing, so that alternative commissioners seek to attract willing subscribers on whose behalf they will then act. Here I propose the establishment of what I have called patient guaranteed care associations (PGCAs). These will be mutual bodies, owned by their members. They will function both as insurers and purchasers of care.

Fourth: the importance of clarity of language about 'choice', quality and outcomes

Words shape ideas. We need much more clarity about what people mean by 'choice' and quality if we are to make progress. For example, we must unpick the meanings of words like 'personalisation' and phrases like 'patient-centred care'. Are these merely labels? Or are they really to be directly linked to instruments for specific change? Is 'the choice agenda' merely an electoral and political obeisance to a general notion of 'citizenship', which is then to be 'interpreted' by unaccountable 'experts'? Or are there to be specific instruments for change, and these within the control of the individual?

I consider the language of these debates, where 'choice' is now a key focus. What is meant by these words? And does everyone who uses them mean the same things by them? We need clarity concerning choice – and the language of choice – if we are to understand why the NHS is as it is. And what is actually being offered to us now. John Stewart Collis once said – he was speaking of the mysteries of physics, but the point applies – that 'We have clapped a name upon an essence in order to conceal our ignorance'. 'Choice' requires economic leverage. And so we must look beneath and within the undergrowth of words for their cultural meanings – and the issues and problems they open up on our behalf. For labels are not thought. Consultation is not control. Information is not necessarily knowledge.

As Raymond Williams said in his *Keywords*, some problems cannot even be focused unless we are conscious of the words and their implications and meanings, in part as elements of the problem.[5] So I examine these concepts of 'choice' and 'personalisation' as words of a problematic kind – inherited within specific British social conditions in the health and social care debate. These words shape ideas, actions and how we consider the possibilities of material realities. They enable or disable the psychological exploration of ideas concerning 'choice'. And of how the individual can securely access a necessarily timely, personal and intimate service. Unless we have clarity about language we will not be clear what we mean by 'choice' and we will not develop those instruments which can make it real.

To make sure that the patient's view and preference is at the centre of all such work we need an awareness of the instrumental devices which genuinely give people sanctions and self-direction. We need to be clear, too, about what it is we are measuring. Outcome measures need to reflect the severity of illnesses alongside the results of treatments. And also the patients' experiences. Yet the language of choice, quality, measurement and outcome is not clear. This needs careful definition. The confusions of language, too, include those between 'customer', 'consumer', 'client' and 'citizen'. The lack of clarity here obstructs the process of facilitating how the individual can securely access a necessarily timely, personal and intimate service which they recognise as 'quality'. Here, too, what counts in making choice real is the consumer being a genuine *customer* with financial power, and with good information. Then money talks and preference walks.

Fifth: structural change leads to cultural change

If such reforms were to come about, a critical issue concerns enabling staff to change. This is a massive cultural challenge. For it is cultures which shape who we are. It is cultures which form how we give service. It is culture which exercises the most significant roles in structuring, sponsoring or obstructing long-term changes. Choice, and its necessary cultural change, asks people to adopt new practices. To share new understandings. To adjust to new relationships. To endorse new realities. To believe in them. To work with them. The most necessary cultural change is to involve people *willingly* in new engagements. This is one of the hardest things to achieve. To take part in change people need a different sense of 'me' before they can fit into a new sense of 'them'. These moral and practical conundrums may be elusive of solution, but they are unavoidable now.

I explore the idea that influential changes are already arising from the English pilot projects in elderly care funding, in which individuals have control over tax-based funding. Greater trust together with mutual learning can be supported in this way, both among users and providers.

I also carefully consider how changes may, too, be achieved by persuasion. Some by powerful employee incentives. And by the contestability of services, and the replacement of some managements. Much fuller publication of information, including reports from consumers, will change the context and its legitimacy. If personal budgets become health savings accounts, and if consumers then join together in mutual purchasing bodies, enormous changes can result. The cost-benefit principle suggests that individuals will indeed take actions when they perceive that the personal benefits exceed the personal costs. This process is one of negotiation, conciliation and reconciliation.

Cultural – and thus structural – change is of the essence to achieve the prevailing objectives of justice in access, and a new balance between the individual and the state. The cultural message of individual financial empowerment by the health savings account would be that we need to think differently about the relations between surface and substance, aesthetics and value, the patients' experience of services, and what they think of them. The HSA can supply the direct mechanisms which can reliably enable and support health providers *willingly* to respond to these messages. The result can be more flexibility at work, freedom from politicised supervision, and a stimulating and creative environment. As well as significant improvements in preventive care. It can include the immediate satisfaction of the customer's wishes, and the prestige which that will bring to the provider and the purchaser. The talents of creative, thoughtful, sensitive staff can, indeed, be the essential complements to the technical or engineering skills of specialists. We can give new value to feeling, emotion, perception and intuition. And to taste and aesthetics, too, as well as to economic and cultural realities.

We need to integrate the knowledge and strengths of many, including the unique knowledge of themselves which only the service-user can have and the technical expertise, professional experience, judgement and know how of clinicians. If the satisfaction of customers with good outcomes is the measure in a free market we shall have an independent source of legitimate value – and a morally superior measure, too.

Seven questions

I thus enquire into these interrelated topics.

1 What is the case for choice?
2 How can choice be made real for the individual?
3 What would count as tests of how successfully individual choice is in place for all?
4 What impact can genuine, financially empowered choice have on effective funding, purchasing, quality, delivery and outcomes?
5 How can an effective market grow and thrive?
6 How can we carry with us in the quest for choice the large numbers of health and social care staff on whom success depends, and who need both permission and incentives for cultural change?
7 How can we confront the disastrously dangerous issue of failures in self-care?

I particularly focus on the following:
❒ individual financial empowerment
❒ mutual, voluntary, competitive purchasing organisations – which I call patient guaranteed care associations
❒ an individual health savings account for all
❒ tax transfers to the poor
❒ establishment of a Disclosure and Information Commission to distribute audited information.

I also examine:
❒ 'The problem of knowledge', or how we can know the wishes of individuals
❒ The importance of clarity of language about 'choice and outcomes'
❒ Extending personal budgets to all services
❒ Cultural changes which will result from structural changes, focused by incentives
❒ Permission for staff to change.

The important linked innovations will be:
❒ A commitment to consumer-driven healthcare, made effective by individual financial empowerment
❒ Incentives and rewards for preventive self-care
❒ Rapid, detailed, audited information
❒ Improved chronic-care management
❒ New IT for self-care, and for purchaser/supplier management
❒ Increased diversity of provision/encouragement of new innovators
❒ Customised care centres
❒ The protection by government of competition and of individual choice.

My concern here is with health, and not just with 'healthcare'. I urge that progress for better results hinges on individual choice being real. That is, being linked to individual control of funds, and to suitable incentives and rewards. This model can diffuse and multiply power, and impact on many desirable healthcare and social objectives. But this will depend on the power structures which people wish for, and on the cultural meanings to which they make an individual commitment. 'Choice' itself can be a deception or a source of hope. The key for 'choice' to be real is for all users of services to hold individual power. And for competing purchasers to seek their willing revenues. User of services, too, should be able to consider and respond both to their own subjective realities and to act to help shift objective structures. New structures and cultures will then become legitimate because of the assumptions and the changed meanings that they represent.

This book is then about how to improve the quality and cost of health and social care for all by empowering consumers with real choices and the power to make these effective, and enabling medical professionals to function well. It considers in detail the three critical factors:

☐ individual financial empowerment and control
☐ consumer choice of both purchaser and provider
☐ the fullest publication of audited information which will enable transparent comparisons to be made and choices to be fully informed.

As with my previous work, *Patients, Power and Responsibility*, I try to see how to make these desirable things actually happen. Such radical changes now have more friends than it might have been thought likely even very recently. There is now every hope of a large-scale transformation of care which will offer a rapprochement for dissatisfied patients and service-users, disenchanted physicians, providers constrained by government, and those innovative providers who can offer increased productivity, higher quality and lower costs. The crisis of funding long-term social care has also lifted the lid on a box of conundrums, as we will see.

The key to innovation is to unleash the individual and mutual buying power of consumers. Professor Regina Herzlinger has led the way in highlighting this argument.[6] The mobility of purchasing power will itself attract other creative and entrepreneurial people who will offer new services and who can continue to improve services. We can do all this without moving away from a system of guaranteed full cover for all free at the point of demand. Here we need precision about language and the instruments of change. Simply declaiming 'choice', 'involvement', 'personalisation' or even a 'market mantra' will not, however, stand or deliver. We need to think carefully and in detail about what 'choice' really means, and how an open market would work. We need to show how desirable transformations would follow funding and other structural and cultural changes. Nothing is going to happen automatically. Equally, we do not want a 'master plan'. We want an evolving, trial-and-error adaptive system. For this is how creative and sustainable innovations happen, to all our benefit.

Existing practices and new IT

New IT has much improved quick and accurate diagnosis and care planning. This expedites treatment, and increases the chance of better outcomes. It can reduce hospitalisation, speed recovery, and expedite follow-up treatment. Modern IT enables more and real-time analysis of clinical practice, and thus much more detailed guidance to patients and to managers. Clearly, it is essential to have clinicians leading and owning innovations, and being closely involved individually. What are the incentives to be which will encourage this? I make suggestions concerning open publication of audited information, and of the direct linkage of rewards to performance. A key variable, too, is how the process of adoption is managed. The successful acceptance and willing use of new IT depends on clinical leadership and on good general management. It is best led by an appreciation of the full benefits in terms of values such as patient safety and best outcomes. This however, still involves considerable new learning both by individual physicians and by managers and staffs. The positive potentials are that fundamental values can be more securely delivered. But new IT can/will/should disrupt some existing practices and query professional boundaries, relationships and status. IT challenges attitudes and cultures by revealing much on which action is then needed. Management here matters. A competitive market would place it at a premium.[7]

Political leadership

We have a clear outline and a lot of practical detail of the dynamic and fruitful ways to reform healthcare (and education) in Britain. It is now a question of political leadership and delivery – notably, by politicians stepping aside, to enable consumer-driven change. And it is also a question of communication, persuasive language, and of bold structural and cultural change. Who will offer this leadership? Who will do this, so that the decisions of those who use the services control what happens to themselves and to the services? Who will help put the direct economic incentives in place so that those who experience the services and their results have control over them, and define what they should ideally be? Which political leader will step aside, and let those who should decide *decide*?

We can all see that some in the NHS, and in academe, certainly do not believe in the financially empowered individual and in 'choice'. Many do not believe in the ideas which these instruments represent. The truth is that many dislike choice on ideological grounds. Effectively, they say, 'You can't have it, because if you do some will get more than others. And that's not fair. Those of you who want to have choice cannot be allowed to have it. You cannot prolong your own life by buying extra cancer drugs. And that's fair. There are those who can't pay, or who have spent their money on other things, or who aren't interested. We officials speak for them. And that's fair.'

I seek to show three things here. First, that we can enable everyone including the poorest and the most ill to have all the benefits to which the middle classes are accustomed. Second, in a free society we should be able to do different things with our own money, and to think in different ways if we wish to do so about what we individually think is 'fair'. And, third, that we can, indeed, get much closer to a situation where we can all hope to have more and better care, if the right incentives are in place. Even so, the attitude of many 'experts' to individuals is one of very guarded approval. I examine why.

Incentives and rewards

The problems of the NHS are not 'unfixable'. Nor are the reasons for its difficulties impenetrable. The systemic causes are indeed known. And creative solutions are not beyond our capacity to fathom and adopt. But we have to ask the right questions. And then to plug in the answers, to connect the wires to real instruments for change, and then to enable the power to flow. We have to make sure that the right incentives guide radical change.

Then we can indeed achieve improvements in equity, access, service coordination, quality and performance, together with individual self-care, self-responsibility, and professional fulfilment. But to do so we have to ask questions about those things which people really care about, and to query those conventional frameworks which do not yet enable these specific individual preferences to be commanding. This book is in part about new ways of looking at such problems. Especially, it urges that we need direct incentives which impact both on the behaviour and decision making of users of services, and on both provider and purchasing organisations and staffs. This includes the fundamental issues of choice and dignity highlighted in elderly care homes by the Commission for Social Care and Inspection in its survey in early 2008.[8]

What do we mean by 'quality'?

It is imperative that we revise our working definitions of quality, to include patients' preferences, values and experiences. For quality is not only or always about 'science'. What do we measure? What do we mean by quality? How do we measure and assess it? We need to take a view if we are going to use incentives to try to get it, whatever it is. We need to consider what underlies quality. The factors seem to be multi-dimensional. There is no one measure. Much is subjective. And different people will value different things. But this does not mean these things cannot be measured. *Au contraire.* Professor Jon A Chilingerian (of Brandeis University and a former senior care manager) has suggested five major measures:

1 Information and emotional support
2 Patient satisfaction
3 Amenities and convenience/environment
4 Decision-making efficiency
5 Patient outcomes.[9]

Death is only part of the story. We want measures and information on many other factors thought to influence outcomes, and their variations. Thus, prior health status; poor patient' compliance'; weak diffusion of medical IT; poorly coordinated care; lack of provider competence; weak clinical leadership; ineffective management practices and unhappy patient experiences. We need measures which tackle each of these, and which incorporate every variable in a model we can use to guide decisions and to improve practices. BUPA, for example, had by 2004 begun to measure the gain in health and well-being from treatment for each of its patients. Now the Royal College of Surgeons has begun a major project studying patient-reported outcomes for four common operations. Some 30,000 patients a year will be covered, with early results to be published in 2009. Professor Bernard Ribeiro, President of the RCS, hopes that the project will grow so that 'every patient undergoing surgery in the UK can participate'. This is an important advance.[10]

The publication of information will influence the transformations in the structure of funding, and of the organisation of 'production'. The cultural changes implied concern for the categories and beliefs about who we are. We need, too, new rules concerning the mechanisms for funding, purchasing and providing so that we can, at last, deliver the promises made over 60 years by the NHS. We need to move beyond the enchantment of the seashell and its promise of the incoming tide to a new reality. Such shifts turn on real incentives and rewards for consumers themselves, and for purchasers and providers who will differentiate and personalise care.

Motivation is the key. Both purchasers and providers should be very directly encouraged to tailor their offers of services, to clearly define their products, to adopt a policy of transparency on quality and on price. To provide specific clinician-information for comparisons to be made. To ease access to services. And to respond to new and patient-defined measures of quality, including individual experiences. We can move rapidly away from centralised and intrusive micro-management, to the realities of both clinical and patient life. We can achieve a comprehensive rather than a piecemeal approach to coordinated and integrated care. Here, not least, in encouraging much more self-care, particularly for those with chronic conditions. And more preventive care, too. Otherwise, very costly failures here threaten to entirely overwhelm the care system.

These issues are central to our hope for the 'personalisation' of services, and for their better coordination. And, too, to our hopes for sensibly controlling costs, and making modern therapies both personalised and affordable. The challenge, too, is how to control curative costs while also encouraging self-responsible choice. Without endangering quality – defined more broadly than just as 'science'. And without storing up more expensive problems for the future. We need to take advantage of new technologies, too. To do so we need information which is relevant to consumers, expressed in plain English, and concerned with the issues that matter to them. Once consumers have information we can already see, in the case of demands to be able to pay for cancer drugs denied by the NHS, that people seek the power to decide for themselves.

The outstanding British example of change along the lines of consumer empowerment is the recent revolution in eye care. Media attention and patient anguish has, too, prompted a review of the policy of denying co-payments for cancer drugs, as this book goes to press.[11] So, too, we are gaining much from the introduction of personal budgets for the disabled and in social care. There, empowered people have successfully controlled these funds and used them effectively. I detailed in my earlier book – in a chapter titled 'With eyes to see: one people in one market for one service' – how such approach revolutionised eye care. Current social care pilot projects further focus this truth. We now have the opportunity to extend this approach and to improve all health and social care (and education, too). These services can then, at last, benefit from the economy-wide changes that have otherwise lifted all boats in markets since 1945.

There are many factors which are opening these new doors. The unprecedented increase in NHS investment has not by itself produced sufficient change. Productivity has not grown, but fallen. There are still insufficient consumer-based definitions of quality, or of their measurement. Here, global information is changing expectations. Clinicians are frustrated by micro-management. Political leadership – notably by Mr Tony Blair as Prime Minister, by the Cabinet Ministers Mr Alan Milburn and Mr Alan Johnson, and by the Minister for Care Services, Mr Ivan Lewis – has helped change the context, too. Liberal MP David Laws has made important contributions. The anguish of patients being denied new drugs has also contributed to a challenge to the legitimacy of the NHS. Consumers have sought more power, too, and do not expect to be denied despite not having clinical expertise.

The Conservative Party Green Paper, *Delivering Some of the Best Health in Europe*, published while this book was in press, stresses important issues here, although it does not propose empowering the individual financially.[12] It very properly urges a drive to transparency and accountability throughout the NHS, based on achieving much better outcomes. It plans the measurement and reporting of both clinically and patient-reported outcomes and experiences, building on the EuroQol patient questionnaire EQ5D, now in successful use by chronic disease sufferers for a decade. It offers a patient choice of provider. And also the introduction of payments by results to reward quality and to offer incentives for provider improvement. It stresses the necessity of 'genuinely useful information', and says that 'Patients with the power to choose their care provider will be able to use information about outcomes and results to hold services to account.' But how? I examine in this book the different means by which this can be achieved. In particular, we need to distinguish between being able to occasionally discipline a system and being able to reliably command a necessarily specific, personal, intimate and timely service, as I said earlier.

This book makes a case for these necessary advances, but also for bolder and larger structural and cultural changes. The most vital stimulus for change will be the financial empowerment of the informed buyer of healthcare. The steam to drive the engine is the user spending their 'own' tax-based funds, making their own self-responsible and cost-aware decisions. Once consumers have information people seek the power to decide for themselves. Here, individual financial empowerment is the be all. These changes can be achieved without disturbing the commitment to universal cover. Indeed, such changes can actually deliver this guarantee.

Will government vanish from the picture?

A major issue concerns the role of government. Government will not vanish, although its role will change. It will exercise essential supervision, on behalf of the customer. It should:

- introduce individual control of tax-based funds in a health savings account
- protect incentives and rewards in a functioning market
- enable competitive purchasing, and protect competition
- establish an independent Disclosure and Information Commission to publish open, detailed, audited information relevant to consumer choice, on issues which matter to the users of services, and in clear English with standardised clinical reporting
- educate on the issue of 'the problem of knowledge' and why we need markets
- monitor the financial status and viability of purchasers, insurers and providers, and audit financial balances and the security of members' funds
- be responsible for the legal accountability of medical practitioners and purchasers
- ensure appropriate risk-adjustment methodologies between insurance/purchasing organisations
- subsidise the poor via tax transfers and thus assure good coverage for all
- supervise professional training and ethics
- establish minimum benefits for all users of services – what I have previously called patient guaranteed care[13]
- stop setting tariffs, and leave these to markets
- encourage purchasers to introduce incentives and rewards for self-care, and give tax deductions to those who achieve health improvement plans.

The dilemmas of social care

As will be seen, both in health and in social care we need bold and dramatic changes. We need a transformation or metamorphosis of an entire system. The key is in situating the right social, moral and financial incentives alongside the right data to achieve the best possible outcomes. And especially including those outcomes – such as the ability to perform the normal activities of life once again –which are most salient to the individual and which give the self-responsible (and price-aware) service-user the greatest satisfactions. These outcomes include not just 'the clinical facts', but the individuals' feelings and how patients interpret these. To see really we need to see it all.

The present governmental review of social care has lifted the lid and opened the box on key conundrums. These once again focus us on how to change and improve all care through consumer-driven controls. The dilemmas posed by the struggle to restructure the funding of social care show that social care and healthcare are inextricably intertwined. Social care has always been means-tested, discretionary and unfunded. By contrast, healthcare has been centrally funded and not means-tested. Nor has it been discretionary, although it has been rationed. The different structures are, in their separate ways, losing legitimacy. And the contrast between the governing principles is itself causing difficulties. The answer is to bring all care purchasing together by every-one holding a lifelong, tax-based HSA.

Both health and social care are becoming increasingly complex and costly. They are often concerned with co-morbidities where customers need help from a range of providers. But as we seek workable answers it becomes clear that the challenge is part of the wider consideration of restructuring funding and of customer power.

Meanwhile, it is difficult to sustain the argument that healthcare and social care budgets should be treated differently in law. People do not understand the legitimacy of such an *a priori* distinction. They do not believe you can fairly divide up and isolate services on different principles. And the claim made that you can do so undermines a general theory of mutual obligation and of self-responsibility on which health and social care is meant to be predicated. Services share the same objectives: to facilitate independent living and individual self-determination. If co-payments can be used in social care, why are they denied in cancer care? Here, issues that have been concealed by the context are being revealed. That context is losing its legitimacy as people pay attention to the results and consequences of some of the social theories of the 'experts'.

In trying to encourage an alternative approach we see that economics is not a separate aspect of society which only matters when you are old. It is integral to these debates concerning how to improve quality and to sustain social solidarity and shared norms. And to all health and social care provision.

How it all works

The NHS is, of course, part of Britain's historical emotion, of national 'belonging' and public memory. It remains rooted in old assumptions, based on the idea that 'experts' know best. Certainly, we want the technical and scientific knowledge that doctors bring. But we want much more than that, as will we see. The world from which the NHS came was one of 'Fordist' industrialisation, the metal-bashing of giant firms with heavy industrial technologies, centralised production and planning, and standardised output. That world is long gone. In the NHS it was the attempt to produce a utopia out of the production process itself. But this book asks us to consider the contemporary world, and what has been achieved by markets, save in health and in education where they have been severely constrained by government. It asks the reader to set aside moral posturing about the NHS and to consider how the system *actually* works. To do so, too, in what is now an entirely different world where people are asking for the greatest possible choices. We need to pry open the past of the NHS, and the source of the ideas in which it is rooted as we try to understand where we have got to now in what the Marxist philosopher Susan Buck-Morss has called 'the dream of mass utopia'. She asks what this idea presented. We ask why, in the case of the NHS (to look no further), it did not actually deliver. Here, the introduction of the welfare state was philosophically complex: 'We understood culture as fundamentally political, operating on the body in a material sense. The machinery of modern power was not so much hidden behind the ideology of mass utopia as it was produced by it. Intrinsic to the politics of modernity was the potential for the abuse of power against the collective, and at the same time in its name.'[14]

This analysis involves us in thinking in economic as well as in social and moral terms. About what to do next. How to empower the individual. How to do so by providing the control over funds. With comparative information, clinical outcome data, and the knowledge of authentic, individual experiences reported by patients. Especially on how people spoke to them, listened to them, and on what worked and what didn't. The incentives required to achieve this agenda and the structural and cultural changes implied are very large.

Metamorphoses

Nature all around can help us. For evolution and adaptive change produced our own lives. Ovid, in his *Metamorphoses*, says: 'How many creatures walking on this earth/ Have their first being in another form?'

We are thus considering the evolutionary and adaptive instruments of reform, rapprochement and revival. To do so we need to step outside the frame of existing NHS culture, and to strike a match against flint. This perspective turns on different ways of thinking and their potential for change. These are integral to the way in which we perceive ourselves, and our ability to change our own lives. We can learn much from natural processes. In nature, such biological adaptation offers and embodies hope. Metamorphosis exemplifies success in evolutionary terms. It brings the adult creature into focus, and on the wing as something new, fully itself, and often iridescent. We are discussing the transformation or metamorphosis of a whole culture, an entire structure and a complete system of art and nature. Metamorphosis has much more than metaphorical potential, much more than a suggestion of subversion. It can help us trace a finger over the portrait and landscape of a more fruitful future. As Kim Todd – the biographer of the biologist, artist and early student of metamorphosis Maria Sibylla Merian – wrote, 'How we understand those flapping wings triggers the flight of our thoughts whose trajectory makes up who we are.'[15]

Opportunity costs

My concerns are to continue to see the world from 'below'. And to resist the idea that the NHS was a good idea which was badly handled. Indeed, I believe it was a bad idea, and that it could not achieve what it set out to do, *however well handled*. It has fundamental philosophical and thus structural and cultural faults, whose consequences many suffer every day. Notably, that the centralist state cannot solve 'the problem of knowledge'. It cannot gather the information which markets uniquely marshal. It is unable to bring together the necessary information to respond to customers and to control and evolve the system. The opportunity costs of the NHS and its bureaucratised and centralised structure have been enormous. Without it, open markets could have evolved and the lost world of working-class mutualism and self-aware self-responsibility and family responsibility been sustained too. Otherwise, free markets have changed all our lives – except in the state provision of health and education which remain exempt from the positive revolutions of the post-war world.

The approach I offer to choice depends on these insights. It seeks to meet the call for a new synthesis of market disciplines and public service models. It can meet calls for a changed organisation, and a different structure and culture. For flatter hierarchies, for creative leadership rather than bureaucratic micro-management, for pluralist competition and for a wider understanding of both risk and of enterprise. Critically, these changes can support the explicit pursuit of quality and outcomes. This is not the same at all as an imposed politicised equality – in which we all join hands to cross the finishing line joint last together. Changes, too, should be significantly defined by the users of services. Such imperatives would institutionalise choice in 'public services', and change the theories and practices of public sector management in fundamental ways. None of these shifts needs to be socially divisive. None of this avoids tight financial controls. None of this abandons moral values. Indeed, it confirms them. Real, financially empowered individual autonomy is, indeed, the key to successful, reciprocal, self-responsible health and social care. The litmus test will be whether reforms are developed, tested and audited by service-users in the market and on their own terms.

The test by voters of politicians should be whether or not they genuinely offer these changes. It is time for the 'big bang'.

Daunting care challenges

This approach will help us to meet the new challenges of care. Every modern society faces daunting dilemmas in care provision. Chronic disease is the greatest and most costly and demanding of all our healthcare burdens. It is an urgent necessity to introduce incentives and rewards to dramatically revolutionise self-care and preventive care. The entire system is challenged by chronic diseases – such as cancer, diabetes, AIDS, arthritis and heart disease. The requirement of good care means helping patients to live with their condition (or conditions), and to self-manage so as to lead a full and active life for as long as they can. Patients have to accept greater responsibilities. But the NHS has infantilised them. They now need control and information. Many have to change how they live, or the system will collapse. The necessity is for collaborative management. This calls for changed attitudes on the part of both the medical adviser and the patient. Prevention and long-term self-care should pivot on incentives and rewards.

The pressures of chronic care, of new demands and rising expectations, and the costs arising from a larger population that lives longer, and which expects the benefits of new technologies – all this asks fundamental questions about what to provide, how to provide it and how to pay for it. We are not alone. We, and other nations, have tried tight central control. We have tinkered with aspects of 'managed [rationed] care' and 'quasi-markets' which were not real markets at all. We have recently begun to see some marginal choice in acute care, and more in social care. But without proper competition we will never meet these challenges *in the system as a whole*. We are now, it seems, beginning to take individual choice seriously as the best means to make changes. A structure set in place over 60 years cannot be replaced overnight. Yet we *do* need *much* bolder initiatives than have yet been proposed by any of the three major political parties. The pilots for personal budgets are much underestimated. They genuinely make the unambiguous case for root-and-branch change in funding, individual empowerment, successful purchasing and pluralist provision. What we have learned from direct payments to the disabled and from personal budgets for elderly social care offers positive guidance. But they are not enough unless we spread them throughout all health and social care.

Structures change cultures. But cultural change is an enormous challenge. It is important in achieving innovation that people can see that ideas can actually be implemented on the ground. For then successes can become best practice. These pilots for personal budgets have shown people who work in health and social care that real and successful action has resulted. Policies based on this new learning can then be set in a stable framework of economic, social and psychological understanding about how and why we can create cultural and service change.

This issue is central to cultural change. Yet, as a speaker to a recent conference organised by the Royal Society of Arts, the Social Care Leaders Learning Set and *The Guardian* said, 'The public sector is still very delivery focused, and the mindset promoted through the current social agenda is new territory. Suddenly, we're asking people to act less like traditional service deliverers and more like entrepreneurs, and that might be a difficult transition to make.'[16] I explore the challenge of cultural change – and of permission to change – which is a fundamental focus and a fearsome problem. But when the costs, risks and benefits of something change, people usually change their behaviour. This is usually a mix of carrots and sticks. And people do think – if not always consciously – about the future as well as the present as they try to anticipate the likely consequences of their actions in an uncertain world. They know, too, that changes are inevitable. And that these adaptations generate new cultural norms. People respond to incentives, and are mindful of future consequences. Rational behaviour and intelligible individual motives, too, are much more widespread than many assume. Intuitive rationality is not the same as being intellectually brilliant. Wise calculations are not limited to economics professors. People know their own interests. Both cultural and structural changes are achievable.

Dynamism or statism?

The inexorable axis on which this book turns is the fundamental, full-stop choice between dynamism and statism. Dynamism is represented by individual financial empowerment, and the impact of economic incentives on structures, cultures, on performance, on self-care and on innovative adaptive change. Statism is represented by a centraliser ideology, by reliance on others ('why doesn't the government *do* something?') and by those 'experts' who claim to know our interests better than we can know them for ourselves. This book rejects the arguments of statist ideologies. And so, too, the arguments of those opinion formers in a number of British academic institutions who over-influence public misunderstandings of the choices between care policies. These have misled us for so long on what the state can and should try to do in 'public services'. Instead, we need to consistently set out a dynamist case for direct incentives for patient empowerment and professional rapprochement, for permission to local staff to change, and for self-responsible customer-driven reforms. This book offers the choice of dynamist rather than statist approaches.

We all seek changes that will be genuinely helpful in everyday life. My approach follows a 'conservative' scepticism about visionary and centrally imposed systems. This is Edmund Burke's preference for order, morality and continuity. But this does not exempt failing institutions from pragmatic, practical, incremental changes which will enable us to support a fairer and more democratic society. I contrast these endeavours with those luminous, synoptic visions and transcendent statist answers – what Buck-Morss called 'dream worlds of mass utopia' – where 'experts' try to control our lives. These allegedly 'liberal' visions include the idea that with even more spending and 'one last push' the NHS can work. Clearly, I do not believe this. I hope to persuade the reader, too.

To focus these issues clearly the introduction of individual financial empowerment and of competitive purchasing is urgent and fundamental. The way for politicians to serve better health and social care is by standing aside from trying to direct services, and enabling the benefits of such purchasing to flow. This will not be attained by an NHS constitution. However, Mr Brown, supported by Mr David Cameron, has now proposed such an NHS constitution setting out patients' entitlements to standards, access, safety and quality. This will not reliably deliver a personal, individual, timely service. Instead, they should let choice, information, comparisons and individual financial empowerment in free markets deliver the essentials. It is only free markets that can achieve the best possible care in the only world we have. We should urgently study overseas models of health savings accounts in particular to see what we can learn from them. They offer an opportunity for individuals to spend tax-based funds prudently, to add savings, and to be aware of the costs of services. To be much more self-responsible. And for producers to have sharp-edged incentives to improve services. It means enabling incentives, signals and information to work to reveal individual preferences and also the costs of our individual actions, not least to consumers. Money and power.

The argument is significantly that only incentives very directly encourage self-help and responsible behaviour, which the state cannot command. As this book went to press there were two developments which underline the importance of incentives. First, the public health minister Dawn Primarolo announced a new incentive scheme offering drug users £200 worth of vouchers to be used to pay utility bills. If they complete treatment and stay off drugs. The proposal, based on an American model, will be run by the National Treatment Agency. If this is an appropriate incentive, why not adopt the same approach offering tax incentives for the individual who adds investment to their own health savings account?[17] Second, Anne Walker, Chief Executive of the government's Healthcare Commission, said that those failing NHS hospitals which did not markedly improve their record on cleanliness and the control of hospital-acquired infections could be closed for business.[18] This is better done, however, by a purchaser making judgements about where to buy services for their willing members.

The best healthcare plan is to avoid illness in the first place. To encourage this we need more innovations in the market. Such innovations are much more likely if we have financially empowered individuals with incentives both to take positive roles in their own self-care and – when they have to resort to institutional care – to demand genuinely customised care.

An excellent example of an incentive-based programme to encourage good self-care is the Pruhealth programme. This shares savings with consumers. The policy is designed to induce and reward changes in behaviour – which putting up posters saying 'Eat more Apples', leafleting dentist surgeries and hectoring does not achieve.

Instead, this insurer has since 2004 offered tangible incentives and rewards to encourage individual preventive care. This actively promotes healthy living, and at the same time reduces the costs of leading a healthy lifestyle. Those who make positive lifestyle changes, or continue to lead a healthy life, have cheaper health cover and incentives. These include cheaper gym membership, access to spas and health screenings, and a choice of hospitals. There are no-claims bonuses, of between 25% and 100%, which are carried over to future cover. Such a model encourages much greater self-care, prompts self-knowledge, transparency and innovation, works with incentives and rewards, and can work alongside the necessity to improve productivity and quality, and coordinated services. Without competition, however, you do not get the fullest possible productivity and innovation. The approach of Pruhealth is of an insurer measuring individual health, predicting a health track, and encouraging self-care, with rewards for hitting agreed targets. It will then be much more likely that people will be healthier, avoid A&E and outpatients, reduce demands on GPs, and save for their own elderly care plan – if there is a health savings account.[19]

My book addresses these issues. It is particularly guided by the hope that at last the promises made to the poor and the unfortunate can actually be delivered.

The 'policy trap'

All this will not, however, be achieved by 'policy wonks'. The economist Steven E Landsburg shows us that 'One of the first rules of policy analysis is that you can never prove that a policy is desirable by listing its benefits. It goes without saying that nearly any policy anybody can dream up has some advantages. If you want to defend a policy, your task is not to demonstrate that it does some good, but that it does more good than harm. And if you are going to argue that a programme does more good than harm you must at least implicitly take a stand on a fundamental philosophical issue. Put most succinctly, the issue is: What does *more* mean?'

I have tried to suggest the standards we should deploy for weighing one kind of cost against another kind of benefit. I have, too, tried to identify the necessary and unavoidable trade-offs entailed by policies. For, as Landsburg says,

> Policymakers need a dose of abstraction to keep their heads out of the clouds. It is easy to get carried away making long lists of pros and cons, all the while forgetting that sooner or later we must decide how many cons it takes to outweigh a particular pro. We can commission experts to estimate costs and benefits, but when the costs are measured in apples and the benefits in oranges, mere arithmetic can't illuminate the path to righteousness. When all the facts are in, we still need a moral philosophy to guide our decisions.[20]

This book is, I hope, a contribution to the application of both economics to health and social care and to a moral and normative theory which offers a desirable landscape for change which will benefit everyone more than the system we presently have in place. For both philosophies and consequences matter. The book is much concerned with how to best deliver care to the poor, to the disadvantaged, to those who are the most ill.

Creative literature shows us that there are almost as many stories as points of view. And the value of revealing and empowering these. Yet choice is still too often just over the horizon. The questions are, indeed, about the scarcest thing in the world, the days of our lives. And especially so for the lower income groups and the many disadvantaged, who have been least well served by the discriminatory NHS and who cannot exit to private services by waving a cheque book. As Gottfried Reinhardt (the German film director and producer) said, 'Money is good for bribing your way through the inconveniences of life'. But do we wish to go on with the present immoral two-tier system, when we could be one people in one market for one service – or, indeed, for a variety of services – as the customer wishes?

These dilemmas enter all of our lives. They are becoming more visible as cultures and expectations change. Niches matter here, as we are discovering with the role of genes in contributing to risk. One insistent dawn is that of therapies tailored to individual cases. Genomics offers unprecedented potentials to actually personalise care, which has until now been statistically determined. That is, that treatments are expected to have some therapeutic benefit for most people. However, a new approach seeks to select treatments based on the genetic profile of the patient. This could not be more personal. It could not be less like the traditional treatment by the average and the aggregate. It takes into account the underlying cause of an illness – both on the basis of the genetic profile of the individual and that of an invasive organism. It considers, too, the individual impact of genetic variation and the response of the individual to a drug. This shift from medicine based on reported symptoms to addressing the condition is changing many basics: diagnosis, prediction and treatment.[21]

We are also expecting to see very large numbers of patients with an interactive, customised website. This will offer each individual tailored information and views of possible courses of action based on an individual's genetic inheritance, care history and risk factors. The machine will 'know you', and reflect your values. As Mark Pearl, co-founder of CareAgents, has said of the Internet, 'Its power lies *not in its ability to aggregate users and cater to all*, but in its ability to cater to individual needs – *to allow users to see uniquely customized views that are specifically tailored for their health needs and interests* [author's italics]'[22]

'Personalisation' here means genome-derived diagnostic tests. Drugs tailored to the genetic code variations which cause or contribute to diseases. And devices that enable us to monitor the functioning of our own bodies. Genes show us more, too, on what contributes to risk. New tests highlight the growing potential of pharmacogenetics – for example, concerning type 1 diabetes and also some forms of cancer. Such diagnosis will personalise effective therapy. As we shift from treating the average, as genetic targeting revolutionises the treatment of common chronic diseases, as the potentials for preventive care grow, as we learn that these interventions will not necessarily be cheap, who decides who decides who will get what and when, and at what cost?

Notes

1 'Public choice theory' has highlighted these problems. See James M Buchanan and Gordon Tullock, *The Calculus of Consent* (Ann Arbor, Michigan, University of Michigan Press, 1962); JM Buchanan and RD Tollison (eds.), *Theory of Public Choice* (Ann Arbor, Michigan, University of Michigan Press, 1972); JM Buchanan, *The Limits of Liberty: between anarchy and leviathan* (Chicago, Chicago University Press, 1975; JM Buchanan *et al.*, *The Economics of Politics* (London, IEA, 1978), JM Buchanan *et al.*, (eds.), *Towards a Theory of Rent-Seeking Society* (Austin, Texas, Texas A&M Press, 1980); Gordon Tullock, *The Vote Motive* (London, Institute of Economic Affairs, 1976) and his *Private Wants, Public Means* (New York, Basic Books, 1970); WA Niskanen, *Bureaucracy and the Representative* (Chicago, Aldine-Atherton, 1971). See also Arthur Seldon, *Capitalism* (Oxford, Basil Blackwell, 1990); Peter Self, *Government by the Market? The politics of public choice* (London, Macmillan, 1993), and Brian Griffiths, Robert A Siroco, Norman Barry and Frank Field, *Capitalism, Morality and Markets* (London, Institute of Economic Affairs, 2000); Milton Friedman, *Capitalism and Freedom* (Chicago, Chicago University Press, 1962; revised edition, 1982); Milton and Rose Friedman, *Free To Choose: a personal statement* (New York, Harcourt Brace, 1980); their *Tyranny of The Status Quo* (San Diego, Calif., Harcourt Brace, 1983; London, Martin Secker & Warburg, 1984; Harmondsworth, Penguin Books revised edition, 1985).

2 On the limitations of voting see Chapter 8, 'Rational revolutions', in Harford, *The Logic of Life*, op. cit. Also, Steven E Landsburg, 'Don't Vote: Play the Lottery Instead', *Slate*, 29 September 2004, www.salte.com/id/2107240/.

3 Speech, Alan Johnson, '*Putting People First*. Launch of new social care concordat', 10 December 2007; 'Personal Care budgets and extra £520m to transform care for older and disabled people', DoH press release, 10 December 2007. On the additional £900,000 provided, DoH press release, 4 June 2008. See www.toolkit personalisation.org.uk. See also 'Johnson outlines new measures to deliver more choice and faster treatment to patients', DoH press release, 15 October 2008.

4 See www.westmidlands.nhs.uk; Joanna Lyall, 'Getting it together', *The Guardian*, social care section, 18 June, 2008, p. 6.

5 Raymond Williams, *Keywords. A Vocabulary of Culture and Society* (London, Fontana, 1976).

6 Professor Regina E Herzlinger has offered this valuable summary of such an approach to create consumer-driven working mechanisms: 'In response to consumer demands, health care providers will create three new types of important innovations: *focused factories* that integrate formerly fragmented providers around the patient's needs for care in ways that improve long-term health status; *integrated information records* that consolidate the many dribs and drabs of medical information that exist for each individual into a cohesive system; and *personalised medical technologies* designed for individual needs. These innovations will be bundled by consumer-driven health insurers. For example, multiyear policies that feature focused factories supported by integrated information records and personalised medical technologies may be offered to people with genetically linked diseases, such as diabetes. These consumer-driven innovations will create better-quality, lower-cost health care.' Regina E Herzlinger (ed.), *Consumer-Driven Health Care: implications for providers, payers, and policymakers* (San Francisco, Calif., Jossey-Bass/John Wiley, 2004), p. 103.

7 Richard M Bohmer, Amy C Edmondson, Gary P Pisano, 'Consumer-Driven Health Care: management matters', in Herzlinger, *Consumer-Driven Health Care*, op. cit., pp. 570–88.

8 Commission for Social Care and Inspection, *See Me, Not just the Dementia: understanding people's experiences of living in a care home* (London, CSCI, 3 June 2008); Janet Street-Porter, 'If this is "care", then I hope I'll never need it', *The Independent*, 5 June 2008, p. 34. See also Dick Skellington, 'Catalogue of disaster', *The Guardian*, society section, 28 May 2008, p. 1.

9 Jon A Chilingerian, 'Who Has Star Quality?' in Herzlinger, *Consumer-Driven Health Care*, op. cit., pp. 443–53.

10 Speech, Dr Andrew Vallance-Owen, BUPA Medical Director, to conference on 'Using Information to Improve Performance', Kensington, London, press release, 'BUPA calls for better measurement of healthcare outcomes', 27 April 2004; www.rcseng.ac.uk on PROQOLID, Patient-Reported Outcomes and Quality of Life Instruments Database; Bernard Ribeiro, 'Outcome data must help health professionals as well as patients', *The Guardian*, society section, 18 June 2008, p. 31. A Vallance-Owen and S Cubbin. Monitoring national clinical outcomes: a challenging programme. *Bristish Journal of Health Care Management*, 2002, 8(11), pp. 412-7.

11 Robert Winnett, 'NHS ban on top-up care to be reviewed', *Daily Telegraph*, 18 June 2008, p. 4, reporting statement by Mr Alan Johnson in House of Commons.

12 Conservative Party, *Delivering Some of the Best Health in Europe: outcomes not targets*. Responsibility Agenda Policy Green Paper, No. 6 (Conservative Party, London, 24 June 2008); David Cameron, 'Delivering some of the best health in Europe', speech to Royal College of Surgeons, 24 June 2008; Robert Winnett, 'We'll scrap targets to save lives, Cameron pledges', *Daily Telegraph*, 24 June 2008, p. 1. See also Conservative Party publications *The National Health Service. Delivering Our Commitment: submissions to the Shadow Cabinet Public Services Improvement Policy Group* (2007), and *NHS Autonomy and Accountability: proposals for legislation* (2007). Also David Cameron Speeches, 'Improving our NHS', King's Fund, London, 4 January 2006, and 'The NHS at 60', after visit to Trafford General Hospital, Manchester, 2 January 2008. Also my discussion in my chapter 'But what are politicians *for*?', below.

13 See my *Patients, Power and Responsibility: the first principles of consumer-driven reform* (Oxford, Radcliffe Medical Press/Institute of Economic Affairs, 2003).

14 Susan Buck-Morss, *Dreamworld and Catastrophe: the passing of mass utopia in East and West* (Cambridge, Mass., MIT Press, 2000), p. 220.

15 Kim Todd, *Chrysalis: Maria Sibylla Merian, and the secrets of metamorphosis* (Orlando, Fl., Harcourt, 2007), p. 38.

16 Lady Jill Pitkeathley quoted in Annie Kelly, 'All fired up', *The Guardian*, Society section, 5 March 2008, p. 5.

17 Alan Travis, '£200 vouchers reward for drug users who break the habit for good', *The Guardian*, 13 June 2008; National Treatment Agency for Substance Misuse, press release, 'New treatment pilot launched', 13 June 2008.

18 More than one in four of English NHS Trusts still fail to meet basic hygiene standards. Healthcare Commission, statement 'Healthcare watchdog to cross-check NHS performance as trusts make declarations on standards', 16 June 2008; Kate Devlin, 'Hospital hygiene as bad as ever', *Daily Telegraph*, 16 June 2008, p. 1; Anne Walker, comment on BBC1 'Breakfast' television, 16 June 2008.

19 www.Pruhealth.co.uk.

20 Steven E Landsburg, *The Armchair Economist: economics and everyday life* (1993; New York, The Free Press, 1995), pp. 50–1.

21 Terry L White, 'Individual Genetic Profiles; the empowerment of the health care consumer', in Herzlinger, *Consumer-Driven Health Care*, op. cit., pp. 707–15; Mark Henderson, 'Novel diabetes therapy paves way for personalised medicine for all', *The Times*, 7 June 2008, pp. 30–1.

22 Mark A Pearl, 'Consumer-Driven Health Care and the Internet', in Herzlinger, op. cit., pp. 428–42.

1

Vignettes and visions

'The prophets who forecast a sterile, uniform future were wrong, because they imagined a society shaped by impersonal laws of history and technology, divorced from individuality, pleasure and imagination. But economics, technology, and culture are not purely impersonal forces ruled by deterministic laws. They are dynamic, emergent processes that begin in the personal – in individual action, individual creativity, and individual desire. And, in our era, they are accelerating aesthetic discovery.'

– VIRGINIA POSTREL

'If it seems too good to be true, it probably is.'

– ROBERT H FRANK

'Governments, the economy, schools, everything in society, is not for the benefit of the privileged minorities. We can look after ourselves. It is for the benefit of the ordinary run of people, who are not particularly clever or interesting (unless, of course, we fall in love with one of them), not highly educated, not successful or destined for success – in fact, are nothing very special. It is for the people who, throughout history, have entered history outside their neighbourhoods as individuals only in the records of their births, marriages and deaths. Any society worth living in is one designed for them, not for the rich, the clever, the exceptional, although any society worth living in must provide room and scope for such minorities.'

– ERIC HOBSBAWM

There is one chief reason why I have written this book: to try to support the case for 'ordinary' people to get the health and social care in a free society which the state has promised them for over 60 years, but which has not been delivered. I offer no challenge to the idea of universal coverage. Instead, I seek to make it real, and to reinforce the British commitment to 'fairness'. Without endorsing what has too often been a force-fed pot-pourri of exalted and coercive moral posturing, soul-saving politicised advocacy, imposed ideology, historical myth, superstition and party-political ritual.

I try to do two things: to put some answers to questions and to put some questions to answers.

That is, to try to answer some fundamental questions, and to put some critical questions to the prevailing answers.

We will not get to the right answers about choice, individual empowerment, autonomy and independence, improved services, higher quality, the necessary innovations, imagination, and productivity gains, self-directed support and structural, cultural and social change which we need until we get to the right questions. We will not get to the right questions unless we understand what counts as an answer. If we are to set targets, too, best that they be set by the individuals who use the services. If we are to reach the most promising solutions, best we rely on continuous and incremental experiment and enquiry and not presume in advance what is best for others.

I ask the reader to consider if we should care more about economics than politics. Do we care more about buyers (or service-users) than sellers (or hospital trusts and PCTs)? Do we care more about the growth of values like self-responsibility, individual respect, tolerance and pluralism? Do we believe that responsibilities – so central to a better life – most positively arise when they are undertaken voluntarily, or can they be imposed 'from above'?

Dynamism or statism?

The crucial overall cultural choice is between dynamism and statism. The first, dynamism, is represented by individual financial empowerment and the impact of economic incentives on cultures and performance. The second, statism, is represented by existing monopoly structures such as primary care trusts (PCTs), A&E and large district general hospitals, and by the idea that the state can know our interests best and that it can run things effectively in the absence of competition and financially empowered choice.

My concern in this book is to encourage people to think again about cultures and structures from a number of different perspectives. And to argue that choice enables competition, which prompts innovation, which – as Virginia Postrel's books illustrate in many contemporary fields – enhances productivity and lowers costs, which produces further innovations and re-combinations, which again increases productivity which generates new investment . . .

Each chapter here turns the kaleidoscope slightly. Each brings us back to the fundamental step of individual financial empowerment and self-responsibility. The pivots are economics and culture. I do not, however, offer a mass of graphs, detailed proposals with full alternative costings, and a phalanx of algebra and geometry, charts and tables. This is not my purpose here, although I hope that economists with more competence will take up the gauntlet. I do not here seek to offer the kind of detail which would satisfy the Treasury, although I trust that politicians will call for this work to be done there. Nor is the book about a 'master-plan', or a finished model, or an imposed hierarchical solution. It is instead concerned with a *process*, and one which is much more akin to the natural world of continuous evolution and interaction than the existing NHS. It is about reaching out to individual choices, and about discovery rather than political purity. We do not need to design every façade and fireplace, every window and tower, each entry and exit – nor do we need to envisage a completed building with all its embellishments. These are the temptations of visionary statism. Instead, we need a dynamist commitment to adaptive innovation.

The case for choice

'Choice' is seen as a catalyst, a source of energy, and of those reconnections denied by the centralised planning systems of the NHS and by its denials of basic information and of choice to consumers. The requirement for reform is, too, rather more radical audacity than is presently offered by any political party. Instead of debating and dis-secting the inconsequential and rather than continuing to obfuscate the issues of real importance or deferring action on them until a later date we should now take major steps towards change. In particular, I propose that we should move towards a generational change whereby everyone invests tax funds in a health savings account (HSA), which they own and which it is in their interests to keep in good repair. This is the policy 'meat' of the book. We could then each add to our HSA and – when we have to use it – we should spend prudently, be aware of costs and of our choices. The wish is to reclaim healthcare from politicians, from specialists, from planners, and from all those who have appropriated our individual decision making. I apply this thinking to such immediate urgent challenges as the funding crisis in long-term elderly care, and to acute and chronic healthcare.

These principles rest on the idea, too, that private provision is inherently superior since it empowers the individual, always provided that powerful purchasing power can be placed in the hands of the poor. This is what an HSA can achieve. Thus, monopoly and tax-funded public services will be replaced by the purchasing of services provided in an open market. As a consequence, taxation itself could be reduced. Indeed, lower taxes would encourage additional personal savings in an HSA. Independence, too, rather than dependence, offers gains in personal dignity and choices, civic and political stability and economic prosperity. We know from opinion polls, too, as I will show, that people like choice. And that, notably, the lower income groups who are the most patronised and have it least want more of it.[1] Tax reductions and tax transfers will fund the HSA. Is choice to be an anthem or an evasion? An accompaniment from our early lives onwards and a vital part of the textures and verities of our thought? Or a promise which we think we have, but with no secure way to retrieve it? It is *not* 'the thought that counts', as in the old English saying. It is incentives and real instruments that can make the thought real. Do we *mean* it?

How can choice be made real?

There is much talk of somehow 'making' the NHS patient-centred or 'personalised'. This is extraordinary. For how could it be anything other than patient-centred? Why else does it exist? 'Personalisation' depends on the control of money, to be able to secure the benefits of personal medicine. We must thus un-pick the meanings of phrases like 'patient-centred care'. Is this merely a label? Or an instrument for specific change? Is it merely electoral and political obeisance to a general notion, which is then to be 'interpreted' by 'experts'? Or is it to be a specific instrument for change and within the control of the individual? Unless we have clarity about language we will not be clear what we mean by 'choice' and those instruments which make it real.

To make sure that the patient's view and preference is at the centre of all such work we need an awareness of the necessary devices that genuinely give people sanctions and self-direction. This, by contrast, with expansionist healthcare 'needs analysis', of enlarged power by the few over the many, of the 'leadership' of 'experts' who plan on our behalf and then 'consult' with us in the margins. The phrase 'patient-centred care' still looks to be in the main a 'consultation' project. Yet as I will show, the expansion of direct payments in social care is leading us towards the proper economic empowerment of the individual. 'Patient-centred care'? No more evasions please. Let's be clear about it: there can be no full patient-centred care without individual economic power. There can, too, be no *cultural* change without *structural* change.

The attempt to substitute 'consultation' for individual empowerment bears directly on 'the problem of knowledge' which I consider in several places. A major problem that arises is what is the source of the necessary knowledge on which to base decisions about what services to offer? In markets there is a daily, incremental referendum. But in public services officials try to guess preferences. They can also thereby hold tight to inefficient organisation. Thus the many complicated, costly and often frustrating consultations, in which people feel they are told that after extensive consultation officials will now act just as they always intended in the first place. However, officials inevitably struggle to gather the necessary knowledge in advance, especially when much of this knowledge is tacit and is only ever expressed by people when they become patients. I explore this significant difficulty.

What would count as tests of how successfully individual choice is in place for all?

We already know the correct conditions in which and by which choice can function effectively. International evidence shows that the essential features for choice to operate include competition; a variety of providers of services; the necessary information by which to make comparisons and on which to found choices; autonomy for providers to respond; and the impact of direct financial consequences for those who fail to do so. 'Autonomy' must mean the individual being financially empowered. And the best means of ensuring empowerment via appropriate purchasing and provision is to have both competing purchasers and competing providers who have to seek willing revenues. Suitable support for retraining for those working in failing providers is also helpful in retaining capacity, as well as encouraging support for cultural change. There is a need for much more information on provider comparisons, on clinical outcome data both by institution and by clinical teams. There is, increasingly, more access to experiences as reported by patients, and patient groups are an important source of outcomes as reported by patients. One development is a site – Patient Opinion – started by a Sheffield GP which offers patients' experiences of going into hospital and invites people to comment on their care. This is one way for people to start to get answers to the question of what happens to 'people like me'. My final chapter summarises these issues and considers ways forward.[2]

What impact can genuine, financially empowered choice have on effective funding, purchasing, quality delivery and outcomes?

There have been important recent changes in the atmosphere under which policy is being conducted. Most notably, policy concerning personal budgets in social care, and the support to the disabled to live fuller and self-controlled lives. Here, the extension of personal budgets in the £520 million *Putting People First* project announced in December 2007 and the *Independent Living Strategy* costing another £1.3 billion announced in March 2008 offer genuinely revolutionary – if still much underestimated – potentials for change across the entire spectrum of health and social care. The government has subsequently pledged £900,000 towards independent living, in a programme for local councils to transform their systems. The care minister Mr Ivan Lewis is helping to create 14 new Action and Learning Sites.[3]

Important, too, are linked initiatives like the *Transition Support Programme* for young disabled children. These steps towards self-directed support for all are vital, and revelatory. They are about people being enabled to escape from disempowerment [being 'cared for'] in a system which still too often exists for itself.[4]

Simon Duffy, Chief Executive of In Control, the social enterprise company which is working with more than 107 local authorities in England in developing self-directed support for consumers, has said:

> Research shows two things: first, people's experience is broadly positive and life is seen as much better; second, there are deep institutional barriers to successful implementation of direct payments. Direct payments work but they are often hampered by wider management and funding systems.
>
> In 2003, In Control was set up as a social enterprise to explore how to co-produce a better system for everyone who needs social care – this system was called self-directed support. In this system everyone is given a clear entitlement to support, sometimes called a personal budget. People can then decide how their budget is spent and how much control they want to take over that budget.

By early 2008 some 80,000 people were also using direct payments – the predecessor policy.[5] These can be much more widespread, into every nook and cranny of the NHS, too. In spring 2008, 107 local authorities were working with In Control to make personal budgets work well, and 450 had given people real money. These included Oldham Metropolitan Borough Council, where 25% of people with long-term difficulties have embraced the scheme. Simon Duffy, one of the moving spirits in these reforms, expects all local authorities to be on board within five years.[6] But if the structure of the entire NHS and social care system is changed to require individual financial empowerment, the pace will clearly radically alter. What is clear is that with just 80,000 or so holders of personal budgets we do see a powerful pilot but not yet a sufficient and unavoidable change for all. We need to raise a *haka* for a bolder game. Otherwise, the system may still spill the ball.

These new approaches to self-assessment, personal budgets and self-directed support offer enormous opportunities for people to make choices, exert control and work alongside carers and families with the informal care which is so morally powerful and valuable. These policies offer an emphasis on self-responsibility and the potential for further radical change. The key here is to move from aspiration to attainment, to move from discrimination to opportunity, to provide accurate and real-time information, and actually to place financial power in the hands of the individual.

Meanwhile, the deficits and denials – in information, in roles, in services, in empowerment – are starkly revealed by these innovative policies. The introduction of these initiatives emphasises as never before how little information there has been available to potential users of services, how difficult people have found discovering, understanding and accessing services, and how disempowered they have been. Not least in ensuring that what they most value is considered.

The chapters that follow thus optimistically emphasise the importance of New Labour's initiatives with personal budgets. These changes to try to personalise that most personal of things – individual care – offer every prospect of dramatic shifts in mentalities and in *all* services.

How can a genuine market grow and thrive?

Central to my policy proposals is that every single person should hold a health and social care fund (a health savings account) for all NHS, social and long-term elderly care provision, just as is being done now with personal budgets in social care. And then to release the power of *mutual* purchasing in member-owned cooperatives as the essential next step. Thus new powers would be released by people taking this newly mobile money to a preferred competing purchasing organisation – which I have called the patient guaranteed care association. The financially empowered patient – and the relevant purchasing body – would insist on personalised services: on very different services and attitudes. The professionals in the membership body would help patients sort out their options. The PGCA would then skilfully and insistently expect to convert these demands into personalised supply. They would focus on personal diagnosis, therapies, coordination of services and integration of care. For example, for chronic diseases, the necessary 'bundle' of coordinated care from different specialists. There would be direct incentives and rewards for doing so. And unless we can deploy these incentives and rewards we face many difficulties. Most notably, the enormous disaster in the failures of self-care and preventive care. And in the effective treatment of chronic conditions in properly coordinated care. PGCAs would use modern IT for supplier-chain management and undertake specialised buying. They would necessarily enable professionals to be much more closely focused on customer wishes. And fund specific wanted services.

Such organisations would be managed and led by people who know how the NHS and social care systems work. They would not be drowned out or diverted by poor information as it exists now, nor by a lack of knowledge of entitlements and options, nor diverted by other blockages in the system over which the isolated individual can stumble and then give up.

Funding is critical. We have to decide if we want to go on with an exclusively tax-based funding system, or to gradually switch away from government funding to a personal savings model. Some of the challenges this would present are confronted in my three chapters on long-term elderly care and funding. Singapore has a successful working system, which offers much better care than in the UK. Shane Frith, Director of Progressive Vision in London and formerly Managing Director of The Stockholm Network, has put the case succinctly: Thus:

> Instead of a government funded or insurance based scheme, Singaporeans save money in accounts dedicated for healthcare. Combined with low-cost catastrophic insurance cover (90% of people should never need to claim upon this) health expenditure is managed by the individual in association with his or her doctor. This avoids the rationing and waiting lists experienced by the NHS and bureaucracy caused by insurance systems. Of course, a state system remains to act as a safety net for those few unable to save money to meet their health needs, but most people are able to manage their health needs without the government.[7]

Professor Regina Herzlinger rightly warns me that Singapore is a one-party dictatorship, and that there are, too, some doubts about the data. Can it all really be done for 6% of GDP? It seems doubtful.[8] Yet, if genuine costs are much closer to our own spending, it is still the case that Singapore boasts enviable outcomes: better life expectancy, better infant mortality rates, and better outcomes. They do it with fewer doctors and nurses. Even with the benefits of access in a small island and an Asian diet the gains seem most likely to be due to innovative approaches, *coordinated* care, and flexibility. The comparisons infer an efficiency lacking in state-based models. The HSA offers an inducement to the individual to be economical. They avoid the snags of partial coverage, high costs and other inefficiencies. In Singapore health savings accounts are treated as equity, as family property. They also avoid the problem of 'moral hazard' since there are no incentives for the hard-drinking, heavy-smoking, un-exercising individual to behave carelessly in terms of personal care and then to pass the bill to others, as under the NHS.

Health savings accounts

Cultural change requires structural change. Funding changes can achieve cultural changes by extension. The health savings account is an individual bank account against the future. This is the way for people to save for their care, and to pay for more routine health costs in cash, thus providing for the future, and lowering premiums on the compulsory accompanying catastrophic insurance, too. Savings would accumulate for future care, including elderly care. Catastrophic insurance would see risks pooled on a national basis and with government subsidy for the poor. The HSA holder would take their fund to a separate insurer who would then make the necessary payments to the PGCA for services purchased on behalf of the individual member. Or the PGCA could be the insurer and purchaser. We need actuaries, economists and insurers to consider these issues, including the pooling of risks between insurers. The essential element, however, is control of funds by the individual. The HSA would empower individuals by offering incentives for cost-conscious behaviour. It is an elegantly simple market-based solution, and one which meets the requirements of equity and access which the NHS is supposed to deliver.

In all healthcare, everything is ultimately rationed. The question is, by whom and how? How we answer is the test of whether we are to live in a society of personal liberty and choice, or one of coercion, hierarchy and command. We must decide whether we are to live by our personal moral compass, or by the command of those who claim to know our interests better than we know them ourselves. Personal care is too important to be left to self-selected 'experts'.

Health savings accounts would make a *reality* of the market. They would:
- change structures, and thus cultures
- increase fair access, empowering the poor and the disadvantaged
- increase public information
- place decision making in the hands of individuals, and stop the political rationing of care
- encourage economy with strong incentives for consumers to be 'cost-conscious'
- ensure that no one would face potentially catastrophic healthcare costs
- reduce the scarcity power of existing providers
- improve existing provider performance, introduce new competitors and foster a more diverse and mixed public/private provision
- permit additional tax-deductible deposits by a member, to encourage out-of-pocket payments and the conscious protection of the fund for future use
- be owned and controlled by the individual.

They would also:
- enable doctors to act for members – either as purchasers or providers – and themselves be free agents, rather than agents of government
- make costs explicit, with doctors advising on cost and clinical benefits
- be based on patient's spending their 'own' money (based on taxes)
- not be dependent on the member being in employment
- assure affordable coverage
- not discriminate against pre-existing conditions
- leave prices to the market

- ❑ compound tax free over a lifetime, and provide long-term cover, including for elderly and social care
- ❑ encourage informed consumerism
- ❑ promote competition and market efficiencies
- ❑ provide a level playing field for all purchasers and providers
- ❑ re-define patient value-based decisions
- ❑ encourage individual accountability, including that of the service user
- ❑ avoid the difficulties of a badly functioning American healthcare market founded on employment-based insurance and over-regulated by intrusive federal and state controls
- ❑ bring in what Tim Harford calls 'the information and incentives of the world of truth'.

How many of these boxes can the existing NHS tick?

The other alternative is a European healthcare financing system, based on compulsory social insurance – the Bismarckian model. These varied systems, of course, struggle with the same pressures of an ageing population, rising costs and new expectations. They are well reviewed by Paul Belien. They do offer better access than the NHS. They should be re-examined as we look again at the necessary structural changes which this book addresses.[9]

Practical experience

There is a large literature on HSAs which will be invaluable as guidance. There is a good deal of practical experience with HSAs in Singapore and the USA from which we could learn a great deal, good and bad. HSAs are a medical savings account which is encouraged by tax advantages, linked to insurance. The adoption of such an approach is a promising route by which we can very significantly increase funding, reduce costs and empower the individual. Tax breaks would fund the initiative. It would also be possible for employers to contribute. Family members, too, could add funds to their own accounts and to those of family members. The HSA would address the problem of moral hazard.[10]

The HSA rules would necessarily include a negotiable 'deductible' or 'excess' (as in car insurance), to encourage prudent healthcare, preventive care and an awareness of costs and alternatives. The funds would be used to pay for medical and social care including long-term elderly care. The holder of a health savings account could pick from mutual competing purchasers in the market. If they had a catastrophic event, they would call upon their catastrophic insurance cover. Otherwise, the fund placed with the PGCA would be a fund invested at compound interest and on which the consumer could call. It would also be possible to add additional insurance for specifics, to increase the available funds if the consumer so wished. Similarly, the consumer could elect to pay an 'excess', as with car insurance, but this would be voluntary.

Government, if it so wished, could adjust the available funds for HSAs, by age, gender, geographical location and tax code – but it should not be able to do so for individual health condition (or genetic background). The HSA would be an important element of a new consumer-driven healthcare system. It could also help to reduce the growth of healthcare costs and increase the efficiency of the services. The account would have equity value, and be able to be inherited by family members. We very desperately need – the words are no exaggeration – a full systemic review of funding, focused on building individual savings as rapidly as possible. We need to be careful about how deductibles are used. This may not be the most efficient mechanism.[11]

There are a number of academic studies of health savings accounts. The case is also well made accessibly by Harford:

> How to give patients choice and responsibility without putting an unbearable burden on them? The best system would be one that compels patients to pay for many of the costs, thus providing an incentive to inform themselves and to make choices that are both in their interests and reasonably cost-effective but which leaves the most severe costs to the government or insurance. This might work, because most medical bills are not catastrophic and so do not need insurance.[12]

As Harford says, the aim should be to give maximum responsibility and choice to patients. They should be required to spend their own money – on where it comes from, more in a moment – rather than that of the government or of insurers. At the same time, they should be protected from catastrophic bills. This insurance is relatively cheap to buy as it is something that relatively few would ever need to call upon. Crucially, the poor would have subsidies to pay for medical care. The most satisfactory approach seems to be threefold:

1   That people should spend their own money to pay for minor costs such as GP visits
2   That we should each insure to cover catastrophic care
3   That everyone should have an HSA from which to pay other medical costs.

Harford has proposed that HSAs could be funded by reducing each person's tax bill. The money would then be invested in an HSA. There would seemingly have to be compulsion here for forced saving, which Libertarians will dislike. But if the system is compulsory, the problem of adverse selection is avoided. For those who pay little or no tax, the HSA would be funded by a tax-based subsidy. Even at the low rate of £1000 invested a year, from reduced taxation or subsidy, Harford estimates an individual fund worth £20,000 by the age of 40, which would buy a lot of care. Catastrophic cover would ensure that it was not all absorbed by one call on the fund.[13]

We currently spend nearly £2000 per capita annually in England, so there is the potential for tax reductions and subsidies to the poor to pay for HSAs. Government figures for the NHS per capita spend for 2006–07 showed per capita expenditure for England as £1915, and for Scotland £2313.[14]

An HSA would offer incentives to the individual to consider different options, including cheaper options. We would cease subsidising providers, a practice which removes any effective choices by consumers. Instead, we should subsidise poorer purchasers. We would thus encourage individual effort rather than control and direction 'from above'. The Singapore model shows significantly lower costs to patients when compared with the NHS. Each individual would then purchase services, priced and offered in the market. A health savings account would cover all care. This would include services required by those with pre-existing conditions. The individual would select from among competing, mutual, cooperative, member-owned purchasing bodies – which I call patient guaranteed care associations – to which they would take their HSA funds. This mutual organisation would cover its costs from these willing individual funds. Competing providers would seek business from willing purchasers. This would be a much more reliable and firmly based business model than that which now exists for NHS or social care. Here, most notably, there is unreliable and underfunded local authority purchasing, and a postcode lottery of eligibility assessment. It is important that appropriate and reliable funding is available for the two greatest users of existing services: children and the elderly. Children and children's services would not be forgotten or excluded. They would be covered by the same system, with the individual savings fund identified for every newborn baby, with government making a tax-based grant to get each one started. The savings account would be held individually. This fund would be placed with an approved purchaser by the parent until the child reached school-leaving age. Regulation would ensure that this happened.

There are many appropriate and effective systems in other countries from which we could learn in restructuring our own system; for example, from Switzerland, which has long had a consumer-driven healthcare system. Or from Australia.[15] I do not try to offer a highly detailed prospectus or 'master plan' here. Instead, I seek to promote a debate about principles which work in a system of self-organising order where we can work out the most successful structure by adaptive change. This is the best way to test and improve the practical details.

If there was mobile money there could also be competing purchasing organisations which would seek to attract these willing revenues. The PGCAs I propose would be the purchaser, on behalf of the individual. These organisations would promptly address a number of crucial deficits with which all workers in the health and care systems constantly but usually unsuccessfully struggle as they try to find administrative and often politicised solutions to what can only be successfully addressed in markets. They would be the representative agent and the broker acting on behalf of the member. They would offer advice and information, and set out possible choices for the individual to consider. They would then purchase a nurturing, specific service carefully related to the individual. They would offer good information, which functions in real time. They would offer a genuine choice between purchasers for consumers – which will not be achieved by the UK policy of practice-based commissioning, which merely shifts work from over-large primary care trusts to monopoly GP practices.

The PGCA would open its doors to willing members and offer a more simplified structure to achieve personalised services. It would offer direct connections between information, advice, funding and independent decision making. The individual or their family would thus be enabled to choose from among competing purchasers and competing provision, where every individual can seek a nurturing but tailored response, or go elsewhere to find it. All these are essential factors in enabling everyone to access services and to manage their own situation.

Advice and advocacy

Advice, advocacy, counselling and user led support is important, too. These are elements which markets uniformly generate, and which the first introduction of direct payments prompted immediately. Here, too, there is a hazard to beware. Advice and advocacy are *not* substitutes for individual financial empowerment. They are an essential element of the whole. We should not, either, make the assumption that people are not capable of choosing, or of learning to choose. Indeed, many people are perfectly capable of being their own advocates – as the direct payment initiatives have fully demonstrated. We should beware advocacy services becoming another professional province and a new dependency.[16] Here it was striking that an article by Stephen Burke (Chief Executive, Counsel and Care) and Cathie Williams (freelance social services consultant) in *The Guardian* recently was headed by a sub-editor 'Coded message. Ambitious plans to transform social care will come to nothing unless people are *told* how to negotiate the maze of care on offer [my italics]'.[17] If people 'must have their voices amplified by advocates', let the individual choose the speaker from among competing purchasers.

With my PGCA model, scarcity power based on provider 'inside information' would reduce. Not only would such purchasers know a lot, but the competitive market would require the publication of much information otherwise denied to patients. Information would be shared, and empowering. Thus markets would correct 'government failure' here. Costs and benefits would then come to the foreground, as would the challenge to providers of having to address prices at the margin rather than just average prices. For it is action on prices at the margin that is essential to improve efficiencies and thus to attract additional demand. This is straightforward basic economics. It is marginal cost – and the extra production at the margin – which generates efficiencies, always provided that the price earned is higher than the marginal cost. That is, producers will keep offering a service as long as the price for which they can sell it is at least as great as their marginal cost – the cost of producing the last unit supplied. Marginal cost is lower than average cost – the producer's total costs divided by the total number of units produced. And average cost continues to fall as the number of units of production increases.

Professor Regina Herzlinger puts this very clearly:

> One reason that average people can reshape whole industries is that markets are guided not by the average consumer but the marginal one. In English this economic jargon means that producers respond to their last customers, not to the average customers. Typically, the last ones to buy drive the toughest bargain; they are the show-me crowd. These hard-nosed buyers are heavy consumers of information and are adept in integrating and using that information.[18]

This is the economics of the downward-slope of the demand curve.

We need to be able to benefit from such economies of scale. NHS and other managements, too, will need to know their costs in an evolving market, and to evolve cost strategies to meet local demand. The efficient provider expands to meet extra demand, which is most successfully and relevantly generated by willing purchasers, and not by planners. To survive in the long run, producers have to sell their output at prices that, on average, are at least as great as their average cost. The surpluses available for reinvestment will increase if a producer can sell one more unit at a price above marginal costs, always ensuring that by doing so they do not have to cut prices charged for units sold to other buyers. The pattern is largely driven by the demand, or buyers, side of the transaction in a market rather than by provider dominance in the present NHS context. Similarly, well managed providers would reinvest this extra yield, to improve services again. This contrasts with the present NHS, where inefficient providers continue to be subsidised by planners and by politicians, while they struggle to gather the knowledge which only free markets can give. Instead, the valuation of services in our own lives would be made by the individual in 'revealed preferences' – and not by planners, by political processes, or by self-interested professionals and pressure groups.

The quest for choice

Such an approach most emphatically empowers the silent and not just the activist, the organised, the pressure group, the special interest.[19] It does more than any other approach to create a relationship of equals – or, at least, to move from the *Animal Farm* world of some being much more equal than others – for the disabled, the mental health patient, those with learning difficulties, those with dementia, the fragile and the disadvantaged. Otherwise, these all rely on 'the system', with all its deficits. The PGCA would enable people to navigate the maze, cope with local authority bureaucracies, and make personal choices. This approach, too, would take people out of pre-assigned categories: 'disabled', 'mental health patient', and so on. They would be *customers*. They would, despite their difficulties in coping with disadvantage, thus experience what most people regard as normal, everyday experiences in every other area of their life – save for health and education where the state has denied all but the middle class critical opportunities. Personal budgets should be extended to every service.

The unending struggle to avoid financial-empowerment of the individual

Meanwhile, many in and around the NHS continue to struggle to find *any* possible solution to what to do about services other than giving people the money with which to take control of their lives. The new horse in this race is an NHS constitution, or an NHS managed like the BBC with its own 'independent' board. This may have a definition of some entitlements and responsibilities. But even if it does so, unless these rights are enforceable at law, and unless attainable via individual financial empowerment, no good will come of it. At least so far as the 'choice agenda' is concerned.

Instead, the proposed jockey is 'public value'. And there will be no financially empowered patient or a silk of choice in the saddle. This is a very instructive debate for what it tells us about what is most valued by some leading NHS figures and adjacent 'commentators'. One instructive report is that by David Levy, *NHS Independence: what's in it for patients and citizens*, published by the Picker Institute as this book goes to press.[20] This highlights the problems hidden within the idea of imposed 'community'.

The Chief Executive of the Picker Institute and the Head of Policy and Communications in an article in *The Guardian* made several suggestions about the possible contents of such an NHS constitution. These deserve close attention. First, an NHS constitution might offer for clinicians 'less fettered clinical independence doing what "they know is right" – rather than being driven by diktat – and, if they are given the commissioning reins, driving the future direction of services'. This would free them from 'targets'. But Dr Angela Coulter and Don Redding do not then take the opportunity to suggest that there should be competing commissioners, and that doctors may indeed avoid being managed by government targets but they can hardly hope to go back to just managing themselves. Commissioners will be in charge, surely? Doctors as purchasers, but subject to the need to attract willing revenues? Yet Dr Coulter and Mr Redding do not say so.

Second, 'The NHS could be similarly driven by patient-focused and citizen-focused objectives, measured where possible through patients' outcomes.' But what can this mean? Individually financially empowered choice? Or more unpriced surveys? Local elections of provider boards? More discredited 'consultations'? This is frequently offered now as 'community empowerment'. But it does not ensure that an individual can obtain a service when they want it. It does not empower the individual. Instead, it seems like trying to force together two pieces of a jigsaw which do not and can never 'go'. It is difficult to insert a squared edge piece into the centre of the puzzle.

Third, these authors do not suggest extending personal budgets to the NHS. Why not? This is the genuinely self-directed and empowered patient focus they surely seek. Dr Coulter and Mr Redding speak, too, of 'co-production', 'which is determined in large part by our own attitudes and behaviours'. Certainly so, and if service-users could control the money and take it to a competing purchaser to buy care on their behalf they could be required, too, to negotiate a contract which would have within it genuine financial incentives to self-management. There could then, too, be significant consequential savings paid into their own long-term elderly care fund as part of their health savings account.

Fourth, they insist on the fundamental importance of accountability. 'A service focused on patients and citizens must engage with, and reflect, what its users value.' Of course. But what does 'engage with' mean in reality? The linguistic linking of 'patient' and 'citizen' is seemingly intended to imply that it will be the current methods of consultation which will be how managers try to find out what people want. However, the only way to gather such knowledge, which is often tacit, is – as this book argues in detail – by giving consumers the power to negotiate and with the backing of economic power. The extension of personal budgets, as health savings accounts, would do this. It will not be achieved by the vagueness of 'wide-ranging public debate to "authorise" the values, objectives, policies and resources accorded to the NHS', whatever this means, if it means anything real at all.

Nor will the certainty of an individual being able to secure a personal, separable, intimate and timely service be set securely in place by 'strong public and patient engagement, nationally and locally, in service design and delivery through meaningful consultation' – unless by this is meant people having the individual economic power that a health savings account would furnish. However, Dr Coulter and Mr Redding appear to suggest instead that we all engage in continuous political agitation and consultation. Is there to be a nation in draughty halls, permanently debating 'service design'? Why does it make sense to spend your scarce time sitting in a cold hall, 'choosing' a heart surgeon or a heart-care strategy until you have a heart problem? And, if you have one, is this the best approach to getting good care?

We do not do any of this when we seek our food in the High Street. Instead, we express ourselves with our purchases (and to the general as well as the particular benefit). Sainsbury's takes my money, too, with no discrimination between me and a man from Jamaica, a woman from Somalia, a child from Grenada, a disabled Chinese in a wheelchair, or a Bristol-born man suffering from dementia who is helped to make his purchase with advice from a family member.

It is correct to say that 'we need a commitment to partnership and shared decision making with individual patients and service-users which can feed back into the effectiveness and responsiveness of services'. But this should not be a call to more political activism. This is not what the great majority of people want to spend their lives doing. And it should not be a prerequisite of being able to get good health and social care. The better means and method is money in the hands of patients. To label the proposals that the Picker Institute makes 'a public value approach' merely diverts the debate. This does not promote individual liberty; they restrict it. The issue is about *personal value* most critically. As the novelist Lloyd Jones says, we here enter onto 'the opposition's field, an unfamiliar ref, nasty changing sheds, a home crowd: that, and an anxiety for how it will all turn out'.[21]

There is, indeed, no excuse for these evasions. Choice for all need not be a make-believe future. It can be fully worked out. It can be one in which there is both a sharing of burdens and also of responsibilities. We have the answer before our very eyes. The disabled, mental health patients, the elderly are all now using personal budgets. Individuals make choice work for themselves. Personal budgets work, as the evidence of pilot projects is already confirming. The point about financially empowered users of services is perhaps most powerfully made by surprise. For example, on behalf of mental health patients. Here power is at its rawest. As novelist Clare Allan has written of her own experiences in this sector,

> Relationships between clients and workers in mental health are different from those in other areas of medicine. For a start, the power could scarcely be more one-sided. Staff have the power to section patients, take away their freedom and medicate them against their will, holding them down if necessary to forcibly inject them. And, more crucially, staff have the power to withdraw support from those who believe they cannot survive without it. However sensitively the issue is handled, it isn't possible to create relationships of equals within such a context.[22]

It depends, to some extent, on how you define equal. And even with evident complexities there is much that can be and is being achieved by such service-users (and by sufferers from dementia, too). When the service-user (or the close family) hold the personal budget the world pivots anew. So, too, does the elusive wish for self-responsibility. If a competing purchaser in a market were to buy services on behalf of many such willing and financially empowered service-users and patients, these could leave the confines of their pre-assigned roles and make self-defined and self-controlled progress in their own terms and in their own lives. However, the limiting roles still too often assigned are perhaps best dramatised by the Tom Shadyac film *Patch Adams* (1998), starring Robin Williams as Hunter 'Patch' Adams. Here we saw that a refusal to accept such categories was critical. Humour, too, is often the best medicine in releasing the individual to be themselves. Adams was himself a mental health patient who transcended what was expected. Lloyd Jones tells us of the view taken by the great victorious touring All Black rugby side of 1905, confronting the shock of England, and illustrating their own open view of innovation and imagination:

> The English saw a thing
> we saw the space in between
> The English saw a tackler
> we saw space either side
> The English saw an obstacle
> we saw an opportunity
> The English saw a needle
> we saw its mean eye
> The English saw a tunnel
> we saw a circular understanding
> The formality of doorways caused the English to stumble
> into one another and compare ties
> while we sailed through like the proud figureheads we were
> The English were preoccupied with mazes
> we preferred the lofty ambition of Invercargill's streets.[23]

The role of politics

The way forward has been made more difficult politically because of the consistent failure of politicians. That is, until Tony Blair and Alan Milburn came along to open up the debate much more fully. Mr Ivan Lewis continues to extend it, as does Mr Milburn. Yet the NHS exists still outside the modern economy in which people strive to seek willing customers and offer added value, continuing innovation and improved services. The way forward is to engage customers directly with cost and value. Yet the NHS still asks people to lower their expectations. In addition, with no prices and no cost consciousness, it also encourages people to think that healthcare is cheaper than it is. The result is that the NHS has failed in its own terms. It is neither free, nor equitable, nor efficient, nor effective, as my detailed discussion will show. It is, however, cheap – unless you happen to be one of those who are denied service or who die early from failing cancer care.

Blair and Milburn, key movers and shakers

It is difficult to make root-and-branch change because people fear it. However, Mr Blair – powerfully supported by Alan Milburn as Health Secretary and by Geoff Mulgan as his Head of Policy – dramatically shifted the discourse. Blair said that the public wanted the 'consumer power of the private sector, but the values of the public sector'. He called for 'new suppliers, injecting new ideas, greater choice, extra capacity and best practice from outside into the NHS'. He and Milburn thus introduced new 'rules' focused on commonly endorsed and apparently consensual standards for approved moral purposes – 'fairness', equal access, better outcomes and so on. They appealed to 'founding values', emphasised the interests of consumers over producers, and took a pragmatic view of change – including significant shifts in working practices and delivery targets, backed up by new contracts, surveillance and controls.

But alongside these centralising measures, Blair moved in the other direction. The prospect of a different kind of cultural change – more choice; fewer targets; personal budgets; effective peer support – arose as Blair realised that the ideals of service in the NHS and in social care have never been delivered despite the self-declared 'public service ethos'. That services are significantly distributed by class. That very serious denials and deficits remain substantial but avoidable. That privileged and professional vested interests obstruct necessary change. That unprecedented new money has not resolved these fundamental problems. That funding alone has not improved productivity or sufficiently changed working practices and attitudes to the users of services. And that in particular the hope of equal access for the poor, the elderly and the mentally ill has been a long-term failing. For a politician often accused of spin and illusion, Blair was especially notable here in appealing to the power of thought and to observed evidence and audit to reframe the debate. He asked people to endorse changes in terms of the legitimacy of the values of fairness, in order to make sense of their own history. He looked at what had actually happened over half a century and urged people to learn from this, and from other people's experiences. To consider what had been done elsewhere and what might be better done in the whole UK. We can learn, too, what not to keep doing here. For example, a doubling of funding in Scotland and Wales 'has led to little improvement in access and even a worsening of access in some areas' according to Professor Nicholas Bosanquet.

Initially, more genuine free choice was small-scale, piloted and restricted to relatively unchallenging aims, such as patients choosing a hospital from a list shown to them. However, as we shall see, the spring tide is now rising rapidly, and reaching beyond those sand-castle ramparts built half way down the beach, notably, in personal budgets for some home-based social care. I examine this in detail in the next chapter. In England the choice agenda has since evolved in a series of incremental landmarks. However, it has not been a smooth path but a switchback, as each initiative has delivered less than ministers hoped. And even when improved information is offered, information is not power. It does not put the patient in control. The constant problem has been a struggle to find real levers which would deliver the promise of genuine choice across the entire spectrum of care.

Lord Darzi, in his governmental review of the NHS, has led the resistance to structural change in the NHS. In his Interim Report in October 2007 he set his face against 'changing the way the NHS is funded or structured'[24] as the think-tank Reform has noted. However, in June 2008 he was reported as saying that that doctors and nurses should treat patients as customers.[25] For this to be real they must control the money. My own consistent and persistent advice to Reform, as a founder member of its Advisory Council in 2001 and since, has been to highlight individual financial empowerment and competing purchasing organisations as the key instruments for structural (and thus cultural) change. It is vital to continue to press for an 'economic constitution' for the NHS. And to do so by deploying economics. There are those who still write as if this was something not being considered by those who are trying to make sense of a 'choice agenda'. As if the prospect of mobile funding has no prospects. As if, somehow, an 'economic constitution' can be envisaged for the NHS without economics itself being part of the structure. As if modern re-thinkers do not need to discuss the potentials for directly linked financial incentives which can radically improve access, equity, performance and outcomes for providers, purchasers and customers alike. Disappointingly, the newest overall analysis of the NHS – which Reform published at the end of April 2008 – does not insist on these issues in public policy. The report, *Demand for a new era: the future of health*, takes us no further on individual financial empowerment. Demand for a *New Era* is a large title and prospect indeed. *But* supply will not essentially change until the conditions of demand change. Yet the report does not say that the only way for the system to be reformed is for consumers to become empowered customers, in control of funds. There is otherwise in this new report much up-to-date and thoughtful analysis on treatments and so on. But instead of clearly advocating individual empowerment in its section under the heading 'Patient Empowerment', the new report states that in a 'Reformed Service' 'Capable people [will] actively manage their health and life styles.'[26] To my regret, there is no discussion of how, nor of the possible extension of personal budgets. No call for leverage from individual control of tax-based funds or tax transfers for the poor. No genuinely radical restructuring of funding. There *is* a call for rights and an 'economic constitution'. But where is the *economics*? Where is the *empowerment*? Where are the *specific devices*? Why no mention of patient fund-holding of any kind? Or of existing personal budgets in disability services, and elderly social care? And of the extension which Mr Gordon Brown himself has hinted at, which Mr Nick Clegg now supports, and which is surely the way forward? Why no foreshadowing of such reforms in chronic and acute care? Why not even a debate about these potentials, even if the ideas are then dismissed? This is a genuine loss. The pioneering biologist Maria Sibylla Merian noted that 'Patience is a very beneficial little herb'. It seems one we must learn to cultivate. But meanwhile there is much unnecessary pain and suffering. Much.

Incentives

To think about incentives sufficiently powerful to achieve a transformation or metamorphosis of an entire system, we do need to think about economics. Economics is the science of measurement. For this we need data. But *which* data? *What* we measure and *when* is a key part of the changing focus of 'the choice agenda' which is highlighting the importance of the experiences of patients. Here, an essential focus is on what kind of information the users of services want – and on which they also report to others. And what it is which they consider the very desirable parts of the whole picture. The challenge is to provide information for comparisons, for personal decisions, for judgements about likely or possible outcomes. An important element is what patients say happened to them. Such reports (on institutions, clinicians, and clinical teams, and the results) are a neglected but necessary driver of change, and of helping patients to navigate the system. We need to link these reports to the power of direct incentives. For, as the economist Steven Levitt and his writing collaborator Stephen Dubner have written, 'An incentive is a bullet, a lever, a key: an often tiny object with astonishing power to change a situation.'[27]

Here, to the reader suspicious of numbers and of economics, let me stress that economics does not stand alone. Nor does analysing the numbers concerning work done mean that everything else is being reduced to numbers. Yet numbers do tell a story, and this is by no means an irrelevant part of the whole. Economics, too, intersects with morality, as Adam Smith – a moral philosopher before he was an economist – well knew. Direct economic *and* moral incentives offer us a social and moral theory which predicts that the structure of rewards can prompt new behaviours. They can help us to achieve more efficient, different and individually effective outcomes. The rewards of incentives (which are not all financial) can motivate more people, and also encourage other talented people to come into the services, too. We all learn to respond to incentives. We are all active decision makers, guided by incentives and rewards. We can use these to urge people to change their behaviour. Incentives involve the individual in trade-offs. So, too, does 'the choice agenda'. We will see how these can interact to positive advantages.

We need to consider, too, how to measure and reward how people respond to incentives, especially as these change. The novelty here is threefold: what to measure (including the story-telling numbers), how to do it, and how to use incentives to encourage competition, imagination, innovation, greater productivity, lower costs, changed services and continuous improvement. The rugby boys from New Zealand showed us how.

New technologies

Here, new technologies are on our side. They can be directly linked both to market incentives and to management action. Innovative, highly detailed, *real-time* information systems offer the potentials of sophisticated technological solutions to analysing clinical and pharmaceutical data (including 'gaming') in great detail. The legitimacy of such integrated clinical information systems and the analysis they offer are recognised by professionals themselves. They permit genuine gains in quality as medical professionals, managers, purchasers and customers respond to the detailed knowledge about practice which new technologies allow. This enables both individual accountability and improvement to be well managed, in collaboration with clinical leadership. I examine this further in Chapter 15, 'Between the data and the deep blue sea'. Again, a structure of individual empowerment would encourage new entries into the system – and of those who understand IT and who know how to tailor services to customers.

Protection against increased monopoly

However, very recently, the NHS has seen a powerful trend towards increased monopoly and the conscious disablement of competition and choice by local managements. Yet a key role of democratic government is to protect competition. In the NHS, the trend towards 'giantism', vertically integrated services and local monopoly (aligned with local government boundaries), remoteness and unaccountability *both* in purchasing and in provision continues strongly. Indeed, in 2006–08 it has grown apace. In 2006–07 the number of primary care trusts was reduced from 309 to 152. The pressures for specialisation – and the gathering of specialists together in large district general hospitals with A&E – is also producing further consolidation. Current NHS hospital numbers are expected to shrink, perhaps to 50. These would be very large institutions with turnovers above £300 million. Choice then will depend on open information, comparisons between clinicians and their teams, any new private sector provision, and on the contestability of managements. But it is not a subject being considered by the Competition Commission nor is contestability being proposed by Whitehall or by HM Opposition – and no doubt a special cardiac care unit in the Treasury would be required if it were. Yet it is an essential 'next step' in reform to introduce such contestability. We should, too, prevent mergers which are against the public interest if they disable competition, which government must protect. It seems that many mergers are driven not only by efficiency demands but by the deliberate preference of Trust and PCT managements to avoid competition and to evade the likely consequences of choice and markets.[28]

Clearly, the economic and cultural incentives for choice and change hardly exist at all in these key areas. And the potential is being much reduced by these PCT and giant hospital consolidations. The contestability of managements – especially where there is monopoly or control by scarcity power, as with A&E and by such local hospital and PCT mergers – may be the only way to achieve value for money and improved outcomes as well as to protect choice. It is a condition, too, of being able to remove managements who are clearly protecting their own position and who are disinterested in choice. We should open the doors to private sector management of such 'public' facilities. We should, too, prevent mergers which are not the consequence of direct and incremental consumer decision making. The risk of very large monopoly-tending PGCAs must be addressed. We could rely on the market to support smaller, specialist purchasers. They could also perhaps be assisted by tax-based subsidies. Regulation through registration could also be used to influence the market. On the purchasing side, competitive purchasers, too, would encourage much greater information, more published detail on individual doctors and clinical teams, and on outcomes – as well as being able to present and use current and cohesive consumer feedback. They would manage the purchasing business with *current* financial numbers as an instrument of present business, and not merely report to Whitehall historical numbers as a mere backwards and inactive observation.

Natural rhythms as models

Clearly, the actual global capacity of the NHS has been significantly increased by unprecedented new investment, even though the service was poorly equipped to benefit from the new money due in good part to the absence of competition over more than 50 years. If we are now to be able to shift the NHS from focusing on the interests of producers to those of consumers as customers we need to think about how organisations and how societies change as well as to very actively promote and protect competition. This is fundamental. Here, we need to move much closer to the natural rhythms of the rest of nature, and away from enclosed systems. For in the present structure NHS planners cannot possibly acquire the necessary knowledge of consumer wishes and they underestimate by several degrees of order the power of innovation, the complexity of the necessary knowledge and the potentials of diversity, flexibility and resilience. For these can only be delivered by un-bureaucratic processes, entrepreneurial processes and adaptive evolution. Indeed, it is only competition and the full power of consumer choice that can enable the NHS to cope with the breakneck speed of technological change, new demands and new expectations for more, better and more responsive services. Unless the NHS accepts and understands this, the bough will break and down will come baby, cradle and all.

Virginia Postrel has discussed the importance of getting closer to natural rhythms, of taking natural forms as our models. The same point is made in a different context by the ecologist Richard Mabey, who emphasises learning from nature and not just 'about it'. He is concerned with innovations which take natural forms and processes as their *models*. He wrote of another inadequate structure:

> The great drawback of exclusively arable systems is that they are two-dimensional. They reduce three-dimensional landscapes to flat drawing-boards, drastically simplifying their ecologies and social meanings. They are wholly managed systems, allowing little space for natural inventiveness or human ingenuity. They are single-minded and single-purposed, contrary to the rules by which living systems normally work. And this reduction, this harmonization, is reflected in the human societies that develop around them. No wonder that arable farming has so often grated with societies operating according to the principles of diversity and opportunism.[29]

By contrast, Dr Coulter, Mr Redding, and those who think like them offer a reductionist and two-dimensional reality. This is a necessarily deadening, wholly managed, homogenised, enclosed system. These attitudes are like the growth rings of a fossilised tree, frozen in time. They represent a particular, statist concept of order. But, as this book seeks to show, there are other non-statist ideas about order which offer us greater potential in a situation of continuous evolution and interaction in response to genuinely empowered choices. The dynamist concept of order enables markets to gather and convey and process or aggregate complex information. This provides people with the incentives to respond in many different ways. These direct lines of communication are much more informative and optimising, and much more efficient than 'consultations' by planners and the hocus-pocus of 'community empowerment' and 'public value'. For market substitutes or evasive mimics cannot discover the truth about values, preferences, costs and benefits however hard they try. Nor do they deliver equity in access.

The economist Tim Harford puts this very clearly:

> In the competitive market, price equals cost; there is no incentive for anyone to produce less (giving up profitable sales) or to produce more (creating products that cost more than anyone is willing to pay). The competitive rule – price equals cost equals value to the consumer – keeps things efficient. The only people who buy products are the people who are willing to pay the appropriate price.

He also says that

> if the right things are being made in the right quantities and going to the people who value them most, there is no room for any gains in efficiency. To put it another way, *you can't get more efficient than a perfectly competitive market* [his italics]. And it follows perfectly naturally from the truth contained in the price system: prices are truly representations of cost to firms, and also true representations of value to customers.[30]

Efficiency is not our only goal, but it is an important one. Economics and incentives are the mechanisms by which to achieve good and fair access for all.

Information asymmetries

Choice is not a tulip speculation. But it does raise the old problem of information asymmetries, which I discuss further later. Commonly, 'experts' have scientific information, about which customers know less. And, as my examination of studies of 'shared decision making' will show, 'experts' can use information specifically to place us at an advantage or at a disadvantage. They can sustain existing asymmetries, or alter these through thoughtful advice and informed discussion, which also admits the patient's own values and preferences. But the control of information, and its interpretation, is for some still a palisade behind which 'experts' can sustain their lives, even to our detriment. So, too, is the mysterious and ritualistic language, the use of Latin tags, the uninviting phrasing of medicine – all of which are effectively professional 'passwords'.

Clinical, academic and management journals widely read in the NHS are notably and powerfully prejudiced against business, and particularly against pharmaceutical companies. The Internet is, however, challenging and changing this 'prison of awe' and of fear, not least in reporting patients' experiences. The net is offering us opportunities to close the gap. But, as I argue, information itself is not sufficient. The individual also needs to control funds. And there should be competing purchasing organisations which seek these willing revenues. This model depends on a key assumption. It is that *we* are the experts on ourselves. We *live* in our bodies. We have to manage with the consequences of disease, and of clinical interventions, good and bad. We die our own deaths. And thus in terms of what counts as a good outcome a key question is what specifically is being measured, and what counts most to consumers/patients/service-users? What counts as an appropriate accomplishment, or outcome, needs to be much more significantly influenced and designed by the preferences and values of the *individual* recipients of services. And to be linked to proper incentives.

Changing the starting point

The key to structural change, as was most persuasively demonstrated by the Nobel prize-winning economist Kenneth Arrow (and as Tim Harford shows), is to adjust the starting position. That is, to give the poor the financial power and the free choice which they have been denied. Instead of interfering with markets we should equip those who have done least well from the NHS to gain the fullest benefits. Thus,

> you can allow the competitive economy to use every skill and every raw material, take advantage of every opportunity to trade, cooperate, educate or invest ... but still get a fair outcome by moving around the starting blocks and letting perfect markets do the rest. The implication is that in a world of perfect markets, the only thing needed to ensure both fairness and efficiency is a 'head start' strategy: a programme of appropriate lump-sum taxes and subsidies that puts everyone on an equal footing. The perfect markets then find every possible opportunity to make everybody better off from their revised starting points.[31]

We may not be able to achieve perfect markets. However, when there are market failures, markets adjust these. When there are political failures, politics evades them. Few current political figures make the case for markets. Politicians want power and jobs, not markets. Yet the former Secretary of State for Health, Alan Milburn – in a series of important speeches and articles – has continued to urge more radical reform of public services. I agree with him that we need to improve equity. He has emphasised a 'new localism' focused on 'citizenship' but he has also suggested that it is economic power which matters. I do not believe that 'a new model of public ownership' with more voting for local health board directors will do this. Such a policy may improve some decisions, *if* elected people are genuinely responsive to consumers. But the critical step is to place financial power in that most local of places, the personal wallet or handbag. Mr Milburn urges that 'resources should follow results'. I try to show how this can best be achieved for all. This, I suggest, is the best means of 'giving people control over their lives and a fairer share of power'. Otherwise, the required content is not quite there.

Culture and structure

Mr Milburn has said that 'the government should give parents their own budgets to make school choice real not rhetorical. Similar policies should extend to old age, health, childcare or training so that people can make the choices that are right for them.'[32] This has placed Mr Milburn very much ahead of any other leading politician in offering a critique of the problems of economy and power with which this book is concerned.

Mr Milburn said recently that,

> The issue is not so much structural. It is cultural. Too many NHS patients still too often feel they are treated like numbers not individuals . . . too many elderly or disabled people still find themselves unable to get the seamless service they want from health and social care. They find themselves in a kind of no man's land stuck between a rhetorical future where the citizen is in control and the present reality that all too often still denies them control.

In addition,

> all too often the poorest services are still in the poorest communities which is why – in survey after survey – it is the poorest groups in society who most strongly want more choices over the services they receive. If we are to achieve our vision of public services personalised to the needs of the individual then we must recognise that big State bureaucracies are invariably hopeless at that and instead that we have to change the distribution of power within the public services to put the user in the driving seat.

Milburn noted, too, that,

> Standards, inspection, devolution, competition, commissioning, incentives – all of these have a part to play in improving public services. But in this next phase of reform it is the distribution of power across the whole of the public services that needs to change. The truth is that the wealthier you are the more power you exercise . . . .. Conversely, despite having higher health need, poorer NHS patients got fewer hip or heart operations than wealthier ones. Our reforms should empower the people who have least power, usually the poorest. So what have sometimes been seen as competing objectives – public service reforms and social justice programmes – should in future be reconciled as compatible one with another. It is not slowing down on reform that will deliver greater equity. It is speeding up.

Thus,

> the governing model in our public services should move from one that is driven from the centre by standards and targets to one driven from below by incentives and users.

Resources should follow results. Schools, for instance, should receive part of their funds according to the value they add to their pupils' education. In turn, health and local council services could adapt the value-added tables that measure how far pupils have improved as part of a radical rethink on how we measure local service performance. The move should be away from assessing inputs and activity rates towards measures that assess outcomes and experiences. And to ensure the focus is on improving the quality of the user experience, the payment of providers should in part depend on how users themselves assess how local services are performing.

This is a very important conceptual lense. It points to a critical strategy: what the left would call 'a hegemonic shift in intellectual discourse'. It describes and critiques a cultural style from 'the inside'.

As the reader will see, I propose a very direct kind of empowerment which will indeed ensure that it is service-users who endorse or amend provider (and purchaser) performance. I entirely agree with Mr Milburn that,

reform should move beyond merely giving individual citizens choice to giving them control. In social care, direct payments budgets already allow some older and disabled people to customise care according to their own need. The next stage is to give far more people the option of their own individual budgets so that rather than having to choose from a pre-ordained menu of services citizens can formulate their own menu. Parents who have children with special needs could choose to have a budget – worth the annual cost of the conventionally provided service – so that they can personalise care according to their specific family circumstances. So too could people who are in training, avoiding the mistakes made with Individual Learning Accounts. And we should not shy from applying the same principle in both health and education. In the NHS patients are already able to choose their hospital. The next stage is to let them choose forms of treatment. An NHS Credit should be payable to patients with chronic conditions – starting with those in the most deprived areas – to give them the choice of direct control over the services they received. In parallel, an Education Credit could be made available to parents with children in failing schools so they could use it to choose an alternative school. Again since the schools that are failing are often in the poorest parts of the country the benefits would disproportionately go to the least well-off.[33]

However, a key point on which consideration of Milburn's ideas pivots concerns the position that culture can be changed *only* by changes in structures. The method of financing healthcare is indeed part of the failing structure. *What Mr Milburn has advocated cannot be achieved without changing structures.*

Health savings accounts: their impact

My proposals for health savings accounts take all these ideas to the next stage. They are the logical extension of personal budgets in social care. They empower the individual. They can enable fair access, the counterbalancing of scarcity power, the publication of much hidden information, and the improvement of services in many respects – including the satisfactions of those who work to deliver them. So, too, to improve self-responsibility, self-awareness and self-care which are as fundamental as any other factors and which the state cannot command. I suggest that the key innovation is health savings accounts. These will make choice and self-responsibility real.

We need policies which address the crucial challenges of funding and delivering contemporary health and social care, including urgently achieving much more effective preventive care, and to ensure that the benefits are available to all. This does not mean providing universal services to those who can well provide for themselves. But it does mean doing all we can to help those who cannot do so. It means, too, ensuring that everyone has the money with which to purchase care which should then be priced by providers. We need an urgent enquiry into the possible benefits from health savings accounts, as a lifelong individual fund for health and for long-term elderly care.

Meanwhile, an inefficient, uncompetitive, poorly informed NHS with inadequate incentives, and no customer control over scarcity power and monopoly services quite unnecessarily costs lives. The issue is in good part to ask where are the boundaries, and how can they be shifted most creatively and supportively to save and improve lives? Not by constitutions. Not by consultations. Not by confabulations. Not by circumlocutions. But by individual empowerment with cash and by direct incentives for decision makers. And by encouraging enterprise, serendipity and surprise.

Appendix: the history

In 2002 the Department of Health launched its first pilot schemes offering patients waiting more than six months for surgery the choice to go to an alternative provider. The offer of choice of where to have a cataract operation was taken up by seven out of 10 given the chance of choice. New services run on a mobile basis raised productivity by a factor of 8. Equity is directly linked to choice. Prior to the extension of choice to all patients, hip replacements were 120% fewer and heart operations were 30% fewer among lower socioeconomic groups than higher ones. In September 2003 Harry Cayton, then the NHS Director of Public and Patient Involvement, launched a national consultation on extending choice beyond elective care. Eight taskforce groups were set up to look at extending choice in children's health, emergency care, maternity care, long-term conditions, elective care and older people's care. In July 2005 the Department of Health published *Commissioning a Patient-led NHS* – which led to primary care trusts being charged with 'effective commissioning' to make choice 'real' for patients. [Department of Health, *Commissioning a Patient-led NHS* (London, DoH, 2005), Com. 6268; followed on from *Creating a Patient-led NHS: delivering the NHS Improvement Plan* (London, DoH, 2005)].

It is the free market which has delivered most improvements in healthcare, and the NHS which has obstructed change. For example, the US led in treatment of lung cancer and gallstones because it adopted production technologies more quickly and broadly, and had shorter hospital stays. Professor Bosanquet reminds us that in the UK cataract surgery was developed against strong professional opposition, and that the NHS has been very slow to adopt such improvements. It opposed the early hospices, and was laggardly in using hip replacement surgery which was utilised more in the US. It is the free market which has delivered most improvements in healthcare, and the NHS which has obstructed change. Nicholas Bosanquet, 'The long-term economic gain from new models of healthcare provision: the opportunities for pharmaceutical companies' op. cit. See also evidence of persistent differences of diffusion rates for medicines between countries, slow UK take-up and failures in equity in Jim Attridge, 'Equity of access to innovative medicines: mission impossible?', *Economic Affairs*, 26(3), September 2006, pp. 17–23; Angus Deaton and Christina Paxton, *Mortality, Income and Income Inequality Over time in Britain and the United States* (Washington, DC, National Bureau of Economic Research, 2001), working paper no. 8534.

In January 2006 the 'Choose and book' programme was introduced whereby all patients would be able to choose from at least four healthcare providers – including one private sector provider – and book online planned hospital care paid for by the NHS. There have proved to be significant cultural, technical and organisational difficulties in the way of the fullest adoption to 'choose and book'. But it is absolutely clear to me that senior civil servants, such as Dr Mark Davies, Clinical Director of Connecting for Health, have done their utmost to make it work. The challenge of 'choose and book' has consequences for the whole organisation. The necessary cultural changes are not only those of integrating new IT or administrative systems, but of changing the whole approach of the organisation, including clinicians showing a *real* interest in such changes – aligning work-flows, operational processes, and customer requirements. By May 2008 55% of NHS referral activity was from GP surgery to first outpatient appointment; 75% of all hospital appointments were directly booked; 90,162 appointments were thus booked in one week in May 2008; 20,000 were booked each day; over 7 million bookings had been made since the inception of the project. In London choice pilots, 66% took up the choice. In the National Cardiac Choice programme 50% took up the offer of an alternative provider. In a MORI Survey in Birmingham, 30% said they would elect to go to a private hospital if available. Dr Davies reported these figures in 'Consumers Transforming Healthcare', his presentation to the Leadership Forum convened by the Cerner Corporation at Great Fosters, Egham, Surrey, on 20 May 2008. [DoH, *'Choose & Book': patients' choice of hospital and booked appointment policy framework for choice and booking at the point of referral* (London, DoH, 2004)].

However, some earlier data on how well 'choose and book' was working was less encouraging. The DoH reported that in July 2007 only 43% of patients remembered being offered a choice of hospital for their first appointment there, a fall from 48% in March that year. [Department of Health, *Report on the National Patient Choice Survey – July 2007 England* (London, DoH, 2007)]. Government spent £11 million on this access survey. In February 2008 *Pulse* magazine said hospitals across England were stopping patients from booking advance appointments in attempts to meet government targets of 18 weeks between GP referral and hospital treatment. The DoH also admitted that hospitals rig waiting lists by making it difficult for GPs to make bookings for patients. [John Carvel, 'Hospitals do rig waiting lists to hit targets, ministers admit', *The Guardian*, 27 February 2008, p. 9.]. King's Fund Chief Economist John Appleby reported that only a third of patients seem to have been offered choice, and a similar proportion only were aware of the policy in the first place. In terms of patients' memories of being offered choice there were variations by sex, age and ethnic group. In October 2007 Health Commission Chief Executive Anne Walker reported that only 11% of PCTs had achieved the target of 90% choose and book utilisation by March 1007. ['IT problems limit choice', *Health Service Journal*, 18 October 2007, p. 6; John Appleby, 'Patients' memory of choice', *Health Service Journal*, 18 January 2007, p. 21, and Appleby and Ruth Thorlby, 'Conflicting data on choice uptake', *Health Service Journal*, 16 August 2007, p. 19; Jon Ford, 'The economics of choice', *Health Policy Review*, 1(1), Autumn 2005, p. 1015; Richard Lewis, 'Reforms in the UK National Health Service: more patient choice in England's National Health Service', *Int. Journal of Health Services*, 35(3), 2005, pp. 479–83; Ewen Ferlie, George Freeman, Juliet McDonnell *et al.*, 'Introducing choice in the public services: some supply-side issues', *Public Money and Management*, 26(1), January 2006, pp. 63–72; Graham Clews, 'DoH aims to empower patients with three-way partnerships', *Health Service Journal*, 13 July 2006, p. 5, and local government White Paper *Strong and Prosperous Communities* (London, Department of Communities and Local Government, 26 October 2006)].

In May 2006 patients could also choose from a national menu of NHS foundation trusts and some independent treatment centres for elective treatment, as well as from local providers.

In July 2006 the Department of Health published a framework document, *A Stronger Local Voice*, to try to increase patient influence on purchasing of services. The Health and Social Care Act of 2001 had already provided for more bureaucratic overview and scrutiny committees. Predictably, the House of Commons Health Select Committee found local scrutiny committees to be constrained by elections, manipulated by council chief executives, and fundamentally ineffective while money remained centrally controlled. [Sasha Strong, 'Sea of Change', *Health Service Journal*, 31 May 2007, pp. 20–1.]. However, these would now be connected to 'local involvement networks'. [This followed an earlier choice consultation in response to the government's command paper *Building on the Best: choice, responsiveness and equity in the NHS – response document 9/12/2003*, published on 1 September 2003 following consultations. This has had little impact. Helen Mooney, 'Government consults ahead of new choice framework', *Health Service Journal*, 24 August 2006, pp. 6–7.]

In August 2006 the Department of Health decided to publish a policy framework on choice in elective care, together with priorities to extend choice beyond elective care. On 13 July 2006 the DoH published *Health Reform in England: update and commissioning framework* (London, Stationery Office, 2006). This followed *Health Reform in England: update and next steps* (London, Stationery Office, 2005) and *The NHS in England: the operating framework for 2006–7* (London, Stationery Office, 2006).

The government's policy of freer choices began on 1 July 2007 with orthopaedic services. Any patient wanting orthopaedic treatment can choose a provider on the NHS Partners Network who can reach NHS prices and standards. This includes NHS trusts, independent sector treatment centres and other approved providers. In the autumn of 2007 the government hoped to extend free choice to general surgery, to gynaecology and cardiac surgery, to ear, nose and throat surgery. By April 2008 it was reported that all specialities are expected to offer choice. The change virtually eliminated waiting in heart surgery. If individual patients controlled their own health savings account and took it to a purchaser the fullest possible benefits from such a programme would be delivered.

In January 2007 plans to amend the Local Government and Public Involvement in Health bill required PCTs and local authorities to undertake joint 'strategic assessments in a potential single local regime for health and social care'. The annual performance rating of PCTs is supposed to be affected by how well local people 'play a full part in the planning, design and delivery' of services – according to the 2006 white paper *Our Health, Our Care, Our Say*, which called for a further shift of acute care from hospitals. [DoH, *Our Health, Our Care, Our Say: a new direction for community services*, Com. 6737 (London, The Stationery Office, 2006); DoH, *Choice Matters: increasing choice improves patients' experiences* (London, DoH, 2006). Also DoH, *Delivering 'Choosing Health': making healthier choices easier* (London, DoH, 2005).]

This elusively meaningless language has not, however, apparently encouraged the objective. A survey by the Picker Institute found, in June 2007, that PCTs do not expect patients' groups to influence purchasing. [Angela Coulter *et al. Is the NHS Becoming More Patient-Centred?* (Oxford, Picker Institute, 2007); Victorian Vaughan, 'PCTs ignoring order on patient group involvement', *Health Service Journal*, 21 June 2007, p. 12.].

Patient comments on treatments were also to go online at the Department of Health. However, the performance of PCTs as 'lean, mean commissioning machines' has been the subject of much anxiety concerning their capabilities and expertise. [See, for example, discussion of the government commissioning documents in Helen Mooney, 'Purchasing power', *Health Service Journal*, 1 November 2007, pp. 6–10 and Mark Britnell, 'On world class commissioning', *Health Service Journal*, 1 November 2007, p. 13.] These have not seemed fit for purpose, even though the Department of Health wants 'world class commissioning'. Some are said to be 'superb'. But many have been slow to respond to changing circumstances, to manage data and costs, to plan ahead and to take initiatives – including 'involving' patient opinion. The Health Commission's annual health check in 2007 reported PCTs as the worst performers 'on the things that matter most'. [Charlotte Santry, 'PCTs score worst on "things that matter"', *Health Service Journal*, 18 October 2007, p. 7.]

In May 2007 the National Audit Office chronicled much wastage, overspending on drugs, and underperformance by PCTs. [National Audit Office, *Prescribing Costs in Primary Care* (London, Stationery Office, 18 May 2007), HC 454, 2006–2007.] Thus the stress – which I believe will not be productive in the existing structure – on the government's new framework for procuring external support for commissioners from the private sector. [See report of PCT Futures Conference, Jo Stephenson, *Health Service Journal*, 25 January 2007, pp. 29–31. Alison Moore, 'A view to a cull: has the PCT shake-up delivered?', *Health Service Journal*, 1 November 2007, p. 16. Also, 'A LINk to real engagement', *Health Service Journal*, 25 January 2007, p. 33.]

On financial performance 19 of the 27 organisations required to take 'urgent action' were PCTs. [Audit Commission, *Review of the NHS Financial Year 2006–07* (London, Audit Commission, 2007).]

On the history of personal budgets in social care see my three chapters on these issues, below.

Notes

1 Julian Le Grand, *The Other Invisible Hand: delivering public services through competition and choice* (Princeton, NJ, Princeton University Press, 2007).

2 Mark Gould, 'Liberation theory', *The Guardian*, Society section, 30 January 2008, p. 5 – interview with Simon Duffy, Chief Executive of social enterprise company In Control. Also, Jonathan Williams and Ann Rossiter (eds.), *Choice: the evidence* (London, Social Market Foundation, 2004). An exemplary example of the claim that administrative changes deliver choice is the article by former Labour Cabinet Minister Stephen Byers on his ideas for empowering parents by administrative changes, but not by the voucher to give parents control over money. Byers said that vested interests resist radical change and protect their own privileged positions. And that giving parents real power would raise standards as well as increase choice. But where is the money to be held? He does not say anything about this. See Stephen Byers, 'Power to the parents: if we want choice for all in education let's change the rigged offer system and expand good schools', *The Guardian*, 3 March 2008, p. 31. See Polly Curtis and Anthea Lipsett, 'Fewer parents getting secondary school of their choice for children', *The Guardian*, 4 March 2008, p. 6; Graeme Paton, Sophie Borland and Aislinn Simpson, 'Children lose out in first schools lottery', *Daily Telegraph*, 4 March 2008, p. 1; SA Mathiesen, 'Power to the patients', *The Guardian*, Society section, 6 February 2007. Other sites offering information include www.iwantgreatcare.org, www.netdoctor.co.uk and www. doctorfoster.co.uk.

3 These followed the Dutch model introduced in 1999. See P Driest and S Weekers, *Het persoonsgeborden budget: Breekijzer of tijdelijke regeling* (Utrecht, Nederlands Instituut voor Zog en Welzijn, 1998). Ministerial concordat, *Putting People First: a shared vision and commitment to the transformation of Adult Social Care* (London, Department of Health *et al.*, 10 December 2007). Speech, Paul Johnson, '*Putting People First*. Launch of new social care concordat', 10 December 200; 'Personal Care budgets and extra £520m to transform care for older and disabled people', DoH press release, 10 December 2007. On the additional £900,000 provided, DoH press release, 4 June 2008. See www.toolkitpersonalisation.org.uk. See also 'Johnson outlines new measures to deliver more choice and faster treatment to patients', DoH press release 15 October 2008. The long but steady lead-up to these initiatives was from the White Paper *The New NHS: Modern, Dependable* (1997) *Modernizing Government* (1999), *The NHS Plan: a plan for investment, a plan for reform* (2000), and *Reforming our Public Services* (2002). These were followed by a stream of other documents including most recently the initiatives for payment by results and the extension of money being passed directly to patients. See Department of Health, *Options on the Future of Payment by Results: 2008/9 to 2010/11* (London, Department of Health, March 2007). Victoria Vaughan, 'DoH to

push choice policy using payment by results', *Health Service Journal*, 23 August 2007, p. 6; Leader, 'What is good for the elderly is good for all', *Daily Telegraph*, 11 December 2007, p. 23. From April 2008 older people could set up or use existing bank accounts into which councils will pay a monthly sum that can be spent on services as the recipient chooses, instead of the decisions being made by social workers. An additional £520 million has been earmarked over the next three years to fund additional help for the elderly. See also Cabinet Office, *Modernising Government* (London, The Stationery Office, 1999), Cmd. 4310; P Webster and C Buckley, 'Blair warns unions of need for more choice', *The Times*, 18 June 2003; 'New blood for the health service', *The Economist*, 23 April 2005, pp. 33–4; Robert Winnett, '"Personal budgets" will give elderly control', *Daily Telegraph*, 11 December 2007, p. 5. See the discussion in my *Patients, Power and Responsibility*. Also, HMG Strategy Unit, *Improving the Life Chances of Disabled People* (London, Stationery Office, 2005). Mr Johnson, however, was accused of abandoning an important aspect of Mr Blair's reforms when he decided to cancel contracts for six proposed new clinics to be provided by the private sector and to close one already open. This reduced patient choice. Colin Brown, 'Blair's reforms watered down as network of NHS clinics scrapped', *The Independent*, 16 November 2007, p. 24.

4 Office for Disability Issues, *Independent Living: a cross-government strategy about independent living for disabled people* (London, Office for Disability and six other government departments, 3 March 2008). See also www.officefordisability.gov.uk. For text of the Disabled Persons (Independent Living) Bill introduced by Lord Ashley of Stoke as a private member's bill and printed by House of Lords on 8 June 2006 see www.publications.parliament.uk. The Bill passed its third reading in the Lords on 25 February 2008. The government's own Independent Living Strategy was cautiously welcomed by the National Centre for Independent Living, regretting that there was no commitment to legislation. Press Release 3 March 2008 at www.ncil.org.uk. See also C Parker, *Independent Living and the Human Rights Act 1998: a paper commissioned by the Disability Rights Commission, the Social Care and Clinical Excellence Institute and the National Centre for Independent Living* (London, DRC, 2004); Disabled Rights Commission, *Discriminating Treatment? Disabled People and the Health Service* (London, DRC, 2004); T Stainton and S Boyce, 'I have got my life back': users' experience of direct payments', *Disability and Society*, 19(5), 2004, pp. 443–54; S Gillinson, H Green and P Miller, *Independent Living: the right to be equal citizens* (London, Demos, 2005); Cabinet Office, PM's Strategy Unit, Dept. of Work and Pensions, Dept. of Health, Dept. for Education and Skills, Office of the Deputy PM, *Improving the Life Chances of Disabled People* (London, Cabinet Office, 2005); A Nocon and J Owen, 'Unequal treatment', *Mental Health Today*, February 2006, pp. 326–30; H Spandler and N Vick, 'Opportunities for Independent Living using direct payments in mental health', *Health and Social Care in the Community*, 14(2), March 2006, pp. 107–15; S Heng, 'Why the Independent Living Bill could be great news for disabled people', *Community Care*, 1627, 2006, pp. 22–3; P Miller, S Gillinson and J Huber, *Disabilist Britain: barriers to independent living for disabled people in 2006* (London, Scope/Demos, 2006); Peter Beresford *et al.*, 'A noble vision', *The Guardian*, Society section, 5 March 2008, p. 3. But for a dissident voice see Donna Dustin, *The McDonaldisation of Social Work* (Aldershot, Ashgate, 2008). See also Peter Beresford, 'Second thoughts', *The Guardian*, Society section, 28 May 2008, p .4.

5 Simon Duffy, 'Personalised care: disabled people taking charge of their lives', *Community Care*, 31 January 2008 at www.communitycare.co.uk; Simon Duffy, 'Progress and challenge', *Community Connecting*, pp. 8–9, at www.in-control.org.uk; Simon Duffy, 'Individual budgets: transforming the allocation of resources for care', *Journal of Integrated Care*, February 2005, 13(1), pp. 1–11; Jane Ahern, 'An adventure that ends in a plan', *Learning Disability Today*, 8(1), February 2008, pp. 34–7; Rosemary Bennett, 'Flexible budget thanks to enlightened worker', *The Times*, 30 January 2008; Mithran Samuel, 'Direct payments and individual budgets', *Community Care*, 29 February 2008. See also DoH, *Our Health, Our Care, Our Say: a new direction for community services*, Cmd. 6737 (London, The Stationery Office, 2006); DoH, *Our Health, Our Care, Our Say: a new direction for community services* (London, The Stationery Office, 2006); DoH, *Choice Matters: increasing choice improves patients' experiences* (London, DoH, 2006); DoH/Dept. for Education and Skills, *Options for Excellence: building the social care workforce of the future* (London, DoH/DfES, 20 October 2006); DoH, *Independence, Well-Being and Choice: our vision for the future of social care for adults in England* (London, DoH, 21 March 2005), Cmd. 6499. See also DoH, *Delivering 'Choosing Health': making healthier choices easier* (London, DoH, 2005).

6 Mark Gould, 'Liberation theory', op. cit. For the original consumer-led initiative 30 years ago see Frances Hasler, 'Questions of Control', Letter, *The Guardian*, Society section, 6 February 2008, p. 4. For story of 40-year-old MS sufferer Gavin Croft see 'NHS pays for season ticket', *Rochdale Observer* at www.rochdaleobserver.co.uk and 'MS doesn't stop Gavin watching his favourite team', Oldham Metropolitan Borough Council at www.oldham.gov.uk.

7 See www.progressive-vision.org/politics/health.htm. For fuller references on Singapore see Chapter 'The messages of the aesthetic environment', note 10. Also, discussion of insurance models in Harford, op. cit., pp. 122–8. The complex problem of 'risk adjustment', and the attractions of incentives for providers to be paid more for treating those who are most ill is examined by Herzlinger in *Who Killed Health Care?* op. cit., pp. 164–6.

8 Personal discussion with Professor Herzlinger in London, 6 June 2008.

9 Paul Belien, 'European Health Care: the cost of solidarity and the promise of risk-adjusted consumer-driven health care', in Regina E. Herzlinger, *Consumer-Driven Health Care* (San Francisco, Calif., Jossey-Bass/John Wiley, 2004), pp. 338–61. See also Brumol Holthof, 'An Alternative to Managed Care: a European perspective on informed choice' in Herzlinger, op. cit., pp. 322–29, and JC Goodman and GL Musgrave, *Twenty Myths About National Health Insurance* (Dallas, Tex., National Center for Policy Analysis, 1991).

10 WG Manning and MS Marquis, 'Health Insurance: the trade-off between risk polling and moral hazard', *Journal of Health Economics*, 1 October 1996, 15, pp. 609–39.

11 Herzlinger, *Consumer-Driven Health Care*, op. cit., pp. 102–3, and *Who Killed Health Care?*, op. cit., pp. 166–7.

12 Harford, op. cit., pp. 135, 247. For detailed scholarly references on HSA's see Chapter '"The "choice" agenda and the "problem of knowledge"', note 14.

13 Harford, op. cit., pp. 135–8.

14 *United Kingdom Health Statistics*, No.3 (Houndsmills, Palgrave Macmillan, 9 June 2008), No. 3., table for England, Scotland, Wales and N Ireland, p. 114; 'Marked differences between UK's four National Health Services', press release, Office of National Statistics, 9 June 2008 gave the per capita spend for England as £1915 and for Scotland £2313. The Office for Health Economics gave an estimate for per capita spend in the UK as a whole for 2007–08 as £2166, and for 2006–07 £1993 (OHE estimate). See Emma Hawe (ed.), *Office for Health Economics, Compendium of Health Statistics* (Oxford, Radcliffe, 20 March 2007), p. 77.

15 For US experience see the US Treasury site www.treas.gov/offices/public-affairs/has and references. Also, Thomas Wilder and Hannah Yoo, *A Survey of Preventive Benefits in Health Savings Accounts (HSA) Plans* (Washington, D.C., American's Health Insurance Plans, 2007, at www.ahipresearch.org. Also, *Understanding the Issues and Proposed Solutions* (Washington, DC, Alliance for Health Reform, 2007) at www.allhealth.org, and JC Goodman and GL Musgrave, 'The Economic Case for Medical Savings Accounts', Paper presented to American Enterprise Institute, 18 April 1994. (Washington, DC, AEI, 1994). For a critical commentary see 'The Truth About Health Savings Accounts', a report by Harvard School of Public Health Research, 2006, at www.thinkprogress.org.

For Singapore, see government publications at sgdi.gov.sg and relevant Ministries. Also, among a large literature, MG Asher, *Social Security in Malaysia and Singapore: practice issues and reform directions* (Kuala Lumpur, Malaysia, Institute of Strategic Studies, 1994); MD Barr, 'Medical Savings Accounts in Singapore: a critical enquiry', *Journal of Health Politics, Policy and Law* (2001), 26, pp. 709–26; Eric S Berger, Carrie Gavara, and Daniel E Johnson, 'The Politics of Consumer-Driven Health Care', in Herzlinger, *Consumer-Driven Health Care*, op. cit., pp. 764–73; P Graham, 'Why We Need Medical Savings Accounts', *New England Journal of Medicine*, 1994, 330, pp. 1752–3; Piya Hanvoravongchai, *Medical Savings Accounts: lessons learned from international experience*, Health Financing Policy Discussion Paper; 52 (Geneva, World Health Organization, 2002); William C Hsiao, 'Medical Savings Accounts: lessons from Singapore. Peer Review', *Health Affairs*, Summer 1995; William C Hsiao, 'Why is a systemic view of health financing necessary?', *Health Affairs*, 2007, 26(4), pp. 950–61; BS Kua, 'Health Care Financing: the Singapore experience', *Proceedings of China's Medical Reform Conference* (Beijing, Ministry of Health, 30–31 March 1994); MK Lin, *Singapore's Medisave Scheme: its rationale, merits and its impact on rising health care costs* (Boston, Harvard School of Public Health, 1991); KH Phua, 'Medical savings accounts and health care financing in Singapore', in E Schreiber (eds.), *Innovations in Health Care Financing* (Washington, DC, World Bank, 1997); KH Phua, *Privatisation and Restricting of Health Services in Singapore*. Institute of Policy Studies, Occasional paper No. 5 (Singapore, Tim Academic Press, 1991); Thomas A Massaro, and Yu-Ning Wong, 'Medical Savings Accounts: the Singapore experience', *NCPA Policy Report* No. 203, April 1996 (Dallas, Texas/ Washington, DC, National Centre for Policy Analysis, 1996); Thomas A Massaro, and Yu-Ning Wong, 'Positive experience with medical savings accounts in Singapore: peer review', *Public Affairs*, 14(2), pp. 267–72; Mark V. Pauly, 'Tax credits for health insurance and medical savings accounts,' *Health Affairs*, Spring 1995, pp. 126–39, and 'Medical savings accounts in Singapore: what can we know?', *Journal of Health Politics, Policy and Law* (2001), 26, pp. 727–32; David Reisman, 'Payment for health in Singapore', *Journal of Social Economics* (2006), 33(2), pp. 132–59; D. Rind, 'Medical Savings Account', *New England Journal of Medicine*, 1994, 331, p. 1158; Warner V Slack, 'The patient's right to decide', in Herzlinger, *Consumer-Driven Health Care*, op. cit., pp. 376–9; V Tweed, 'Medical savings accounts: are they a viable option?', *Business and Health*, October 1994; E Zabinski, TM Selden, JF Moeller and JS Banthin, 'Medical savings accounts: microsimulation results from a model with adverse selection' *Journal of Health Economics*, 1991, 18, pp. 195–218.On Switzerland, see the recent detailed analysis by Herzlinger, *Who Killed Health Care?*, op. cit., Chapter 8; also, Herzlinger and Ramin Parsa-Parsi, 'Consumer-Driven Health Care: lessons from Switzerland', *Journal of the American Medical Association*, 292, 10, 10 September 2004. On Europe, too, see survey by Paul Belien, 'European Health Care: the cost of solidarity and the promise of risk-adjusted consumer-driven health care', in Herzlinger, *Consumer-Driven Health Care*, op. cit., pp. 338–61, and JC Goodman and GL Musgrave, *Twenty Myths About National Health Insurance* (Dallas, Tex., National Center for Policy Analysis, 1991). For a recent patient report comparing some care in France and the UK see John Collyer, 'So where would you rather be ill?', *Daily Telegraph*, 9 June 2008, p. 19. Germany has a social insurance system established by Prince Bismarck in 1883 on a national basis. Care is funded by a blend of statutory health insurance, taxation, and private insurance, with additional co-payments. German healthcare insurance is employment-based. Some 90% of Germans are covered by compulsory health insurance, which is paid for by employers and employees. The balance of civil servants (who have a separate scheme) and high-income individuals have identical access, although the latter pay into their own private systems. Unemployed people and those on benefit are covered by the state. Hospital provision is diverse, and there is choice of doctor and of hospital. Some 51% of beds are in the public sector, another 30% are provided by private, not-for-profit organisations, and the balance of 14% are in private, profit-making institutions. Germany has twice as many doctors and three times as many beds per head of population as in Britain, which offers the spare capacity necessary for choice, and for efficient competition. All classes of people have the government guarantee of access to good care. Outcomes and user-satisfaction are much better than in the UK. See also *Saving the health of the nation: an introduction to Health Savings Accounts*, DVD by The Stockholm Network, London 2008. www.stockholm-network.org.

France has a system structured on a compromise between egalitarianism and classical liberalism, insisting that all have equal access to good care while ensuring that choice and competition are maintained. The basis of funding is compulsory social insurance, which covers 99% of the population. This compulsory insurance pays for half of total health expenditure, and about a quarter of costs are covered by out-of-pocket payments. Private insurance and voluntary mutual funds cover the rest. Again, there is much more choice, and a similar guarantee of access for all. There are virtually no waiting lists (except for transplants). French hospitals are public, private not-for-profit, and private for-profit. The private sector offers about a third of all beds. There are twice as many doctors and beds per head of population as in the UK. The government closely regulates the system.

See OECD Electronic Publications, Paris, *OECD Health Data 1998: a comparative analysis of 29 countries*, and *OECD Health Data 2001: a comparative analysis of 30 countries* (10th edition); Anna Dixon and Sarah Thomson, 'Choices in health care: the European experience', *Journal of Health Services Research and Policy*, 11(3), July 2006, pp. 167–71; David Marsland, *Welfare or Welfare State Contradictions and Dilemmas in Social Policy* (London, Macmillan Press, 1996); *Seeds of Bankruptcy* (London, Claridge, 1988); 'Methodological inadequacies in British Social Science', in S Cang (ed.), *Feschrift for Elliott Jaques* (Washington, DC, Cason-Hall, 1992); 'Not cancelled – postponed: a revolution in healthcare', *Health Business Summary*, 13, pp. 4–9, 1994; 'Public service plus: the role of the independent sector in health care', *Health Summary*, 13, pp. 8–132, 1996; E Jabubowski, *Health Care Systems in the EU, A Comparative Study. European Parliament Working Paper*, SACO 101/revised. Brussels, European Parliament, 1998; World Health Organisation, *World Health Report 2000* (Geneva, WHO, 2000); R Freeman, *The Politics of Health in Europe* (Manchester, Manchester University Press, 2000), 'European Policy Research Unit Series'; David Smith, 'So how do you want to pay for it?', *Sunday Times*, news review, 2 December 2001; Reform, *Briefing note*, 11 December 2001 (Reform, London 2001); Karol Sikora, 'New ideas needed to revive the NHS', letter, *The Times*, 20 February 2002; David G Green and Benedict Irvine, *Health Care in France and Germany: lessons for the UK* (London, Civitas, December 2001) contains interesting material comparing the British, French and German systems, and reports interviews with French and German patients. But see also letter from Hilary Bramley, an NHS-trained nurse who has worked in the French health service, 'NHS care row', *The Independent*, 25 January 2002.

On insurance, see Deepak Lal, *A Premium on Health: a national health insurance scheme* (London, Politiea, 2001); Sheila Lawlor, Greg Baum, Jean-Louis Beaud de Brive, and Deepak Lal, 'A National Health Insurance Scheme' in *Systems for Success: models for healthcare reform* (London, Politiea, 2004); David Laws, 'UK health services: a Liberal agenda for reform and renewal', in Paul Marshall and David Laws (eds.), *The Orange Book Reclaiming Liberalism* (London, Profile Books, 2004), especially Introduction by Paul Marshall, Chapter 1 'UK Health Services: a Liberal agenda for reform' by David Laws, Chapter 2 'Liberalism and localism' by Edward Davey, Marshall and Laws. Also Jessica Asato (ed.), *Introducing Social Insurance to the UK* (London, Social Market Foundation, December 2004).

16 For this trend see Bob Sang, 'Don't let's forget, we're in it for the long-term', *British Journal of Healthcare Management*, 2007, 13(4), pp. 122–5 and 13(5), pp. 160–1.

17 Stephen Burke and Cathie Williams, 'Coded message', *The Guardian*, Society section, 5 March 2008, p. 6.

18 Herzlinger, *Consumer-Driven Health Care*, op. cit., p. 12.

19 See my address, 'Empowering the silent patient', to Socialist Health Association annual conference, Holloway, London, 19 November 2005, at www.sochealth.co.uk.

20 David Levy, *NHS Independence: what's in it for patients and citizens* (Oxford, Picker Institute, 2008); Angela Coulter and Don Redding, 'Voices of Reason', *The Guardian*, Society section, 12 March 2008, p. 6. Mr Redding continues to use the general language of 'participation', 'inspection', 'user involvement' and 'the consumer interest'. Don Redding, 'Two cheers for the Care Quality Commission', *The Guardian*, society section, 11 June 2008, p. 4. No cheers for Mr Redding. On 'involvement' I refer him to Lloyd Jones, *The Book of Fame* (London, John Murray, 2008): 'In Chicago, Billy Wallace and Jimmy Hunter visited the meat-works which boasted they used every part of the animal, except the squeal: ". . . the pig goes in one end of the machine and comes out the other as hams, sausages, lard, margarine and binding for Bibles . . ."' p. 169. The pig participates, and is involved, but not empowered. See also Anna Dixon and Arturo Alvarez-Rosete, *Governing the NHS: alternatives to an NHS board* (London, King's Fund, January 2008). When the NHS Confederation published a document in June 2007 which emphasised sensitive responsiveness to patients there was no discussion of financial empowerment. NHS Confederation, *Great Expectations: what does customer focus mean for the NHS?* (NHS Confederation, London, 2007). See also Brian Edwards, *An Independent NHS: a review of the options* (London, Nuffield Trust, 2007); BMA, *An NHS Constitution for England* (London, BMA, 2008); Gordon Brown speech on NHS at King's College, London, 7 January 2008; Alan Johnson, Ministerial statement on 'NHS Next Stage Review', speech, *Hansard*, 4 July 2007, col.639.

21 Lloyd Jones, op. cit., p. 170.

22 Clare Allan, 'Out of the ward, and out of the control of others', *The Guardian*, Society section, 5 March 2008, p. 6.

23 Lloyd Jones, op. cit., pp. 82–3.

24 A. Darzi, *Our NHS Our Future – NHS next stage review interim report* (London, DoH, October 2007).

25 Sarah-Kate Templeton, 'Laggard doctors "put block on" on new treatments', *Sunday Times* news section, 22 June 2008, p. 7.

26 Nicholas Bosanquet, Andrew Haldenby, Helen Rainbow, and Michael Pullinger, *Demand for a New Era: the future of health* (London, Reform, 30 April 2008), p. 17.

27 Steven D Levitt and Stephen J Dubner, *Freakonomics: a rogue economist explores the hidden side of everything* (2005; London, Penguin Books, 2006), p. 126. The discussion of incentives throughout this book is invaluable.

28 See DoH, *The NHS in England: operating framework for 2007–08* (London, DoH, 11 December 2006), and *The NHS in England: the operating framework for 2008–09* (London, DoH, 13 December 2007). See also Ann Rossiter, *The Future of Healthcare*. Introduction (London, Social Market Foundation, May 2007). For studies offering contrary perspectives see C Bojke, H Gravelle and D Wilkin, 'Is bigger better for primary care groups and trusts?', *British Medical Journal*, 10 March 2001, 322, pp. 599–602; Robert Town, 'The welfare impact of HMP mergers', *Journal of Health Economics*, 2001, 20(6), pp. 967–90; W Anderson, D Florin, S Gillam and L Mountford, *Every Voice Counts: primary care organisations and public involvement* (London, King's Fund, 2002).

29 See Postrel, *The Future and Its Enemies*, op. cit.; Richard Mabey, *Fencing Paradise: reflections on the myth of Eden* (London, Eden Project Books, 2005), p. 76. Also Irwin Stelzer, 'Brown can't afford to abandon his long term view of a great Britain', *Daily Telegraph*, 9 April 2008, p. 20.

30 Tim Harford, *The Undercover Economist* (London, Little Brown, 2006;Abacus edition, 2007), p. 67. On the unwisdom of vertical integration see Herzlinger, *Who Killed Health Care?*, op. cit., pp. 171–2 and *Market-Driven Health Care*, op. cit.

31 Kenneth Arrow, *Social Choice and Individual Values* (New York, John Wiley & Sons, 1963); Harford, ibid., pp. 73–4.

32 Alan Milburn, 'Be bold, Gordon, trust the people', *Sunday Times*, 16 March 2008, comment, p. 19; www.timesonline.co/uk/politics.

33 Alan Milburn, 'The next stage to public service reforms', speech to Progress, London, 16 January 2008. See also Milburn's speeches 'Older people's services', statement by Secretary of State for Health, House of Commons, *Hansard*, col. 882, 23 July 2002; 'Empowering citizens: the future politics', speech to the Global Foundation, Sydney, 2 May 2006; 'A 2020 Vision for Britain's governance', St Chad's College, University of Durham, 24 May 2007, and 'A few bold steps to save Labour', *Sunday Times*, news section, 1 June 2008, p. 19. For speeches on charities legislation, House of Commons, *Hansard*, 26 June 2006, cols. 40–52, and *Hansard*, 25 October 2006, Report stage.

2

Why choice? Two concepts of order

'If, after all, men cannot always make history have a meaning, they can always act so that their own lives have one.'

– ALBERT CAMUS

'We have found all the questions that can be found. It is time we gave up looking for questions and began looking for answers.'

– GK CHESTERTON

'Choice' is both moral and instrumental. It is moral because to take choice away from individuals in this most sensitive area of life – the provision of healthcare – undermines an individual's dignity as a free, human person. Enabling choice is also central to 'the power of change' as well as signalling an understanding of the unique nature of all people. Pope John Paul II had a good way of putting the moral aspect of a free economy in saying that it was compatible with the anthropological nature of man. If we do not have choice, our dignity as persons is diminished – though we may wish to use our free choice to submit to the authority of others.

'Choice' is democratic. It interposes the individual – their personality, history, experience and wishes – as the essence of a clinical decision. It offers this as a counter to the decisions of external authority. Choice suggests that for many questions there is no 'right answer'. Instead, it signals individual identity and mobilises personal ideas of authenticity. It privileges necessarily changeable subjectivity about the most personal things in the world. This idea has many symbolic, practical and cultural consequences. It concerns the individual fulfilment of each of us, and the personal trade-offs each of us must inevitably make. The issues include the notion that the more choice we have the greater our self-responsibility. Choice is integral to an economic and a social structure which can encourage self-responsibility and self-care, neither of which can be achieved by attempts to impose them centrally. Indeed, the reliance on trying to do so is proving disastrous and costly. Reform is thus one critical pivot for preventive care. It is linked directly to incentives, to information and comparisons, and to the idea that since we each have only one life we should learn to make choices about it. We are then concerned with how to enable the expression of individual purposes and preferences, by contrast with the offer of impersonal services and impersonal standards. Individual commitment, aspiration, trade-offs, values and self-knowledge are essentials, too, in being able to gain the fullest benefit from treatments.

Choice is not only about 'efficiency' and 'value for money', although in a genuine market it can assist both of these imperatives materially. It is about authenticity. Choice is about making a service individual and special. It involves us all, too, in the creative trial and error processes where societies evolve successfully by experimentation and adaptive responses. To make things and individual experiences special is one of the tasks of health and social care, as it is also one of the principal tasks of markets. When served in open markets, individual choices increase the possibilities for others. There is a constant ratchet effect. Choices change ideas, and create ever more ideas and options which can be re-combined to make further possibilities. Choice generates unequivocal improvements, which cannot have been predetermined by planning. They arise from experiment and from the impact of previously unexpressed tacit knowledge, too. These gains are contingent, and incremental. They recognise the uncertainty of the world, and welcome trial and error as the means to reveal new possibilities. The expression of values, the negotiation of trade-offs, the ideal balance varies from person to person. Imagine, too, the choices soon to be presented to us by genetics and the consequent treatment opportunities for diseases which at present are untreatable or which are discovered too late, let alone the increasing sophistication of diagnostic methods. Here is the prospect of many controversial controls and of increased rationing ('managed demand'), or changing funding. Who decides? Who decides who decides? Whose expectations, perceptions, tastes, emotions, thoughts and policies will integrate the individual, and the opportunity? There is no longer any one best way. Yet unless we are very alert, impersonal standards are too easily disengaged from individual purpose and preferences. The essence of 'choice' in markets is who decides *who* decides. Who do we *assume* has the right to be in control?

As Virginia Postrel says,

> Rather than trying to erect an impersonal standard, removed from individual purposes, we can turn to more subjective definitions, truer to the way people actually use 'look and feel' to define themselves, and their surroundings. We can decide *for ourselves* what is authentic for *our purposes*, what matches surface with substance, form with identity. We can define authenticity from the inside out. This approach to authenticity challenges the ideal of impersonal authority, replacing it with personal, local knowledge.[1]

This kind of openness in choices about healthcare is very threatening to many professionals, and to NHS staff who have claimed to know what was best. Indeed, they have known our own best interests better than we have known them for ourselves. The NHS is one of the constructions of what was a proposed 'mass utopia' in post-war Britain. This visionary idea has, indeed, been one of the driving forces of modernisation. It is, however based on the contradiction between democracy and sovereignty which originated in the French revolution. It is based on the idea that 'experts' can know our interests better than we can. Of course, the shaman, the witch and the oracle go back to the earliest times. But in the modern era this idea is deeply political. It derives from propositions which, since the French Revolution, have privileged a vanguard party leading the falsely conscious masses.

The proposition is that 'the general will', expressed via government (or a vanguard political party), can substitute for the traditions of civil society. Thus the power of 'the people' is said to be best exercised by our leaders. Often, 'the party' and not the individual or the state becomes the sovereign agency of 'the masses'. The party and the state become one. The state is then its own end as an instrument of universal 'liberation'. These ideas now have many fewer adherents than formerly. But the 'expert' who 'consults' us stands in this tradition. Let me cite here not a figure from the liberal economic right. Let me cite the Marxist 'Frankfurt school' philosopher Susan Buck-Morss. She says:

> From the perspective of the twentieth century, the paradox seems irrefutable that political regimes claiming to rule in the name of the masses – claiming, that is, to be radically democratic – construct, *legitimately*, a terrain in which the exercise of power is out of control of the masses, veiled from public scrutiny, arbitrary and absolute. . . . It makes no difference whether the model of their legitimacy is the liberal claim of political (formal) democracy based on universal, mass suffrage, or the socialist claim of economic (substantive) democracy based on the egalitarian distribution of social goods. Either way, as regimes of supreme, sovereign power, they are always already *more* of a democracy – and consequently a good deal less.

That is, they use power democratically derived to impose their own ideas.[2]

These ideas have lost cogency and persuasiveness, although they are still being defended under the guise of a 'new localism', more 'patient involvement', increased public 'consultation' and 'a say' (even 'a greater say'). A 'new localism' may encourage innovative people to create new ways of working at local level, and to put individual requirements (not 'needs') at the centre of their work. But the fear is that a 'new localism' and an emphasis on 'patient involvement' are diversions – actually palisades against continual creative discontent. So, too, the idea of the NHS being 'run' by an independent board. Such structures would still marginalise individual satisfaction and self-definition, for these are disruptive of planning as it is conceived in public services.

Two concepts of order

We see here the contrast between two concepts of order. Indeed, two concepts of the nature of creative order itself, and of how we each see the world. One is of central control in a traditionally static framework, contrasted with one of a society as creatively self-organised, developing by trial and error experiment, welcoming innovation, expecting advantageous surprises. These two conceptual possibilities represent powerful opposing cultural and political images. They represent distinct and contrary ways of looking at the world, at people, at human nature and at cultural possibilities. The statist believes that technology enslaves us, that economic and market changes make us insecure, that popular culture coarsens us, that consumerism depends on people being cheated, and that the forces of change must be disciplined, by bureaucracy and by a Webbian or Fabian elite which knows our interests best. The dynamist supposes instead that trial and error without vastly intrusive systematic planning, an open society of choice and freedoms best support creativity, enterprise and the benefits of necessarily unpredictable discoveries as the key to human fulfilment for all. The choice about 'choice' thus concerns two conflicting views of progress, of the nature and sources of order in a self-organised or a bureaucratically constructed society. It is about two views of the nature of human life, of human potential, of who can learn to choose, and of who will make the trade-offs which are unavoidable in life. By whom? On whose terms? On whose behalf? The issue here, as ever, is who decides? And *who decides* who decides?

This is, in effect, a clash of civilisations. We are thus looking at the prospect of huge cultural changes. There is a vast canyon to cross. And you cannot change a culture by a new law. Some change will be achieved by demonstrable benefits seen in pilot projects. Some by persuasion. Some by powerful employee incentives. Some by contestability of services, and the replacement of managements. Some by much fuller publication of information, including reports from consumers. In all this the staff are essential partners in change. We should not assume that providers know best. Equally, we should not think that the people running the present system are necessarily bad people. Many are very good people who do their best to give a good service, despite the often inadequate resources. The challenge is not the language of hyperbole, but of negotiation, conciliation and reconciliation. But with the *context* set by direct economic incentives. It is, too, for staff to agree that they not the 'experts'. They may have technical knowledge. But our bodies and our lives are our own. *We* are the experts on our own lives.

This is indeed a massive cultural contrast between the centraliser and the dynamist. There are those who believe that hierarchical control should rule, and that an ideology could and should construct a comprehensive and sufficient set of answers to how to live life. And there are those who vest their faith in adaptive, trial-and-error evolution, innovation and fruitful surprise. It is a choice between knowing best and listening best. This choice offers very different views of the potentials of governments, of individuals, and of the nature of knowledge and ethics which guides policy and services and supports the idea of the individual living their own life.

The choice *is* both instrumental and moral. It distinguishes between the language of 'self-improvement' and the rhetoric of positively directed human perfectibility. We have to decide *who* we are.

Notes

1 Virginia Postrel, *The Substance of Style: how the rise of aesthetic value is remaking commerce, culture, and consciousness* (New York, HarperCollins, 2003; Harper Perennial edition, 2004), pp. 113–14.

2 Susan Buck-Morss, *Dreamworld and Catastrophe: the passing of mass utopia in East and West* (Cambridge, Mass., MIT Press, 2000), pp. 2–3. Buck-Morss – a critic both of Western capitalism and Soviet communism – thought that mass 'dream-worlds', of which the NHS is surely one, 'were compatible with terrifying assemblages of political and economic power: world war machines, machines of mass terror, violent form of labour extraction. But it was the structure of power, not the democratic utopian idea, that produced these nightmare forms.' And, as the old dream worlds dissipate these power assemblages continue to exist, she believes that 'the whole idea of what constitutes critical culture and practice may need to be rethought'. p. 276.

3

Language, and smuggled goods

'Before you begin building these great systems, let us make sure what the bricks are made of.'

– GE MOORE

'Let no one suppose that the words doctor and patient can disguise from the parties the fact that they are employer and employee.'

– GEORGE BERNARD SHAW

Language matters. There is much talk of patient-led services, of giving power to the people, of us having a say, even 'a greater say'. Of a 'new localism', of us entering 'a post-bureaucratic age', of 'consumer choice'. But what does this all mean *in practice*? Discussion of choice is increasing. But where are the instruments to make it real? To make any progress we need to be very clear about what politicians of all parties mean by *effective* 'choice', and how it is to function instrumentally in terms of improving *individual* access to public services.

The language and the instruments need to be clear. We need to unpick such slippery incantatory wording as 'passing power as close as possible to the people'. And to rescue language from what, to borrow from Sir Francis Bacon, we might view as 'a deceit of eye'. If financially empowered choice is to animate the action we need to be sure that we all mean the same thing by 'choice'. For there can easily be slippage in the meaning of words, which then recasts the terms of debate. The attempt to be more precise about the language of choice concerns the attempt to link language to reality. This is a problem with which many struggle now. When choice can, it seems, mean very different things. It can mean being in control, or it can mean being 'consulted' or involved – conflicting representations compete for our support.

These different offers in fact represent different political models. Choice can mean a new localism, or choice imposed in consultations by a concept of 'community'. It can mean the individual instead being able to go elsewhere with a tax-based fund.

A key issue is whether choice can be real, and how. In addition, it is insufficient to 'experience' these issues as intellectuals. This distorts the view. For what matters to the individual most is when they are immediately and bodily engaged with all their vulnerable corporeal senses in concrete, immediate, physical and psychological experience in healthcare. This is when empowerment matters.

We have been warned to be aware. As the Marxist philosophy Professor Susan Buck-Morss has written, 'When the structuring topology between words and the world undergoes a seismic shift, it may happen that truth cannot be said. Certain phrases, certain discourses become inaccessible, while others may re-emerge with new power. To speak of a crisis in language sounds idealist, yet it can be a profoundly concrete historical experience.'[1]

With these perspectives in view, we should consider what is meant by 'people'? What is meant by giving people more control over their lives? Is this just hocus-pocus, or is actual financial power to pass to the individual? Or just to another collectivist summation of 'the people'? If power is passed to an individual, in what form? Will the state genuinely empower the individual, and then stop its social engineering and await the accumulated results of incremental and individual decisions? What does 'a new focus on patient engagement and empowerment' and the 'personalisation of services' actually mean? We are all members of a community. But is empowerment at the level of the commune sufficient?

Dr Angela Coulter's and Don Redding's hopes for improving 'public value' in 'the local healthcare economy' but without individual financial empowerment may be attractive to some. But many would surely like to be able to be sure of a personal, necessarily intimate, separable and timely service when they want it. And to prefer not to have to spend their evenings and weekends in draughty halls 'consulting' about strategies and blueprints and reconfigurations. Or even hopefully voting every fifth year for better care amid a confusing bundle of almost identical general election promises from convergent political parties on foreign policy, transport, schools, laws, pensions, healthcare and so on. And, the election having passed, then having no prospect of sanctions for a number of years. I *would* like to be reliably well treated when I come to A&E or have access to a GP when I come home from work or be visited by an intuitive and sympathetic elderly care worker in my own home and at a time which suits my life. I would, too, like to see *my* doctor, the same doctor every time, when I go to see the GP. Similarly, investment in railways may give me better-looking trains or 'public value' and 'public ownership' (if this is what you want). But I'd also like one to arrive on time regularly, offer me a seat, and arrive safely at the promised moment and for a sensible price.

And so what does passing power 'as close as possible' to people actually mean? There is nothing closer than an individual's own hand, or pocket, or wallet, or handbag. Does it mean this? Or something else entirely? Is 'choice' to be deployed as an economic concept, giving the individual power over the health and social services they choose to use? Or is 'choice' just an instinctive centraliser's euphemism for user empowerment really meaning an increased role in local politics? Is 'choice' a proxy for something called 'the new localism' – with powers delegated to local bodies, and with users having 'a greater say'? Thus, is it 'choice' as 'community', as 'public value', as competing minorities voting, as vocal pressure groups yet again grabbing more resources in a continued beggar-my-neighbour process? We need to have in place a meaning represented by 'choice' that does not merely raise expectations but which actually describes real processes of change and of individual control. The words must not merely be political theatre, nor must they represent confusing evasions.

Consumer, customer, client and citizen

We are not, however, alone in this bumpy railway carriage. Professor George Jones (Emeritus Professor of Government at the London School of Economics) has discriminated between the four confusing words, 'consumer', 'customer', 'client' and 'citizen'. They are often misused, although they reflect different assumptions – just as they mirror basic distinctions concerning major disparities of power. It is important to have this clarification since those opposed to the individual as an empowered customer in the NHS spread confusion. They do so, as Professor Jones notes, by using the word 'customer' as if it were the same as 'consumer', and by attacking consumerism as if it were 'customerism', as he calls the two alternatives. It is 'customerism' which we want if it is individual empowerment we wish to achieve.

'Consumer' is the overall term which applies to all individuals. We all consume. We use a variety of goods and services, from various suppliers. But we are not thus necessarily empowered. No one ever says, 'The consumer is always right.'

'Customer' is the word when we have a *true* choice of supplier and are willing to pay to obtain our choice of service or provider from among multiple suppliers. The word 'customer' encapsulates several kinds of relationships, notably including a direct economic connection.

'Client' is what we are called when our 'needs' are assessed on our behalf by a professional 'expert'. Not necessarily empowering.

'Citizens' is what we are known as when we vote and pay taxes. But these two acts do not enable us to be sure of a service. Again, not empowering.

As Professor Jones says:

> Customers, clients and citizens are all individuals, consumers of goods and services, some provided by the public sector, some by the private sector, and some by the so-called independent and voluntary sector, and a few co-operatively. The enemies of consumerism denigrate the concept of consumerism by calling the consumers customers, and attributing to consumerism the elements of customerism. Government contributes to this conceptual confusion by talking sometimes of putting the consumer at the centre of public services, and at other times of putting the customer at the centre.[2]

The present book seeks to empower the *customer*, who is to hold the funds.

We should beware of smugglers, as very different objectives can be wrapped in apparently friendly sounding words. The confusion of 'patient-centred' care with consumer power, for example, is notable contraband. Later, in my chapter '*My* body, but *your* decision? 'Concordat', and shared decision making', I examine another important aspect of this conundrum. In particular, returning financial empowerment to the individual is not at all the same as passing powers to local government, to other elected bodies, to local 'experts', or to some other 'representatives', agencies or gatekeepers. We should instead focus the searchlights on the customer as the key in the equation, and the customer should be financially empowered. Without this, choice is no choice at all. We should, too, remark the use of the word 'need' repeatedly in NHS and social care discussions. The important distinction, which we should underline, is between 'needs', which experts decide for us, and 'wants', which are our specific individual preferences.

The false arguments of the protectionist producer/provider approach

We should address what Professor Jones has called 'false trails', the false arguments of the 'protectionist producer/provider approach' (as he calls it) to divert us from the customer agenda of true choice. Professor Jones has himself carefully considered these trails. The following notes cite his thoughts on the seven false trails, and my own reflections.

1   **The public is not well informed.** In this book I show why these asymmetries of information have been deliberate on the part of the NHS. And I stress that the problem of knowledge can be solved only in a market. In addition, we, the consumers, are ultimately the experts on our bodies and our lives, advised by the technical and scientific knowledge of professionals. We will also see that the public likes choice, especially those who otherwise have had none.

2   **Consumerism will raise expectations, and increase demand.** This is why it has been suppressed. The NHS has also entrenched monopoly, whereas choice and competition increase responsiveness, and expand competitive supply.

3   **Consumerism will produce a two-tier system.** We have this already. And enormous inequalities persist under the NHS. Indeed, under the NHS they have worsened. The middle class has advantageous access, and financial exit as well if they wish it. The evidence suggests that far from 'cream skimming' in competition, diverse provision and choice ensure that even poorly performing services improve. Choice over some elective care, for example, rapidly collapsed otherwise inveterate waiting lists, except in Scotland, Wales and Northern Ireland where the policy was not introduced – although Wales is now trying to catch up.

4   **Consumerism will harm the poor.** Not if financial empowerment and competition remove barriers to access. We could also introduce additional supplementary subsidies to their health savings accounts (the equivalent of weighted vouchers for the poor, which Professor Julian Le Grand has suggested). Thus empowered choice would make a reality of individual preferences, especially among the poor. In addition, an effective market would ensure that even those who take no interest in services will benefit from the results of better, cheaper, more responsive services which markets discipline.

5   **Consumerism is wasteful.** Economic evidence post-war suggests the opposite to be the case. It is hard to argue, too, that consumerism causes wasteful services when we have the evidence of so much waste and also of unnecessary suffering because of the way the NHS has operated. 'Planning' by 'experts' has not avoided enormous waste, or the lost opportunities of an open market. Efficient competition curbs waste.

6   **Consumerism will damage the public ethos.** Professor Jones says here that 'This argument is usually a cloak concealing the interests of public sector professional organisations and trades unions. It is a reactionary stance against the interests of consumers, and it curbs innovation.' Moreover, 'The best public service ethic is that producers/providers ensure their decisions are shaped by the desire to anticipate and meet their consumers' preferences. Then they will be serving customers.'[3]

7   **Consumerism threatens collective choice.** Greater local democracy would enhance collective choice *if* representatives responded to the imperatives that choice represents. Then consumerism would strengthen citizenship.

More on these issues in a moment. But first something more on words themselves.

Cultural messengers

Words are cultural messengers. We need to focus very carefully on the words 'consumer', 'customer', 'client' and 'choice'. And especially on the conditions in which choice works; on how it can be instrumental and not merely aspirational. Again, we need to move away from averages and aggregates, from collectivities and communities, to focus on individuals and particulars rather than on grand abstractions, to place the individual centre stage. We need to be clear about the meanings of the words now in confused currency, about the implications of such fundamental concepts as 'choice', and of the words which purport to describe its meanings.

For 'keywords' (to use Raymond Williams's term) carry many silently enfolded cultural signals. These are political, economic and social messages. They need to be 'read', just as a novel, a play, a film or a painting, to be decoded and unpicked for messages. To be seen for what they are, and what they intend and imply. They are of empirical, tangible and conceptual interest. They subtly reflect individual values and valuations. They offer ways of seeing and guidance to ways of living. However, an apparently shared vocabulary often conceals entirely different understandings about words, concepts and central processes in the culture and society of our lives. This can make discussion of policy a matter of misunderstood misunderstandings. This is not always accidental. We should be alert to the meanings of keywords: about what they 'say', for example, about who is to manage and supervise our lives and how.

Raymond Williams pointed out in his *Keywords* that the meanings of words are inextricably bound up with values.[4] And that without clarity in the cultural role played by these concepts we will not appreciate the issues and problems hidden 'inside the vocabulary'. Nor can we have an open, informed, honest and productive debate in which the true choices are understood. Words like 'choice', 'price' (or value for money) and 'market' – and attitudes to them – are not merely descriptive. They are indicative of forms of thought, of ways of thinking and feeling, of dynamist or statist assumptions.

The great dividing line, indeed, is not between individual freedoms and local accountability on the one hand and increasing central controls on the other. It concerns the individual being in control of money. Verbal precision here is no mere pedantry. It is not trivial. And so we need to be very much clearer about what is meant by the 'choice agenda', and how it would work. We do not yet all use the same words for it with the same meanings. The risk is that it will be a deception at the centre of our lives. We do need more precise words and instruments, and to use these to reveal the likely shape of future policy and events.

The start of personal budgets in social care has enormous (and much underestimated) revolutionary potential. They help us to enquire about what individual choice means *in practice*. This examination takes us beyond the language of consensual pragmatists to start to transform healthcare purchasing and provision. It also opens up crucial difficulties that exist for those who are self-funding elderly care already, as well as for those struggling with local authority accreditation regulations and diversionary tactics to deter demand. I devote three chapters to savings, funding, and the choice agenda in long-term elderly care: 'Are you being personal, or what?', 'To see the statue in the marble', and 'The picture in the frame'.

I have urged a move towards consumers joining mutual, member-owned purchasing bodies. The reasons are clearly summarised by Professor Jones:

> Consumers are disorganised individuals, in a weaker position in society than service producers/providers, who are more powerful, well-organised, richer and better located to exert effective influence. Their voice counts for more than that of lone consumers. They are strategically better placed in their businesses to advance their interests against those of consumers. And trade unions often unite with employers to protect jobs and to preserve practices that suit their convenience, rather than serve the interests and needs of the consumers of their products and services. The trade unions of the middle class, the professional bodies, are in this category of producer/provider, who know better than consumers what they need and want. Because of their organisation these producer/provider groups are better able than consumers to influence government.

They are listened to as representative stakeholders, presenting an informed and coherent argument, which is harder for a mass of individual consumers to do. So these producers/providers, employers, trade unions and professional bodies exercise a dominant influence in both the public and private sectors.[5]

Authenticity

These challenges present very difficult dilemmas. To find answers we need to consider the stressful daily work of the NHS, the relevant economics, and the value of using some theory to illuminate practice by posing questions. Free market first principles, especially those which can encourage consumer-driven reform, are essential. The important thing is to be clear about the first principles of consumer-driven care. There is health and social care news every single day. Any book is likely to be rapidly out of date, at least in terms of these detailed events. This is why in 2003 I published my book *Patients, Power and Responsibility*, to try to set out the first principles of consumer-driven reform. Professor Herzlinger's innovative works have done so, too, and for many years.[6] My previous work offered a structure and a means by which to assess this daily news. And, by the by, to interrogate proposals for change put to us by politicians who suggest that the currency of care is votes. The case for consumer-driven reform has significantly strengthened with a further five years of experience. The first principles were correctly stated and remain entirely valid, as they should.

I am here especially preoccupied with authenticity, and with freeing us all to be subjective. I suggest that we can and should invest in enabling people to choose for themselves, to develop an authentic sense of themselves by which to guide their own decisions about health, long-term care, savings and outcomes as customers. This is not the kind of authenticity which has been identified – painfully for us all – by politicised discourses such as that which is represented by the NHS. It is a political myth that systems must be 'designed' or have a creator. The unexpected evolves best in adaptive change. Value is subjective. Dynamism is creative, positive and to be welcomed. Risk is unavoidable, because we are alive. People want to accept no more risk than is necessary. But the problem is to discover what this might be. Information which is really knowledge, reputation, advice, hard work, talent and luck all come into this.

'Equality', too, is a dangerous delusion if by it we mean the same genetic inputs and the same care outputs for us all. Instead, we should have equal *access* to care.

What works best for an individual can only be discovered through concrete experience. Personal meanings and personal values in healthcare are fundamental. These are necessarily based in the particular as it appeals to the individual. It is for people to make their own trade-offs among the alternatives they face and discover. That way lies self-responsibility and the hope of preventive care. This means taking people seriously as competent interpreters of their own lives. It means ceasing to treat people as categories and statistics. We are none of us average. This case, indeed, has been made not only by economic liberals *but also*, surprisingly, by such Marxist historians as EP Thompson and EJ Hobsbawm. But do their public sector followers believe them?[7]

The debate about personalisation and care opens up more widely into one of how to help everyone to save and self-fund, as I have said. And of how people can make their individual purchasing decisions really effective through collaborative, mutual purchasing organisations – patient guaranteed care associations. Such a reform will, I believe, enable those on lower incomes at last to receive the care which is taken for granted in many other modern countries, including – as the evidence shows – some in the former Soviet bloc in Eastern Europe.[8]

Keywords and phrases in these debates reflect the history which has shaped where we begin. Well understood, properly deployed, suitably appreciated they can unlock many of the potentials of a better approach to health and social care. Yet, as the Irish Anglican bishop and philosopher George Berkeley said, 'We must get behind words, and consider the things themselves.'

George Orwell wrote in 1946 that 'If thought corrupts language, language can also corrupt thought. A bad usage can spread by tradition and imitation, even among people who should and do know better.'[9]

You can hide things in vocabulary.

Notes

1 Susan Buck-Morss, *Dreamworld and Catastrophe: the passing of mass utopia in East and West* (Cambridge, Mass., MIT Press, 2000), p. 240.
2 George Jones and Catherine Needham, 'Debate: consumerism in public services – for and against', *Public Money and Management*, April 2008, 28(2), pp. 67–77. I owe this reference to Professor Michael Connolly. Other loosely used and undefined terms include 'care pathways'.
3 George Jones, ibid., p. 72.
4 Raymond Williams, *Keywords: a vocabulary of culture and society* (London, Fontana, 1976).
5 Jones, op. cit., p. 67.
6 See Regina E. Herzlinger (ed.), *Consumer-Driven Health Care: implications for providers, payers, and policymakers* (San Francisco, Calif., Jossey-Bass/John Wiley, 2004); *Market-Driven Health Care: who wins, who loses in the transformation of America's largest service industry* (Cambridge, Mass., Perseus Books, 1999); *Protection of the Health Care Consumer: the 'Truth Agency'* (Washington, D.C., Progressive Policy Institute, March 1999); *Who Killed Health Care? America's $2 trillion medical problem – and the consumer-driven cure* (New York, McGraw Hill, 2007), and many articles referenced in these books. See also Richard L Reece (ed.), *Innovation-Driven Health Care: 34 key concepts for transformation* (Boston, Jones and Bartlett Publishers, 2007).
7 See Richard Sennett, Preface to Alessandra Buonfino and Geoff Mulgan, *Porcupines in Winter: the pleasure and pains of living in modern Britain*. London, The Young Foundation, 2006.
8 Nick Bosanquet, Andrew Haldenby and Helen Rainbow, *NHS Reform: national mantra, not local reality* (London, Reform, February 2008).
9 George Orwell, 'Politics and the English Language', 1946, in Sonia Brownell Orwell and Ian Angus (eds.), *Collected Essays, Journals and Letters*, Vol. IV, *In Front of Your Nose, 1945–1950* (London, Secker and Warburg, 1968).

4

The ticking clock: six policy recommendations

'In general I believe that [the value of competition] is a necessary condition, albeit not always a sufficient condition for economic welfare. Regulation is sometimes necessary as a surrogate for competition. I believe that the promotion and protection of competition should be given greater prominence as a policy objective.'

– SIR [NOW LORD] GORDON BORRIE

'Doctors really must get typewriters. This lady is suffering from something unreadable.'

– JUDGE TUDOR REES

Successful reforms depend on direct incentives. And on the NHS itself being prepared to change. On people accepting a shifting role. And on staff being granted *permission* to change. The issues are cultural as much as political. Structures are cultural. A viable, evolving, market-based system is possible only if incentives and rewards are introduced and then if people willingly endorse change. All this necessarily includes major revisions to structures as well as attitudes. That is, if services are indeed to respond to the preferences of consumers. However, 'Beware choice!' Certainly beware the word if it stands alone. We should beware using it by itself; it will only really be meaningful if we link it to incentives and levers by which it can be individually effective. Thus, we should use the phrase 'individually financially empowered choice', if we mean choice to be real. When you read 'reform' proposals which do not include these words, enquire within carefully and sceptically.

If we wish to modernise the NHS and social care and to empower 'choice' (for short!) and benefit from competition there are specific policy recommendations which could form a new framework. I have outlined these, but it may be helpful at this point to summarise them.

As my proposed health savings accounts imply, we need to carefully re-examine a number of key structural issues. These include taxpayer subsidy, the administrative mechanisms, the role of insurance, the creative possibilities of tax relief and so on. It is not my purpose in this book to try to work out the details of this series of mechanisms in every respect. I have previously addressed these questions at length in my *Patients, Power and Responsibility*. In my chapters on long-term elderly care I do try to address details. But otherwise I am seeking to encourage the reader to think about why these cultural and structural changes are necessary and, indeed, the only solution. There are clearly some major steps that we should take.

As I have already argued, one key was most persuasively demonstrated by the Nobel prize-winning economist Kenneth Arrow (and as Tim Harford shows). This is to adjust the starting position. That is, to give the poor the financial power and the free choice which they have been denied, with the introduction of health savings accounts. Instead of interfering with markets we should equip those who have done least well from the NHS to gain the fullest benefits from them.

Thus:

1 The tax-based funding of health, social care and long-term elderly care should be brought together.

2 Every person should hold a lifelong health savings account. Ideally, this fund would be based entirely upon personal savings, as in Singapore. Every holder of an HSA would be encouraged to add to the initial tax-based investment, with tax incentives to do so. Non-taxpayers and other low-income groups would continue to receive support. Hypothecated funds from taxes would be paid into personalised accounts. However, a key feature of HSAs is that once your personal fund reaches a set level your required payments can reduce and possibly even cease. This provides a real incentive to be frugal with expenditure. In terms of social and elderly care funding, the HSA would end the discrimination typical of the NHS towards the elderly and other groups by ensuring that everyone had economic power. It would also be a means for encouraging ways to expand revenues via additional, voluntary co-payments. If the holder negotiated a bi-annual 'health plan' there could also be incentives for achieving specific objectives such as changing lifestyles. This would directly impact on preventive care, as we saw with the discussion of Pruhealth.

3 Competitive purchasing organisations in localities should offer their services to individuals who would decide where to place their HSA. These would be mutual, cooperative, member-owned organisations – my patient guaranteed care associations.

4 Competing provider organisations should offer a pluralist response to competitive purchasing.

5 The management of existing monopoly institutions should be regularly contested. Notably, in A&E services and large district general hospitals, PCTs and teaching hospitals where specialists are clustered and where doctor training is exclusively approved. These managements should be contestable on a periodic basis. It is not only politicians and policymakers who should be subject to challenge and recall. As this is increasingly an issue as many more hospital trusts and PCTs merge, apparently to avoid competition.

6 Rapidly audited information should be promptly published to empower comparisons. I have urged the establishment of an independent Disclosure and Information Commission.

Choice would *be* choice by being backed in every individual case by money. It would be ineluctable, unavoidable and a permanent factor in a market. It would require both *competing* purchasers *and* competing providers to seek willing revenues from the actual users of services. Money would be mobile. The individual would express preferences both by joining a mutual, cooperative purchasing organisation (a PGCA) and by negotiating about specific service (and costs) with that organisation. Choice would not depend on a list of centrally directed priorities, which can be and, indeed, are being actively ignored by PCTs. Choice would be particular, specific, individual and powerful. It would offer the greatest incentives to change in cultures, purchasing and provision – as well as in lifestyles. The incentives for the organisation would be that if chosen it would flourish by satisfying those who use it and who work within it. Or it changes, retrains, and retools with the help of an official 'failure strategy'. Or it really fails, fades and is forgotten. Eric Hoffer says in *The Ordeal of Change* (1963) that 'There can be no freedom without the freedom to fail'.

Crucially, we must stop being frightened to let really failing organisations actually fail if they cannot be improved or transformed. It is absolutely vital in a growing economy and a changing society that there is movement, which includes organisations closing down which no longer fit the purposes of the consumers. Fossilisation cures no one. Failing organisations must start afresh, with a new culture and new values. New organisations must have the opportunity to come in, offer services and access cash flows. One of the great weaknesses of public services is that the inept are protected. As the present reforms take effect – and as recent increases in funding level out – the weaker providers will come under greater pressures as they find it difficult to meet demand. When they plead to the state for help this must be given in such a way as to avoid embedding even more disincentives to reform and to respond to consumer choice. In a market they would have to compete for help. The effects of financially empowered choice must not be 'mitigated' for political reasons, although it is certain that in the absence of a properly functioning market they will be. There should be pluralist competition in response to financially empowered demand. Cash flow or cash ebb.

Then there is the issue of 'equality'. This is neither desirable nor possible as a politically imposed view of the world. But we can try to achieve equal access to services. Trying to impose a politicised equality by the NHS does more to cheat the poor than restrict the better off. It has proved difficult for the NHS to achieve equal access to services. My proposed PGCAs offer the best hope of this.

We might note, too, that much of what the NHS now tries to do is not about life or death conditions, but about lifestyle choices. For example, it is wonderful to be able to get a new hip, but you do not die without one. The removal of tattooing may help some with mental problems, but the difficulty is self-imposed. Fertility services can help many, but they were never part of the original idea of the NHS and the case for this being a burden on taxpayers looks very slight. Indeed, Aneurin Bevan said that he thought that once a backlog had been cleared, demand for services would fall. If we each had an HSA we could decide for ourselves, and bear these costs, although the incentives would be to be more frugal and prudent.

In brief, do not obstruct the evolution of the market, but set up the conditions for a genuine market with all its advantages. Enable organisations to innovate. They do this most when they are under the most intense competitive pressures. If not, many do not ever do so. To do these things:

❐ Empower the customer with both knowledge and information, the power to make comparisons, and money to make personal choices effective
❐ Move from limited choice and the recent introduction of personal budgets in social care to a health savings account for everyone
❐ Make purchasing locally competitive
❐ Make individual funds mobile, to enable the purchasing tools to evolve effectively
❐ Protect competition
❐ Require a minimum level of catastrophic insurance
❐ Measure and publish the patients' experiences
❐ Cease to subsidise providers
❐ Ensure pluralist provision and end the predominance of monopoly providers and purchasers

- ❏ Use direct incentives that will change structures, cultures, behaviours, purchasing and provision
- ❏ Halt the drive towards a national tariff for all services. Let local negotiations agree prices, on every element of service costs including staff incomes. Competitive purchasing and provision is how to reduce costs and waste
- ❏ Substitute empowerment for politics.

Politicians and civil servants want power and money. They do not want a market. Yet we face the conundrum that it is only politicians who can make politicians stand aside. However, their social and economic context is itself changing. Not least because of the unexpected consequences of some political initiatives, notably in personal budgets for social care.

5

The seven uninvited guests: 'markets', 'risk', 'competition', 'customer', 'profit', 'price' and 'demand'

'In our own time the division between the high-born and the base-born has become a fiction, transparent to every eye. But the distinction between the lowly manual world and the lofty intellectual one continues – no longer as lord and serf, but as officer and subaltern, party cadre and party member, expert and everyone else. Even after the rights of property have been unmasked, those of intellectual labour remain.'

– RL HEILBRONER

'We must, for the most part, choose how to act as individuals on the basis of moral beliefs which are merely fairly grounded, but when we make these choices we are exercising our freedom, whereas when governments choose, they are diminishing freedom.'

– JOHN MARENBON

'. . . although competition is uncomfortable if you are on the wrong end of it, it is pleasant to be on the right end, as the customer.'

– TIM HARFORD

'The efficiency criterion dictates that we measure all gains and all losses in terms of willingness to pay and measure one total against the other.'

– STEVEN E LANDSBURG

'How selfish soever man may be supposed, there are evidently some principles in his nature, which interest him in the fortune of others, and render their happiness necessary to him, though he derives nothing from it, except the pleasure of seeing it.'

– ADAM SMITH

The law tells us that 'ignorance is no excuse'. But we do not make this a principle in health and social care debates, as we should. And so there are many uninvited guests.

Notably 'Markets', 'Risk, 'Competition', 'Customer', 'Profit', 'Price' and 'Demand'. If we are to make genuine progress in reform we must seat these friends, and with a warm welcome.

The health savings account introduces these into the debate. And they then together introduce self-responsibility, which centralisers otherwise find so elusive. They introduce the idea of saving. And they ask people to make relative judgements about expenditure. 'But we cannot possibly do that!' you may say. Yet we do so already, do we not? Isn't this what rationing represents? 'Ah, yes. But that's different.' How? 'Well, we experts make these decisions, of course.' Ah! Even so, there is no way to side-step affordability. As the increase in revenues declines this will become clear again to an NHS that has recently experienced unaccustomed investment. We need some mature discussion about 'Markets', 'Risk', 'Competition', 'Customer', 'Profit', 'Price' and 'Demand': about what these represent, and how they can help us. History helps us. Markets make do and mend. Risk *is* life. Competition raises all boats. Empowered customers hold funds. Profits are the result of customer preferences. Profit (or 'surpluses') can be redistributed as lower costs or more services. Demand is the expression of otherwise distributed knowledge, which NHS 'consultation' seeks to discover but fails.

These friends are neither ghouls nor ghosts. They are specific. They ask the individual to make a considered trade-off. They are the non-political but democratic devices by which resources are allocated according to individual preferences. They measure the weight to which each individual gives to a choice. These then are an expression or a form of payment, and of income to the successful provider. Price rations scarce goods. But it does it openly. This sounds simple. But it is not always understood within the NHS and in social care where many still try – unavailingly and with many contortions (of which 'public value' is another new runner) – to find a political substitute. However, unprecedented new investment in the NHS has done nothing to resolve the enigmas that both officials and service-users have to face. We need different understandings if we are to move forward.

Markets

There are a number of points to be made about markets, but the most important are these five.

First, they are the bedrock of democracy and freedom.

Second, far from being the enemy, they are the most powerful mechanism ever developed for achieving human objectives and in matching scarce supply with priced demand. If we want to achieve quality care for all, and to encourage self-care and self-ownership, it is time to put them to proper use. It is time, too, to stop criticising 'quasi-markets' as if they were real markets, and then blaming untried free and real markets for the deficits of the pretend version.

Third, markets do not represent a choice between humanity and selfishness. Instead, they do most to raise standards and provide quality care. Where there is any 'market failure' in healthcare – some uncertainty, moral hazard, adverse selection, asymmetry of information – this is more swiftly corrected by action in markets themselves. When there is 'government failure' politics makes these much more difficult to correct.[1]

Fourth, in terms of health and social care it is the exclusion of the poor from markets which has been to their disadvantage, rather than the so-called conspiracy of markets which has damaged their health and social care. Markets, too, are non-coercive. And if we equip the poor with tax-transfers, markets will empower the silent and the disadvantaged. Markets do not require us to be saints or prophets or political activists, as Adam Smith pointed out more than 200 years ago. Markets take people as they are, and competition serves the general good.

Fifth, free markets force you to tell the truth and reveal information about individual priorities and preferences, demand and costs – which leads to a more efficient economy. As the economist Tim Harford has said,

> In a free market, people don't buy things that are worth less to them than the asking price. And people don't sell things that are worth more to them than the asking price. . . . The reason is simple: nobody is forcing them to, which means that most transactions that happen in a free market improve efficiency, because they make both parties better off – or at least not worse off – and don't harm anyone else.[2]

A few moments reflection on how we live 'ordinary' life tells us much which we should relate to healthcare and its organisation. We all know that as consumers we do not buy goods or services, *as such*. We buy particular *characteristics* of goods and services: price, quality, timeliness, convenience, colour, size, and so on. Influences on decisions include taste, income, preferences, the seasons, information, habits and traditions, and other objective and subjective factors. The incentive for the provider is to seek our custom. It is our decision as to whether they succeed.

Market forces determine supply, price levels and the cumulative impacts of buyers and sellers. Providers try to meet consumer preference. They must protect their income, and also the interests of their purchasers and their staff. They dare not be careless about their reputation and their competitive position. In an NHS monopoly, however, the customer cannot go round the corner to a competitor, save for those who see the same doctor privately and for a fee.

In a proper market the only way to protect the essentials for survival is to deliver a good service, in whichever sector of the market an organisation chooses to supply. They must continuously innovate, control costs, invest, take feedback seriously, and stretch to try to increase satisfactions. Markets thus ensure quality, and variety, too. Markets are not necessarily only about private profit, though any provider must make some kind of surplus to survive. Markets do not require every action or exchange to be profit-making. There are numerous institutions where we see the expression of this impulse: in families, among friends and neighbourhoods, in charitable, church and voluntary associations. We see this among carers – who are one of the biggest providers of welfare, in a moral economy – and in provision for children, the elderly and the sick. The argument here, too, and by the by is that these institutions are a more appropriate outlet for our moral obligations than are coercive state institutions. But, unfortunately, they have often been undermined or displaced by the state.

So far as the poor are concerned, the NHS has functioned as a particular kind of cultural 'market', or as a class structure in itself. Social and linguistic clout brings better service to specific individuals. Consider attitude, accent (even in a 'call-me-Tone' world), education, and all the messages concerning class and expectations which these carry to professionals in healthcare. This structure of class and culture has created what for the poor and the inarticulate have proved to be impassable barriers between themselves and good, ready, prompt, routine and reliable access to care. They have competed less successfully than the middle class for artificially restricted funding and rationed services. The middle classes take less time to get on to a waiting list; they wait less time on waiting lists. They pay a smaller price in terms of pain and early death. And they can evade uncomfortable barriers by writing private cheques. The issue is to ensure that everyone irrespective of income can participate in these benefits.

I have offered illustrations of how this is already achieved specifically in UK healthcare in the deregulated optics market, and how it can more widely work to the individual and mutual advantage of us all. In particular, this is seen in the high street with the revolution in optical care where we are one people, in one market, for one quality service. I described this in detail in my *Patients, Power and Responsibility*. Markets like this, too, in Dr Irwin M Stelzer's phrase, offer us 'an anchor when the gales of special privilege hit the ship of state'.[3] They proffer protection from vested interest. However,

> The lack of faith in markets leads to meddling which produces inefficiencies that we can ill afford; the sumptuary mentality gives policy-makers licence to impose their values on everyone save themselves; and the anti-risk attitude deprives society of innovations that it needs if productivity is to continue to provide an impetus to continued inflation-free economic growth.[4]

The proof of these notions can be seen round us in the huge changes in our society since the 1940s. It is easy to underestimate these very significant – and widely diffused – economic advances, because they are now so familiar and unexceptional. But we should properly identify the sources of prosperity, freedom and choice. The advances in living standards (for all the short-term unreliability of some markets – but which rapidly adjust, unlike political markets or government-failure) have been long term. They have been diffused and truly enormous changes. We are all better fed, clothed, housed and more independently mobile than we were. Social distinctions and class bias have reduced, and minorities are less disadvantaged. These advances make the point that they are the result of initiative, dynamism, enterprise, choice, personal aspiration, desire, optimism and voluntary cooperation in the marketplace. As Stelzer has noted, 'Rapid growth has historically been accompanied by rising living standards for all groups, making economic growth perhaps the most successful of all anti-poverty programmes.'[5]

Indeed, the whole history of England has been one of consistent and continuous enterprise, of markets and of market forces. These, prior to 1948, were regarded as legitimate, valid and mutually advantageous. This was, indeed, a history of creativity and dynamism, responsibility and risk taking, opportunity and social mobility, mutual and cooperative self-organisation. Markets were and are marked by the wide spread of ownership and opportunity through trial-and-error adaptation, feedback, self-help and mutual aid. Many working people – and many poor and disabled people, too – have successfully made personal judgements, exercised choices and improved themselves. This has been true not only of the old 'Labour aristocracy' – previously well-organised in the 'craft unions' – but of those formerly considered merely as labourers where in fact many are indeed highly skilled. One such, a tiler and a member of my own family (Mr Robert Cooper), said to me recently: 'I don't want or expect anybody to pay for me or my family. I expect to pay my own way. I'm not a businessman. I'm a worker. I work with my hands, not with a telephone. And I stand on my own two feet.'

This reflects an old English attitude, that if something needs doing then the best person to do it is you. If there's a problem, deal with it. Don't go bleating to government for a grant or a social worker. People are not all fools, and public policy should not assume that they are. They are well aware of how markets actually work, of the relationship between choice and service – as the dynamism of the revolution in eye-care has shown. They know that there is an inescapable connection between action and outcomes. And that self-responsibility and deeper satisfactions are necessarily intertwined. Secondly, prior to the monopoly NHS and its statist structures, many working people made forward-thinking and personal provision for their own families, and on a very impressive scale in the marketplace.

As we learn from William Beveridge, the preface to the original rules of the Hearts of Oak Benefit Society (June 1842) – begun in a meeting of a handful of unknown individuals in a back room – said: 'Providence has given to no man an indemnity from affliction, disease and death; it is a duty, therefore, that every man owes to himself and family, to provide against these exigencies and that distress which inevitably attends their visitations.' These initiators were 'individuals not satisfied with what they were getting from existing institutions and therefore making a new institution to meet their needs, as men always can in a free society'. This ability (which itself enunciates the prime colours in life – learning to choose, to organise in mutual aid, to protect oneself and family against sickness, unemployment, old age and the other risks in every life), together with the richness of its history, is much underestimated. Scholars like Professor Alan Kidd have shown this, and Beveridge himself stressed it and urged its once-and-future role just at the moment when the Social Service State was coming into being.[6]

Risk

Whichever way we move, there is a risk. But life is risky, which is a part of its fascination and its challenge. If we are to improve health and social care we need a different attitude to risk, notably in supporting people to innovate, giving people permission to improve by varying services. Indeed, the traditional certainties (taxes; death) are disagreeable. Berlin told us that all choices have costs – we cannot have it all.[7] Playwright Tom Stoppard said that 'Life itself is a gamble at terrible odds – if it was a bet you wouldn't take it.'[8] And in Adam Wildavsky's famous commentary, we should not chase the illusion of a risk-free society, since this would prohibit many wealth-enhancing activities, and deplete the vital resources which alone can combat and compensate for hazards. Ultimately, what safety can be had is secured by taking risks since this allows knowledge to build up, and adaptations to occur in a necessarily uncertain (and, personally finite) world.[9] Ivan Illich, in Limits to Medicine, argued that modern medicine is one of our biggest risks. For him it had become a threat to health – by undermining our ability to cope with death, sickness and pain. For death, pain, risk and sickness are part of being human.[10] Or, as Dr Petr Skrabanek commented: 'Since life itself is a universally fatal sexually transmitted disease, living it to the full demands a balance between reasonable and unreasonable risk.'[11]

The business of risk assessment is very complex. All forms of endeavour involve risk. In business, market conditions shift constantly. Natural hazards intervene. There is a constant effort, too, to shift risk. In medicine, risk – or its probability – is not always measurable. Even when it is, it is not always easy to comprehend. Again, trade-offs are at issue, too. And the users of services find it difficult to understand. So, too, for many doctors. Economists write about 'uncertainty' in terms of unpredictability or imperfect foresight and knowledge. There is here a world of estimates and guesses, predictions and prayers. The individual has to choose among several possible actions and among a number of possible outcomes. There is an attempt, with advice, evidence – if it exists, which is often a large presumption – and advocacy to offer some calculations of chances or probabilities, especially if the course has been followed many times before. Thus we seek to reduce uncertainty and improve outcomes. Here, the ability to make informed comparisons is important, which is one of the basics of improved choice.

Statistical probabilities, however, do not always help patients decide. What is going to happen to *me* is their question? Where do *I* stand on the graph? What actually happens may be different from what they expect. In addition, since this is the only time that the individual is likely to have a particular treatment, probability theory may not be as much help as they would like since the actions are unlikely to be repeated for them.

It is, however, their values which should guide their choice once they have received all possible guidance. Arthur Seldon and FG Pennance put some of the issues thus:

> . . . the British economist G.L.S. Shackle has developed a theory of which a bare outline is as follows. The individual who has to make a choice focuses his attention on the best and the worst possible outcomes for each of the possible actions. He may think that some outcomes are more likely than others. The best and the worst possible outcomes for each possible action can be converted into values corresponding to the outcomes that seem equally likely. For each set of converted best and worst possible outcomes, a point can be plotted on a gambler's indifference map for each possible action. The point (or points) falling on the highest indifference curve then indicates the best possible action (or actions). A point on a higher indifference curve is preferable to a point on a lower curve, because for the same loss a larger gain is possible.[12]

In medicine, doctors tend to frame their interpretation of data in ways which promote procedures they prefer. Thus the emphasis on the role of biomedicine as the solution to health problems. This arises from what is well-known as the 'framing effect' – of how questions are put and data assessed. Often the data can be honourably interpreted in different ways but the biomedical answers have been preferred by doctors.[13] Second, the conceptual tools are not always easy for the layperson to use. There is NNT: the number necessary to treat. There is the further concept of 'the standard gamble' – balancing the negative utility of a particular outcome against a risk of sudden death.[14] There is then the notion of 'time trade-off', concerning the value of improvements by comparison with the amount of life expectancy an individual is prepared to forgo to achieve them.[15]

The NNT is the inverse of the absolute benefit of intervention. It has been argued that this can give an indication of the likelihood of actual benefit from treatment.[16] Dr David Misselbrook cites Chatellier, who points out 'what is the clinical meaning of a number needed to treat for five years to avoid one clinical event for the average doctor? Some doctors will probably consider that this number represents an important health benefit, whereas others will consider the benefit as only moderate or slight.'[17] These are difficult concepts for the individual to consider when trying to decide on high and low probabilities, benefits and detriments, good or not-so-good outcomes, and 'what might happen to me'.

These are all mathematical models, with which doctors are familiar. Yet even doctors can confuse statistical significance with clinical significance.[18] And the ordinary individual probably doesn't think in these terms, of absolute risk, relative risk, and NNT. Patients want to know: 'What are *my* chances, doc? What's going to happen to *me*?' What patients know and think concerning risk is thought to be based on a polarity model – high-risk or low risk – mixed up with destiny, luck, fate and forces outside individual control but which might determine the future. Incentives may not reach into this world at all. Misselbrook points out that the SAVE trial shows that if doctors give captopril after a myocardial infarct then the death rate will fall from 24.7% to 20.4% over three years. This gives an NNT of 23. That is, 23 people have to be treated over three years in order to save one life. This genuine benefit requires 22 to be treated with no benefit. Misselbrook advocates a different measure, PPB or personal probability of benefit, which is the inverse of NNT. Thus, the PPB for this treatment would be 1 in 23 over three years. For conditions with a large NNT, only a small minority will benefit from treatment, whereas the detriments of treatment potentially apply to each person treated. Few patients know these terms or are aware of these issues. But, as Misselbrook says, 'One could argue that if we do not explain the low probability of benefit to patients then they are not giving informed consent to treatment.'[19]

Misselbrook tells us that 'lay models of probability are not based on maths, but upon an innate sense of personal significance within the universe'.[20] And 'John Smith is not the slightest bit interested which group is at risk. He wants to know if he is going to have a heart attack. *And we cannot tell him!*'[21] This is what makes it so difficult to change behaviour by talking about populations, or to do so by offering individual incentives. Framing effects have a big influence on patients' choices, but unless the individual can personalise the issue he or she may take no notice of educational materials. Individual doctors can offer some guidance on the personal probability of benefit. But it is a complicated mathematical card. In the end, however, as Misselbrook says, 'Only the patient can determine what is the best buy for them. Proper medical goals should therefore normally be seen as patient-defined and subjective. Outcomes that patients want are more important than outcomes that doctors can measure.'[22] And they are much more likely to do so when considering how appropriate advice is to their individual interests than by reference to the theoretical 'population' which planners consider.

Risk assessment in medicine is very problematic. It is reliant on numerical probability information, which many doctors do not understand or which they can misinterpret. And there is some evidence that patients are at least as likely to assess risks as well as 'experts'.[23] As Dr Richard Smith, then editor of the *British Medical Journal*, concluded: 'This is the way that the world is going. It's called postmodernism. There is no "truth" defined by experts. Rather, there are many opinions and theories of the world. Doctors, governments, and even the *BMJ* might hanker after a world where their view is dominant. But that world is disappearing fast.'[24]

Competition

This gets socially embedded markets enthused. Competition is a process of discovery. It diffuses power. It provides incentives for discovery and supply. It generates efficiencies. It encourages responsibility. It widens freedom and opportunity. It prompts imagination and innovation. It reduces costs. It is self-correcting. It is embedded in a framework of laws and institutions, of property, contract and organisations. It directs private effort into public benefit. It fulfils moral and social purposes. It lifts all boats. Of what other methods of economic management can any or all of this be said?

As the economist Arthur Seldon wrote, 'Competition in its fundamental social, dynamic purpose is a device for discovering demand and supply (in their everyday sense, i.e. what people want and how to give it to them) rather than merely responding to existing wants and techniques.' And: 'in general it is better policy to exert power so that it harmonizes with human proclivities (as expressed in market forces), not against them.'[25]

I have already urged the ethical interdependence and coincidence of fairness and economic efficiencies. And the desirability of competition *of itself*. Here, many people part company. Those with an ideological commitment to a particular, redistributive view of 'fairness' fear that there will be losers, or individuals who suffer poorer care because of competition. However, the opposite is, observably, the more certain truth.

By making payment among competitive offers of goods individuals secure a personal service. The concept of equality of treatment – a long-standing ethical demand – is then more achievable. It has not been shown to be deliverable from the centralising promise of the state intervening on behalf of the individual. It is, indeed, in state monopolies where there is ordinarily inadequate capacity, lower standards, insensitivity to customer wishes, inconvenient access, poor communication, and inadequate means of complaint and redress. Government failures are very difficult to correct, unlike those in markets. Where there is a state monopoly there is a single producer with a single product and with no close substitute available for all. Similarly, for long there was also a situation where there was a single buyer, the state. It is in those situations where the desire of good access for all has been more usually denied.

Indeed, the lack of competition is more normally associated with failure to give good access to good care. Here, the incentives for efficiency are less pressing or less motivating. Corporate goals are set and directed from above instead of by local management responding to demand. Satisfying the consumer (as opposed to the Chancellor) is unnecessary, for he or she cannot hit back at the manager's wallet. These deficits (and opportunities) are only invisible when looked at through ideological spectacles. Competition, by contrast to state interventions, provides an efficient allocation of resources. A mix of competitors have typically shown themselves more likely to offer a greater variety of services at lower cost and with more focus on consumer preferences. This is not the case when there is a single dominant firm, or a government monopoly of funding, purchasing and providing. When this latter is the case, government sets prices, decides on products or services, concentrates economic power and does not deploy direct incentives. Instead, it relies on political direction and on centrally set targets and priorities. There is no challenge to the incumbent – which is 'No. 10'. True, there are periodical elections, but there has been little choice between health policies. And voting does not *in any case* secure a specific, personal service to the individual. Even if policies differ, which commonly they do not. By contrast, competition improves standards and increases opportunities. It protects both the necessary rivalry and fair access, while promoting economic efficiency and individual choice. Those organisations, institutions and managers who lose the competitive race will be the losers – and not the patients who presently suffer from delays, denials and dilution of services. For these will transfer to better providers. Those who must improve to continue offering services which people will willingly choose or avoid will be those poor providers who can no longer attract users of their services.

This makes the point that competition has two different meanings. In most aspects of life it can mean personal rivalry, with one person seeking to outdo his known competitor – for example, for a job, or for a sale. But in the wider market, going beyond the single individual, the situation is much more impersonal. For no one participant can determine the terms on which other participants in the market can achieve access to goods, services, or to jobs. Everyone must take prices as given by the market, which (save for conditions of monopoly or duopoly, which are regulated by government) no individual can control, although all participants determine price by the combined effect of their separate actions. Of course, when government itself is the monopoliser, as in much British health and social care, we are cut off from these benefits. For half a century government has been the chief and often the only buyer of the products of many enterprises. This has been a serious restriction on voluntary exchange, by reducing the alternatives available to individuals in a free society, and the access to care they otherwise could have secured in an open market and with the freedom to spend more of their own money.

So the proposition is that competition is more successful than monopoly, or regulation, in generating services that people want, at prices more closely related to costs, and that these costs/prices are minimised by competitive pressures. If we want prices to be low but also have quality services that are value for money, it is competition which controls both. In addition – an important point for those seeking equality – *within any given distribution of income* competition maximises welfare. If incomes are made more equal by tax-transfers into a health savings account, competition will equip the individual to do as well as any other in securing healthcare services. In our recent history, too, the successes of competition include changes in social mobility, among other favourable social changes. Vigorous competition contributes to social mobility, and to the escape from a sense that one is doomed to live out life in inherited economic circumstances. This has done much to break up the rigidities of class, which the NHS has otherwise reinforced. Competition increases organisational mobility, too. Inertia, indeed, is radically insufficient as a recommendation in a market. Competition prevents the accumulation and abuse of monopoly power – in public or private hands. Thus, too, it makes unnecessary the costly bureaucratic endeavour of governmental regulation of prices, output, investment, and consumer targets – as a substitute for empowered individuals making choices. And it frees us from the impossible task of seeking by administrative means to try (unavailingly) to capture tacit, local and personal knowledge in 'policy', in trying to aggregate guesses about individual preference into instructions for all.

We should notice, too, that it is rigid societies which are the most unequal, and which offer the least potential for the correction of this situation. An open society of dynamic change offers social mobility, changes in status and new opportunities. In this sense, a society which shows inequalities and diversities, and yet expects these to exist but to be changeable, is to be preferred to a system of hierarchical controls. In this sense, inequalities are necessary, and inevitable. We see these in our society, but we also see the floor level constantly rising. To argue that there is more poverty than there was 20 years ago is to regard poverty as a form of hypochondria, for poverty is a relative concept, and the floor has risen greatly in many countries. Standards have risen very significantly. Choice and competition are at the heart of this. We know that inequality, wide income differentials and poor health often coincide. Mr Alan Johnson announced in June 2008 a £34 million plan to tackle health inequalities, in a statement on 10 June 2008. But statist approaches have not changed these relationships.

Non-capitalist societies – and hierarchical systems of centralised provision within capitalist societies – have greater inequalities. And these tend to be permanent because they are so difficult to correct because of inertia and the power of special interests. Competition, by contrast to central control, enables us to discover information – who will serve a particular customer best; who offers which services from among the alternatives; who will provide the best standard of care, or the most effective care. This remains to be discovered, and rediscovered. The answers are neither obvious, nor permanent and stable. Competition enables us to see which services emerge and which cannot be – or are not yet being – bettered by rivals. This occurs with price, too. It is competition which uniquely generates the information that people need to make decisions.

Of course, in human affairs, total predictability is not possible. This uncertainty disturbs some. Competition does not provide the certainty which government has seemed to promise. But this certainty is not actually attainable, *either* by central control *or* the adaptive workings of markets. The attempt to achieve certainty itself destroys the potential for improvement. And so dynamism and competing services are the better means for the protection of consumers, when they have choices. Competition works best, and it is ethical. It meets the conditions of a society of liberty and self-responsibility. It is vital, too, to appreciate that it is dynamism which has always shifted boundaries, broken the mould of outdated authority, shaped new possibilities by adaptive inventions and by market emulation. Static authority is a poor guide to the future. As Thomas Kuhn pointed out, revolutionary events occur when the weight of new observation has discredited a previous paradigm – and this contradictory evidence itself depends both on scientific logic and social, cultural and aesthetic influences.[26]

The challenge for competition here concerns outcomes, the narrow funding base, the expectations of political and managerial controls, how much continuing government subsidy there will be, in the short term and in the longer view, and at what level. It concerns, fundamentally, cultural challenges: to ourselves and to our self-responsibility, and to what Foucault called our 'gaze'. That is, to what we admit as possible, legitimate and necessary. At one point, the NHS looked right, to some people. Then suddenly, it doesn't. We have reached this point.

What would happen if real competition came to the NHS and to the local government funders and providers of social care? Initially, I would expect old loyalties, inertia, some resistance to travelling (but much less than has been thought – as a British Medical Association study showed).[27] However, once health savings accounts began and consumer cooperatives were really in business, this would change. Then there must be no ministerial insistence on 'a steady state', nor on protecting 'the local health economy' (to borrow the King's Fund's favoured statist language). The vigour of new competition and of creative purchasing should be realised, and new entrants be permitted to seek the large savings-based revenues available from willing consumers.

Meanwhile, to artificially depress or to politically disregard price as a mechanism of guidance or knowledge is the surest means to inflate demand and to choke off supply. This attitude is the parent of shortages and waiting lists. And since price and supply are inextricably linked centralised rationing is the necessary handmaiden of price denial. Its marching fellows are the whole and costly diversionary state panoply of rules, inspections, policing, restriction, control and 'consultation'.

As Arthur Seldon wrote,

> the 'social purpose' of pricing is to make you think twice before using scarce resources and denying them to other uses that may be more urgent and productive. In principle this is as true of education, medical care, housing, pensions, as of roads, land for car-parking, water, or any other commodity or service hitherto supplied 'free'.[28]

Customer

Some healthcare workers – such as a relative of mine, Mrs Iris Hackett, a retired hospital almoner in Hackney with whom I discussed this issue recently – say that people are not customers; they are patients. This is the authentic voice of the past speaking. The distinction is between a customer who can escape from an unsatisfactory provider and a proposed beneficiary (or patient) who has no individual power to bargain or escape. This is the difference between the sovereign consumer and the supplicant applicant. Which is why I suggest that if there is to be genuine, attainable choice, individuals must have leverage over an individual fund, as customers. They should be subscribers to cooperative purchasing organisations, as customers. They will be seen by competing purchasers as customers. They will be able to move between these, taking their health savings account with them as customers. This power over money, together with open information about services, makes them a customer, rather than a passive recipient and consumer of services decided upon by others. My almoner relative in East London is right: you are not a customer if you only pay indirectly by taxes. The money has to be disentangled from the close grip of the state. It has to be in your control.

Profit

What a dust storm is associated with the word for a surplus of income over outgoings or expenses! Yet every venture (whether calling itself 'not-for-profit' or not) needs to create a surplus, unless a venture can survive as a loss-maker by subsidy or gift. Classical economists regarded profit as the recompense for risk taking. It encouraged people to take risks, to put in energy and effort. Others described it as the rewards of entrepreneurship, or the rent for special knowledge. More recently, it has been considered as the result of uncertainties and the yield from unpredictable change. Profit (or a 'risk premium') is present in all kinds of human activity. It is an element that enters into the rewards of all endeavour to some extent. In terms of health and social policy, the two chief issues (and one rider) concerning profit (or 'the increment of value') are:

1   It is not that we do not want it, but who gets it and why
2   There should not be monopoly profits
3   That there should be a reasonable and guaranteed return on investment: for example, for long-term care of the elderly, where stable and new provision is urgently required to meet demographic trends. Similarly, for research in drugs, where the innovator is permitted to recover large costs and a profit under licence. It can cost £350 million to get a new drug to market. Of every 10,000 compounds screened for their effectiveness, only one is likely to emerge in the final marketplace. Typically, this takes 12 years, from initial synthesis to market authorisation. By then the patent has more than half expired, leaving a limited period to recoup costs. Without patents and high initial prices there would be no inducement to develop medicines. Fortunately, the system works or we would not have had the benefits of antibiotics and anaesthetics, which have transformed medical practice, the status of doctors, and patient benefit. Do we want to discourage drug companies from innovating (for example, to save those who are HIV positive) by refusing them a yield from many years of costly research? Surely not, if we want dangerous problems solved.[29]

On the first point, profit in healthcare should go to reward providers who give satisfactions to patients, encourage investment, lower costs to consumers and improve services. For the primary economic function of profit in a market society is allocative rather than distributive. And we want to encourage the good provider to do more. Payment in accordance with efficient production is necessary so that resources can be used most effectively. This incentive, too, seems – from everyday observation – to reward effort, encourage activity to satisfy service-users, and serve as a morally and politically suitable alternative to compulsion and coercion. We need to be able to demonstrate that its deployment in healthcare yields appropriate redistributive justice, as we have seen in optics. But one of the difficulties in persuading people to consider these questions is the idea – an enduring perception and prejudice – that no one should profit from giving care. Even though much of this individual care is an entirely *private* benefit for which a charge can properly be made. Even though profit (or 'surplus') is essential to remain able to give *any* care at all. However, in the patient guaranteed care association, remember, any surpluses will go to the account of the individual *as a member* – along with all other members – rather than to the individual *as a producer*.[30] Granted, this still represents the state interfering in the relations between people. And it relies on some notion of fairness which overrides the entitlements of some to the advantage of others, in order to acquire the resources to improve the opportunities of the poor. It does so by relying on the notion that somehow medicine is different.

However, there is a balance to be struck here between the statist system we now have and a freer dynamist society. I do not see how this redistributive action can be avoided, in order to shift us towards a freer society, even if this expression of fairness is claimed to be different in degree from socialist redistribution. Socialist systems enforce a political view of 'positive freedom' to limit the freedoms of different individuals facing some different and some similar difficulties, with different resources and different personal goals. It cannot be denied, however, that to improve the position of some we necessarily worsen – by taxation – the position of others. This is, of course, to impose a solution rather than depending upon voluntary cooperation. I am uncomfortable about this (as Robert Nozick tells us we should be). But we may have to do it, to make some progress towards the evolution of services on a different basis. However, we should be aware of what we are doing. This, in itself, is no easy task.

Price is an instrument of discovery. As Stephen E Landsburg has said, 'Economics is the science of competing preferences'. By contrast, ideology is the science of imposing preferences by manipulating the political and economic system. But 'payment for product' enables distribution to occur impersonally, and without the need for coercive authority. It effects cooperation and coordination without compulsion. It encourages diversity, experimentation and the diffusion of innovation. It enables people to extend their capacities. It leads, too, to less inequality than other systems of organisation, as the post-war history of liberal capitalism demonstrates. And by distributing decision making it offsets the centralisation of political and economic power.

'Profit' (or surplus, if you like) is essential if we are to see investment, and the survival of the best provider. In my proposals the 'dividend' of any surplus will be owned by the subscribing members of a patient guaranteed care association, and held individually to their accounts. Any profit held by a producer would be used for investment, the improvement of services to purchasers (or, in a PGCA, to subscribers), and the reduction of costs. This directly connects detail and democratic principle. Democratic control thus exists over the rationalities of production, purchasing, distribution and exchange. We could notice, too, that those who can charge what the market will bear – demonstrating that they give customers satisfactions – have fewer money worries than those dependent on government for tax allocations. We should also appreciate that the only alternative to state care is not necessarily for-profit care. Much voluntary charitable and not-for-profit care is typical throughout Europe (and more so, too, in the USA than is commonly credited). The hospice movement in the UK is a powerful example of how people look after themselves and those for whom they care and without the state. Here, we should discourage those who demand state funding for hospices. They are a wonderful charitable endeavour and this moral basis should not be corrupted by welfarist 'give-us-grants-ism'. They represent the organisational creativity and voluntary action manifest in working-class self-ownership and mutual aid. They should keep clear of the state.[31]

Much vital care is provided in people's homes by outreach teams, rather than in residential institutions. Now 72% of hospice funding comes from donations, charity shops and fundraising drives. The hospice movement was founded in 1967 when Dame Cicely Saunders opened St Christopher's hospice in Sydenham, South

East London. It embraced the physical, spiritual and emotional aspects of patients' suffering. The movement grew during the period of the political suzerainty of the NHS, demonstrating that despite its claim to be the compassionate intervener in our lives, the state neglected these fundamentals. There are now in the UK 208 inpatient NHS and voluntary hospices with 3029 beds, 334 home-care support teams and 243 day-care units. Hospice care is free, and has radically changed the way in which death and dying are approached.[32] This, too, underlines two truths: first, that individual initiative can make huge differences; second, that public service is not only or necessarily delivered by organisations dominated by so-called 'public service trade unions'.

So profit is an operating surplus, to ensure that an organisation can remain able to provide services. It (and competition) does not *of itself* produce inequalities. On the contrary, it raises standards and reduces inequality more successfully than the alternatives. It is essential if providers are to invest and to innovate. For without prices, productivity and margin there is no framework of competitive discipline. There is only guesswork. The NHS conducts this with planning, consultation and regulation. In this form of consultation pressure groups compete to establish the priority of their own 'needs', and individuals insist on their 'rights' irrespective of cost. This is how the NHS attempts to predict the consequences of proposals for service development. But this is a task which can only be undertaken effectively in a market of discovery. This, of course, means accepting and welcoming the surprises markets bring. For results will only be determined and thus known when consumers express their preferences with regard to price, quality and other facets of services offered to them. And which they judge for themselves. This will only happen when consumers can decide how much power to give their preference, instead of having someone else's guess about it granted to them – whether they are 'consulted' or not. Which services, at which prices, at which level of quality, in which combination, are matters which cannot otherwise be 'rationally' determined in advance. The necessary dynamic relationship is between the provider and market knowledge as it is at a given moment. This more informed estimate of current and possible consumer behaviour only arises from the provider facing a consumer who has free choice, and by a consumer facing a priced choice for which they have to make payment. Profit is one element that shows how well people are being served.

On the point concerning monopoly profits, this is a question for regulation – as I discuss when considering A&E services, which are a 'technical monopoly'. Managements must be contestable. Contestable markets deter profiteering. Although in theory all monopolies are at hazard from innovation, in practice it seems that practice does not always seem to make perfect.

Those who see the world through statist spectacles have a difficult challenge to meet. How can they prevent change, and persuade us that all requirements can be met without uncertainty? If they are unable to do so, some incentives, some rewards, some measures are necessary as indicators of success. There is no statist argument against dynamism and profit. Unless, in principle, you think that the firm which makes a profit from discovering and producing a drug which saves people from desperate suffering – for example, from AIDS – is doing something illicit, in principle. There are such people. But it is difficult to have any kind of rational debate with them.[33]

Price

A signal. Notably so, too, when it is absent. What to produce, how much, when and for whom? Our old 'friends' the 'expert', and 'consultation'? Or price as the vital functionary in offering answers in a market, based on the cumulative decisions of empowered service-users? All markets are to some extent imperfect. This is among their advantages. For it is by continuous experimentation, guided by prices (and by advertising, which is a vital element in 'reputation') and by the signals consumers thus give that the system of voluntary exchange reaches out towards an ever unstable but progressive optimum.

Prices of complex products give and also gather much information, which is itself confirmed by other players in the market such as agents. Price rations goods, too, and is changed by elasticities of supply and of demand. Marginal prices are a key to efficiency, as I have earlier discussed. Without prices, NHS 'experts' struggle unavailingly to guess the equilibrium level of demand at which the totality of demand and supply tends to be equal. 'Experts' guess (it is sometimes called 'consultation') – or they determine by political or managerial prejudice – how much supply the public ought to get, and how to allocate purchasing power between possible alternative services. By contrast, the free market itself constantly adapts to further and incessantly useful change. Price is a key comparator. It pictures the value an individual gives to a service or a good, by being willing to meet it. It distils all the relevant information that sums up the individual economic and social contexts which influence supply and demand with regard to a particular good or service, when determined in a competitive market. Professor Norman Barry has said that 'it would be a very optimistic theorist who assumed that an imperfect state, controlled by utility maximisers (officials) much less constrained by price, could significantly improve on this'.[34]

No one has been able to invent any better way of distributing resources than through prices. There is, too, no such thing as a genuine demand without a price. But some of us have been persuaded that this isn't so. Thus, patients inevitably demand whatever is 'necessary' for their treatment, with little or no sympathy with or understanding of the concept of cost, or of competition for resources, or, indeed, of who will pay. We vote for 'more', with no thought of costs. Yet when making purchases in our 'ordinary' lives we all know we must link price and quality, and consider the trade-offs. Unless we do so in health and social care we shall continue to see governments chasing a fleeing bandwagon. There are prices in any and every system, hidden or explicit. The important issue is to use price explicitly to allocate scarce resources, to encourage people to consider self-responsibility, and to use it for the measurement of demand. This is the necessary link between price, quality, opportunity cost, innovation, investment and choice. There are many different kinds of prices, too, including those effected by the delays, dilutions and denials of the NHS.

To achieve radical reforms we should embed and protect (rather than suppress and secrete) price information, to benefit from the signals – and bargaining power – which price uniquely encapsulates and enables. A price is specific, and much more meaningful than 'the fog of figures without individual identity' with which we otherwise struggle.[35] For the billions regularly cited in NHS debate give no information on the comparative cost, price and value of services, and the competing alternatives which could be offered. Indeed, the billions are as likely – indeed, more likely – to conceal the misapplication of resources as they are to show us consumer satisfactions. Price, as it could function in health and social care, is an example of the most basic problem of social organisation: of how to coordinate the activities of large numbers of people, to make best use of scarce resources, and to ensure that all can benefit from opportunities.

A key question for *any* healthcare system is: where do you place price in the system? This is an absolutely fundamental question. Do you place it in the system as a general tax, with services 'free' at the point of supply? It is still a price. Or at the point of entry into a health savings account? Or by compulsory insurance with some co-payment? Or at the point of use? Or some of each? My argument is that if you want to encourage self-responsible living, and if you want to help people build savings, then priced services and (probably with a voluntary and negotiated 'excess' as an element of the HSA) offers the best chance to do so. We shall have to face this question. For price is the only known effective mechanism for matching demand with supply. And the only known mechanism for setting prices efficiently is a market. This idea, however, does not necessarily mean payment for critical illness interventions or for A&E services at the time of use, though it cannot exclude – save in dreamland – prepayment of some kind, either by taxation, or by tax transfers to subsidise the poor, or by cash savings or some equity release, or by an efficient combination of these including catastrophic cover by insurance. This is a necessary thought alongside the stress on the value of individual cost-conscious preference.

As Milton Friedman wrote,

> Fundamentally, there are only two ways of co-ordinating the economic activities of millions. One is central direction involving the use of coercion. . . . The other is voluntary co-operation of individuals – the technique of the marketplace. The possibility of co-ordination through voluntary co-operation rests on the elementary – yet frequently denied – proposition that both parties to an economic transaction benefit from it, *provided the transaction is bilaterally voluntary and informed*. Exchange can therefore bring about co-ordination without co-ercion.[36]

This book discusses how to achieve these necessary conditions, and whether or not the service-user must be congenitally ignorant and incapable of choices. I say more on this key issue in my chapter 'Between the data and the deep blue sea'.

By urging this case for choice it should be said that this is not to argue that all 'values', being 'subjective', immediately release the individual from responsibility. They do not. We are each, in priced and cost-conscious choice, *more* accountable for our actions, choices, judgements and the expression of our 'values'. Price in a system obliges each of us to make relative judgements between *costed* opportunities. Price is, too, an essential tool *for government*. As Arthur Seldon says,

> The task of government, *which it cannot perform because it deprives itself of the information*, is to decide the good that its allocation of funds will do in all alternative uses. Every human activity can do more good with more resources. . . . But that is not the important decision for government. It has to demonstrate that the money would not do more good elsewhere. It must therefore show that additional ('marginal') utility in all possible uses has been equalled so that no more 'good' can in total be done by transferring resources from where they do less good to where they can do more. The result is that all the interests are unconsciously ganging up to force government to continue old activities when they could increasingly be financed by individuals – with the additional advantage that they would know how much satisfaction they received. The financial acid test of most 'public' services is whether the people for whom they are supposedly intended would pay for them. Let government and subsidised 'public' services be judged not by politicians and lobbyists but by the people for whom they are intended.[37]

Where pricing mechanisms exist in healthcare systems they are, in the main, concerned with constraining burgeoning expenditure. Research over a lengthy period has shown, too, that when opinion polls calling for more expenditure on the NHS are personally linked to prices, levels of demand vary significantly.[38] The practical experience of HSAs makes the same point. What we want is to have a price system which enables choices to be meaningful, and to relate price, choice and quality for the individual to consider. A static price – like a fixed fee per day spent in hospital – is not a price *mechanism*. It is just an additional tax. Incentives are necessary to encourage providers to price their services efficiently and competitively. But in the NHS prices are either unknown or their occurrence and levels hidden, or where known they vary by surprisingly large margins. Imposing a national tariff of prices is no answer either, for it deliberately disables the market and prevents its evolution.

Resistance to the transparency of prices has several sources. First, it will be uncomfortable for those within the NHS who have managed without prices 'very nicely, thank you'. Second, price seems to some to be unfair since the ability to pay (under the existing NHS/private system) reflects the distribution of incomes, which some view as improperly unequal, at whatever adjusted levels. Thirdly, politicians have always preferred alternatives, such as allocative budgets, by which to sustain *political* controls. This has suited 'experts' and planners, too. They act as proxies for consumers (who have no choice) and agents for government. They can spend these budgets, while demanding more ('underfunded') to meet current demand and even 'unmet needs'. Under the NHS, government, broadly, has agreed the total spend, and left the professionals to sort out the local spending, manage risk and resolve local political difficulties.

However, recently, much increased targeting on priorities has made this a less comfortable cushion. Now, if we are to move to the efficient allocation of scarce resources and empowered choices, prices need to be explicit and set at competitive levels so that they reflect and enable providers to recover all costs. The cost-conscious consumer, the self-responsible consumer, the financially empowered consumer, the 'knowing' consumer, is no longer a creature of the distant future. This cultural change can now enhance supply, and require consumers to choose *both* between different health services *and* between health services and other goods and services. Remember, rather little healthcare is about life-threatening conditions. Much of it is now about lifestyle, about individual choices, not 'rights'. Government will have little to do on the supply or the demand side but to make the rules. The real world, at last. We can have price mechanisms, of course, which encourage dynamism, innovation and the continuing evolution of services. Or we can have political mechanisms, which hinder all this. Each has to cope with an increasingly complex modern economy. 'You pays your money and you takes your choice'. Or, in the NHS, you don't.

Friedman eloquently describes the choice between markets and centralising measures and their results:

> The central defect of these measures is that they seek through government to force people to act against their own immediate interests in order to promote a supposedly general interest. They seek to resolve a conflict of interest, or a difference in view about interests, not by establishing a framework that will eliminate the conflict, or by persuading people to have different interests, but by forcing people to act against their own interest. They substitute the values of outsiders for the values of participants; either some telling others what is good for them, or the government taking from some to benefit others. These measures are therefore countered by one of the strongest and most creative forces known to man – the attempt by millions of individuals to promote their own interests, to live their own lives by their own values. This is the major reason why the measures have so often had the opposite of the effects intended. It is also one of the major strengths of a free society and explains why governmental regulation does not strangle it. The interests

of which I speak are not simply narrow self-regarding interests. On the contrary, they include the whole range of values that men hold dear and for which they are willing to spend their fortunes and sacrifice their lives. . . . It is a virtue of a free society that it nonetheless permits those interests full scope and does not subordinate them to the narrow materialistic interests that dominate the bulk of mankind.[39]

Demand

Demand is another facet of price. It is a commitment. It concerns the amount of available spending power. It expresses desires and relative judgements, or total and marginal utility – the judgements by an individual of the value of extra benefits. In rationing, as in the NHS, we meet the frustration of demand. In my proposals we confront the empowerment of individual demand. In economics demand has lots of complicated curves and functions. These concern how quantities produced depend on a number of variables such as price, income and tastes. Demand concerns utility, scarcity and choices. The theory of demand is at the core of the theory of value, together with the theory of supply. In considering how to improve health and social care it can be a friend of the best. It summarises the quantity of a commodity or service for which consumers wish and are able to pay for at a given price at a given time. Without the ability and willingness of someone to pay, the wish is not the father of the child. Without a price being met there is no supply.

There are, too, many other related aspects of demand. It is affected by price, quality, service and the prices of related or substitutable goods. Individual preferences between alternatives also influence demand. So do our incomes, our expectations and our ambitions. Demand is a 'function' of all these factors. We can see that without prices it is little wonder that demand easily overwhelms services. And that the NHS has not been able to gather the necessary knowledge for appropriate actions, including sufficient supply. It is no surprise that other administrative forms of demand management – notably, rationing, deficit, denial, waiting lists and new rationing and blocking institutions like NICE – have all been used by government to intervene and to 'guide' or suppress demand. The absence of good public information is both a necessity in a rationed NHS as well as a consequence of this situation.

But should anyone be able to make just any demands on the system? Few would say so. But with no prices the incentives are to demand consistently. As Lord Ralph Harris suggested, the attitude then is to say, 'If it's free, put me down for two.' No one wishes to deny good care to anyone, when it will help them. However, we know that general practice in particular is overwhelmed by many people whose concerns are social, psychological and personal without them being conventionally ill, at least as determined by the biomedical model. The difficulty is how to respond to those four groups presenting at the GP offices – identified by Groves as 'the dependent clinger' (dependent on constant advice), 'the entitled demander' (threatening and cajoling), 'the manipulative help rejecter' (for whom nothing will work), and 'the self-destructive denier' (the smoker with lung cancer; the obese gross eater).[40]

Misselbrook discussed this labelling, saying,

> What the four groups have in common is that they're not playing the game. Our view of how the social contract of healthcare works is to have the patients come to us when it is medically necessary, to follow our advice, to get better, and to be grateful to us. This is the social role of the doctor, adjusted to suit the doctor's needs. If the patient doesn't conform to this social role they become our heartsinks.[41]

This may be so, but the costs are still real, and someone has to bear these. The PGCA will be asked to work out relationships with each patient, encouraging the individual to consider, addressing the issues of demand, and its cost. There is no avoiding this issue. At present its displacement onto the shoulders of GPs is one of the burdens that is breaking the system. Labelling patients as 'the dependent clinger', or a heartsink patient, does not resolve the difficulties of the individual – they may be irresolvable – and it does not sort out who is to bear these costs. And so they are piled onto the GP, which is not a recipe for success. We need to think more deeply about labelling, about social constructs and about education. But costs are costs, and we need to sort out what these truly are, and who is to bear these. If we wish as individuals to make what others regard as antisocial decisions, we should bear the costs. But we cannot all demand every test, insist upon every drug, demand antibiotics for the 'flu or for every self-limiting complaint, expect constant 'counselling' in a system to shield us from the risks of life, expect the time of others when it suits us, take as long as we want, live anyway we wish, and expect to pass all the costs onto others. If we insist on a long menu of 'rights' without any responsible thought and any consideration of opportunity cost, we will find there is no one there at the end of the telephone line. At present, we fudge the issues. When heated, fudge melts.

... And then there is charity

On a transfer design on every tea cup in every respectable Victorian cottage: faith, hope, and charity. Take the last of these. True charity and compassion can *only* be individual; it is not something that the state can express or make real. When expressed in an individual life it has moral power. To many the word charity smacks of handouts. But charity is one part of the great trilogy of optimism – along with faith and hope – which was slip-printed onto Victorian porcelain. Charity and compassion are *personal* expressions. They are not ideas which can be captured in state law and regulation. Charity is the mark of a good society because it is the mark of many people *voluntarily* taking an interest in others, making a commitment to others rather than being coerced. It has been an important and valued part of our historical traditions. It is one expression of the proper use of dynamist freedom, with the individual directing part of their effort to helping the less fortunate, and in voluntary rather than compulsory action. Tax policy is again seeking to encourage it. As mentioned, the hospice movement is an outstanding example of the truths it represents. These directly contradict the ideas on which the NHS is based: that the state should take over ultimate responsibility from the individual; that resources should be distributed according to 'need' and defined by 'experts'; and that services should be free of any obligations or of any consideration of the consequences of one's own behaviour.

Charity offers the idea (and the opportunity) that *an individual* should do something, and not continuously demand that *the government* do something; for example, about the obesity of the individual concerned. And that by coming together locally, or by acting individually, we can take positive actions for ourselves which make the lives of others better. Private charity has an enormous heritage of achievement, including the provision prior to 1948 of immense investment in health facilities.[42] We should resist it being rolled up into the grasp of the state by the allure of subsidies and the transfer of resources by political markets. This is a major risk as long-term social care changes and is 'commodified'.[43]

Patient?

A dictionary definition: 'Patient or patience. Calm endurance of pain or any provocation; forbearance; quiet and self-possessed waiting for something; perseverance ... Game, usually, for one person, in which object is to arrange cards in some systematic order.'[44]

We may be it. We may have it, patiently. But many prefer to use the words 'service-users'. This is clearly more accurate. It is less patronising. It is more active. We do, however, continue to use 'patient' as shorthand. Patient is understood by everyone. But, for example, the disabled are service-users and not necessarily patients. Pregnant mothers-to-be are not patients. They are not ill. Pregnancy is not a disease. Equally, children in care (and those using mental health services) do not necessarily view themselves as patients. Not only are they entitled to be listened to, but many expect to take an active role in decision making. This has been a legal duty, too, under the Children Act for the past 11 years.[45] But the public understands the language of 'patient'. Whichever the language, all must be empowered as citizens in society, with personal autonomy and control over their lives.

Equally, the stress on patient *guaranteed* care is essential. The word helps as a reassuring shorthand for building support for market-led reform. But I mean user-led, service-user guaranteed care, and I hope I will be forgiven the inaccurate brevity of the word 'patient'. We must, at all events, use vibrant and accurate language. And begin with the important word 'guarantee', which underlines a legally enforceable contract for care for everyone, irrespective of class, background, income, gender, ethnic origin, disability or age. The language of purpose is patient guaranteed care. Markets are our most secure guarantee. We have been patient about the deficits for too long.[46]

Notes

1 See, for example, political failure in pensions policy and the very significant resulting difficulties. Philip Booth, 'The young held to ransom – a public choice analysis of the UK state pension scheme', *Economic Affairs*, 28(1), March 2008, pp. 4–10. See also Vincenzo Galasso, *The Political Future of Social Security in Aging Societies* (Cambridge, MA, MIT Press, 2006).

2 Tim Harford, *The Undercover Economist* (London, Little Brown, 2006), Abacus edition, 2007, p. 62.

3 IM Stelzer, *Lectures on Regulatory and Competition Policy* (London, IEA, 2001), p. 184.

4 Stelzer, ibid., p. 194.

5 Stelzer, ibid., p. 176; see also WJ Baumol, SAB Backman, EN Wolff, *Productivity and American Leadership: the long view* (Cambridge, MA, The MIT Press, 1989); T Startup, *In Poor Measures?* (London, Social Market Foundation, 2002); P Spicker, *Poverty and the Welfare State: dispelling the myths* (London, Catalyst, 2002); J Daley, 'Poverty of aspiration is what keeps people poor', *Daily Telegraph*, 28 August 2002, p 21. For an alternative view, but which makes no distinction between absolute and relative poverty, see H Glenerster, 'Social Policy', in Anthony Seldon (ed.), *The Blair Effect* (London, Little Brown, 2001), pp 382–403. Glenerster seems not to appreciate that poverty has decreased on an *absolute* scale, despite a broadening disparity of income. The two things are different. General prosperity in the past half-century has seen the standard of living increase three- or fourfold, and the liberal capitalist economy has proved itself the best creator of prosperity and the least harmful of production systems. As Professor N Barry has said, 'The success of capitalist economies is not to be measured solely by their ability to produce wanted goods and services but by the rise in standards brought about by competition.' N Barry, op. cit., p. 33. See also [The Black Report] Dept. of Health and Social Security, *Inequalities in Health: report of a research working group* (London, DHSS, 1980); and G Davey Smith *et al.*, 'The Black report on socio-economic inequalities in health 10 years on', *British Medical Journal*, 301, 1990, pp. 73–7; *Joseph Rowntree Foundation Inquiry into Income and Wealth* (York, Joseph Rowntree Foundation, 1995).

6 William Beveridge, *Voluntary Action: a report on methods of social advance* (London, George Allen and Unwin, 1948), p. 14; Alan Kidd, *State Society and the Poor in Nineteenth Century England* (Houndsmills, Hants., Palgrave Macmillan, 1999). Also, references in chapter 'The present reforms "coherent and right"', note 17.

7 Isaiah Berlin, *Four Essays on Liberty* (London, Oxford University Press, 1969).

8 Quoted by P Johnson, 'Ten commandments while we ride the financial rollercoaster', *The Spectator*, 13 July 2002, p. 24.

9 A Wildavsky, *Searching for Safety* (New Brunswick, NJ, Transaction, 1988).

10 I Illich, *Medical Nemesis: the expropriation of health* (London, Marion Boyars, 1976), revised as *Limits to Medicine* (London, Marion Boyars, 1995). See also re-review by R Smith (the editor) in *British Medical Journal*, 324, 2002,

p. 923; David Misselbrook, *Thinking About Patients* (Newbury, Petroc Press, 2001) especially Chapter 1, 'The Biomedical Model'.

11 P Skrabanek, *The Death of Humane Medicine* (London, Social Affairs Unit, 1994). Consumers systematically underestimate personal health risk. ND Weinstein, and WM Klein, 'Resistance to Personal Risk Perceptions to Debiasing Interventions', *Health Psychology*, 1995, 14(2), pp. 132–40; Weinstein, 'Accuracy of Smoker's Risk Perceptions', *Annals of Behavioural Medicine*, 1998, 20(2), pp. 135–40. 'People differ in their attitudes to healthcare. They also differ in their aversion to risk. Take diagnostic tests for the detection of cancer. The more frequent the tests, the higher the costs. But medical science cannot tell us how frequent exams should be. That's largely a value judgement, and people's values differ. In general such exams are not promoted by a risky event. They are largely influenced by people's preferences'" Goodman, op. cit., p. 229.

12 Arthur Seldon and FG Pennance, *Everyman's Dictionary of Economics* (1965; revised, 1975), reprinted in volume 3, *Collected Works*, op. cit. See pp. 654–5. This is an outstanding guide in its field. It is much more technically sophisticated than my more frugal and bare use of economic concepts, and it achieves its ambition to be expressed 'in plain English'. See also Eamonn Butler, *The Best Book on the Market: how to stop worrying and love the free economy* (Chichester, Sussex, Capstone, 2008).

13 Misselbrook, op. cit., p. 19.

14 J. von Neumann, O Morgenstern, *Theory of Games and Economic Behaviour* (Princeton, NJ., Princeton University Press, 1953).

15 G Torrance, 'Social Preferences for health states: an empirical evaluation of three measurement techniques', *Socio-Economic Planning Sciences*, 10, 1976, pp. 129–36.

16 G Chatellier *et al.*, 'The number needed to treat: a clinically useful monogram in its proper context', *British Medical Journal*, 312, 1996, pp. 426–9; G Davey Smith, M Egger, 'Who benefits from medical interventions?', *British Medical Journal*, 308, editorial, 1994, pp. 72–4.

17 Misselbrook, op. cit., p. 19.

18 Misselbrook, op. cit., p. 138; D Smith, M Egger, op. cit.

19 Misselbrook, op. cit., p. 19.

20 Misselbrook, op. cit., p. 101.

21 Ibid.

22 Misselbrook, op. cit., p. 86.

23 R Fuller, 'Are choices irrational or doctors and patients misinformed?', *British Medical Journal*, 324, letter, 2002, p. 215; J Ashworth, *Science, Policy and Risk* (London, Royal Society, 1997).

24 R Smith, 'The discomfort of patient power.' *British Medical Journal*, 324, 2002, pp. 497–8.

25 Arthur Seldon and FG Pennance, *Everyman's Dictionary of Economics* (1965; revised, 1975), reprinted in volume 3, *Collected Works*, op. cit. See pp. 130, 246.

26 T Kuhn, *The Structure of Scientific Revolutions* (Chicago, University of Chicago Press, 1962).

27 N Hawkes, 'Public prepared to give up on NHS and travel abroad,' *The Times*, 1 July 2002, p. 6.

28 Arthur Seldon, *The Future of the Welfare State*, originally published in *Encounter*; reprinted in Robert Schuettinger (ed.), *The Conservative Tradition in European Thought*, 1970; then reprinted in volume 6, *Collected Works*, op. cit. See p. 51.

29 'Medicines priced high to recoup research and marketing cost', *The Times*, 13 August 2002, p. 4.

30 This unites means and ends. JTW Mitchell, the cooperative leader, urged: 'My desire is that the profits of all trade, all industry, all distribution, all commerce, all importation, all banking and money dealing, should fall back again into the hands of the whole people. Quoted CS Yeo, in C Levy (ed.), *Socialism and the Intelligentsia 1880–1914* (London, Routledge & Kegan Paul, 1987), p. 58. The PGCA approach achieves what is realistic in this project, but without the Marxian overlay of 'class-struggle' which Yeo's analysis offers.

31 Keep clear of the state. Mr David Cameron has urged that charities be allowed to earn 'substantial fees' from delivering public services as part of a shake-up of Britain's voluntary sector. Nicholas Watt, 'Cameron wants to see charities paid market rate for public services', *The Guardian*, 4 June 2008, p. 11. Also, Craig Dearden-Phillips, 'Stated aims', *The Guardian*, society section, 28 May 2008, p. 10.

32 See, for example, the views of D Hinchcliffe MP, then Chairman, House of Commons Health Committee, in J Revill, 'Entente not so cordiale', *British Medical Journal*, 324, 2002, p. 1239, and ex-Secretary of State for Health Frank Dobson MP, 'The last thing the NHS needs is another dose of the private sector', *The Independent*, 28 January 2002. Also, House of Commons Select Committee, *Inquiry into the Role of the Private Sector in the NHS*, First Report of Session 2001–02 (HC 308), 14 May 2002.

33 A Frean, '35 years of palliative care', *The Times*, 28 August 2002, p. 8.

34 However, see JH Tanne, 'Mortality higher in for-profit hospitals', *British Medical Journal*, 324, 2002, p. 1351.

35 N Barry, in J Blundell and C Robinson (eds.), *Regulation Without the State: the debate continues* (London, IEA, 2000).

36 Friedman, *Capitalism and Freedom*, op. cit., p. 13; italics in original. On the key coordination of services see 'Teamwork the key to better patient care and sustainable health services', 1 March 2008, at www.usyd.edu.au.

37 Seldon, *The Dilemma of Democracy*, op. cit., p. 77; italics in original.

38 R Harris, A Seldon, *Choice in Welfare* (London, IEA, series 1963, 1965, 1970, 1978, 1987).

39 Friedman, op. cit., pp. 200–1.

40 J Groves, 'Taking care of the hateful patient', *New England Journal of Medicine*, 298, 1951, pp. 883–5.

41 Misselbrook, op. cit., p. 126.

42 D Green, *Working Class Patients*, op. cit.; F Prokashka, op. cit., D O'Keefe, 'Charity versus the state', in A Seldon, *Re-Privatising Welfare*, op. cit.

43 AJ Culyer, *The Economics of Charity* (London, IEA, 1973) analyses the charity market.

44 J Coulson *et al.* (eds.), *The Oxford Illustrated Dictionary* (Oxford, Clarendon Press, 1978), p. 618.

45 R Morgan, Children's Rights Director, National Care Standards Commission, has emphasised this approach. See R Morgan, 'Learning to listen', *The Standard*, NCSC, 2, summer 2002, p. 9; J Richardson, C Joughin, *The Mental Health Needs of Looked-After Children* (London, Royal College of Psychiatrists, 2000; N Stanley, 'What young people want', *Community Care*, 15–21 August 2002, pp. 36–7.

46 I am grateful to Professor Donald Winch, who taught me economics at the University of Sussex nearly half a century ago, and to Arthur Seldon, who added to my understandings. I know that Arthur would agree with my arguments, and I hope that Donald might.

6

The present reforms: 'coherent and right'?

'Conductors must give unmistakeable and suggestive signals to the orchestra – not choreography to the audience.'

– GEORGE SZELL

'Progress is merely a metaphor for walking along a road – very likely the wrong road.'

– GK CHESTERTON

'That practice makes perfect is not necessarily so. Practice makes permanent . . ..
Incorrect practice, bad practice, will eventually produce permanent bad habits.'

– CHARLES HUGHES

How far along the road are we in achieving an 'economic constitution' for the NHS that will make choice real? Individual responsibility depends on enforceable contracts. But an NHS constitution as proposed by Mr Brown and Mr Cameron is a political document. It will state general moral aspirations. But it will not then be the basis of actions at law by individuals who are unhappy with the service. We will not be able to redeem these generalised promises in court. Yet the need is for enforceable contracts, enhanced competition, appropriate direct incentives, attention to consistency, and the protection of competition for willing revenues so that we can achieve the yields of market forces. These generally serve us better in an adaptive society than do political promises, however newly polished. An NHS constitution will not, it seems, be an economic constitution.

My colleagues at the London think-tank Reform said in their recent report on *NHS Reform* that the present changes in the NHS introduced by the government are 'coherent and right'.[1] That is, that they are moving us towards an 'economic constitution'. I have advocated exactly this shift in several previous books, as I have done in each of the national healthcare posts I have held. But is it truly happening across the span of health and social care? And if not yet – as I suggest – what are the signals in the wind, and what might we do to strengthen or challenge them?

The key issues remain these two: where is individual control over funding? Where is competitive purchasing? Without these, the NHS reforms are, indeed failing, as the fourth annual Reform report itself shows in some detail. And without these we will not and cannot achieve the necessary shift towards an economic constitution. There need to be direct incentives for a proper market to emerge. The present reforms do not yet give the individual financially empowered choice, save in the still limited if changing situation of empowerment in social care. And here, in June 2008, only some 80,000 people have personal budgets. This is still a very slight shift when seen in the big picture of the NHS and social care as a whole. Personal budgets do not yet introduce competitive local purchasing save on a small scale. They do not make payment by results a full reality.

The Reform report itself shows clearly that the problems are complex, and not responding to the treatment. Many life-threatening diseases, many chronic conditions, many personal difficulties are not being addressed properly and in a coordinated manner. The catalogue could hardly be more considerable: critical deficits in cancer care, stroke care, chronic care, mental health, fracture care, dementia care, end-of-life care, maternity services, general practice, infant mortality, and many others. All these services remain much under par by comparison with comparable countries, and even in some respects by comparison with some former communist bloc eastern countries, as I document below. It is not difficult to see the blockages. Critically, there is no competition in purchasing. And so instead of taking the lead in the flagship NHS policy of 'practice-based commissioning' the PCTs in charge are often obstructing the policy. They are also diluting what limited patient choice of elective care does tentatively exist.[2]

Failing primary care trusts

There are no pearls without grit. And without the necessary incentives, the controlling culture and structure is not changing. The NHS organisations charged with making purchasing work are resisting changes. Or they are not equipped – intellectually or in terms of management ability or conviction – to lead these. The providers they were to renew or replace are, instead, in command. Both purchasers and providers are protected from appropriate competition. And the challenge of private-sector provision has been radically diluted by them. It is now minimal. Politically motivated vested interests, as Reform notes, continue to steer the ships. There is opposition to change from GPs, consultants, national professional bodies, and from many PCTs. The focus on prevention and public health remains fuzzy and to little effect. No surprise there. The policies rely on hectoring, and not on incentives and rewards.

The proposed reorientation from secondary care to primary and integrated care is, too, making very slow progress. Hospital doctors retain their cultural and political clout. PCTs do not have the management capacity, even when they have the will, to lead the changes. Practice-based commissioning is intended to devolve some of the purchasing work to GPs from PCTs. However, many GP practices have used new budgets to pay for the direct provision of their own services, and have further limited potential competition. Some have bought services from outside firms which some partners of the same GPs also own. A long-term view is necessary but unusual. Monopolies in A&E or its management are not contestable at all. Yet A&E deals with a little over half of all NHS hospital work, and some 80% of all treatment events begin in general practice.

Even with the intense political emphasis on 'the community', PCTs have not sufficiently encouraged innovation in 'the community'. Many necessary partnerships with local bodies are often behind-hand or non-existent. PCTs are poor at gathering and using information. The policy of contestability in offering patients a choice over the hospital in which they can have elective care is failing. The PCTs have 'failed to reach their full potential' because the lack of competing purchasers makes it so. Again, the economic incentives are insufficient.[3]

Increased monopoly

A key role of government should be to protect competition. Yet the trend towards 'giantism' and local monopoly (aligned with local government boundaries), remoteness and unaccountability *both* in purchasing and in provision continues. In 2006–07 the number of primary care trusts was reduced from 309 to 152. The pressures for specialisation – and the gathering of specialists together in large district general hospitals with A&E – is also producing consolidation. Current NHS hospital numbers are expected to shrink, perhaps to 50. These would be very large institutions with turnovers above £300 million. Choice then will depend on open information, comparisons between clinicians and their teams, and the contestability of managements. But it is not a subject being considered by the Competition Commission nor is contestability being proposed by Whitehall. Yet it is an essential 'next step' in reform to introduce such contestability. We should, too, prevent mergers which are against the public interest if they disable competition, which government must protect. It seems that many mergers are driven not only by efficiency demands but by the preference of avoiding competition and evading the likely consequences of markets.[4]

Clearly, the economic and cultural incentives for choice and change hardly exist at all in these key areas. And the potential is being much reduced by such PCT and giant hospital consolidations. The contestability of managements – especially where there is monopoly or control by scarcity power, as with A&E and by such local hospital and PCT mergers – may be the only way to achieve value for money and improved outcomes as well as to protect choice. It is a condition, too, of being able to remove managements who are clearly protecting their own position and who are disinterested in choice. We should open the doors to private sector management of such 'public' facilities. On the purchasing side, competitive purchasers also would encourage much greater information, more published detail on individual doctors and clinical teams, and on outcomes – as well as being able to present and use current and cohesive consumer feedback. They will manage the purchasing business with *current* financial numbers as an instrument of present business, and not merely report to Whitehall historic numbers as a mere backwards and inactive observation.

Central micro-management and 'government failure'

Meanwhile, local mergers continue and the DoH continues to bombard the system with short-term targets. These override any efforts to set local priorities. Purchasers continue to marginalise private sector provision. Local relationships persist in reflecting provider dominance and cultural leadership. And despite – or perhaps because of – intense central micro-management, clearly focused and locally deliverable objectives are not in place. Spending growth is unlikely to continue, despite proposals to consume 11% of GDP on the NHS. Nor are NHS surpluses an answer, for they are a short-term illusion as we will see below. We may well need to spend more on health and social care as the population ages, but this is an issue of personal savings as well as tax-based services. I explore these questions in my chapters on long-term care. It is not the government's money, but ours. It should be returned to us to invest in our own health savings accounts and the like. There will be no growth in the productive economy, too, unless public sector spending levels very significantly fall. And, as Simon Heffer recently emphasised, too, a policy of 'sharing the proceeds of growth' (the policy of both HM Government and HM's Opposition) will not work if there is no growth.[5] The problem is government failure. It seems unlikely that politicians can fix a problem which they do not recognise until they ask the right questions.

Meanwhile, the NHS fog persists. We do not even know, in detail, what is actually happening, line by line, on costs. There are no coherent financial line-by-line measurements or cost management structures which a proper business would recognise as necessary. We do not know whether or not the unprecedented new money has been spent to good or bad effect to impact on outcomes. Outsourcing and compulsory tendering remain fragile at best and small beans at worst. The Healthcare Commission, which has previously been critical of PCTs, showed in its 2007 'Health check' that these organisations – intended as the critical drivers of reform – were not improving practice-based work. Nor is there enthusiasm among many GPs for the changes. A survey issued by the DoH itself showed that only just over half (57%) of GPs were supportive of the practice-based commissioning policy. The Audit Commission was also critical of progress.[6] Once again, as in previous NHS reorganisation, enormous efforts and huge sums of public money have been spent on trying to do 25% of the necessary job of reform, but without appreciating why and how this cannot be done. It would be much better – and perhaps no more of a struggle if we followed the lesson of the incremental and piloted path this book describes – to try to achieve the entire task by evolving a proper market.

Much of this detail the annual Reform report does in fact recognise. It says this of the reforms – which I suggest stop far short of individual financial empowerment and the use of competition: 'Each of the reform programmes is either far behind schedule or in actual retreat. They have lost coherence, in that reforms that should have happened together – in particular a more flexible and commercial supply side has not been matched by a strong demand side.' And: 'The fact that PCTs are not leading reform can also be seen in the evidence of the obstruction of both practice-based commissioning and patient choice.'[7]

I therefore respectfully dissent from my colleagues that the present reforms are 'coherent and right'. I draw the robust conclusion that what is instead necessary to achieve the objectives of major changes is *competitive purchasing instead of PCT monopoly*, and *individual financial empowerment*. Further, there needs to be much improved data by which service comparisons can be made, and the coming together of the holders of health savings accounts in local competitive purchasing via mutual, cooperative organisations. In a word, a market. These organisations will then only be able to survive by attracting the willing and mobile revenues of individual holders of health savings accounts, and by effective purchasing which changes the culture. They can play a crucial enabling role in bringing about the necessary competition among both purchasers and providers.

'The forces of conservatism'

We can see from the available public evidence that we are not, indeed, likely to achieve the necessary economic and social objectives by the complex, bureaucratic, expensively managed, re-jigged, unambitious and consciously obstructed local structures of the present reforms. Professor Bernard Crump, Chief Executive of the NHS's own Institute for Innovation and Improvement, has recently pointed out that even such a simple but essential change as getting doctors and nurses to wash their hands between patients is difficult to achieve. But this is essential to improve patient safety, care and consistency. Professor Crump said that some hospitals are simultaneously among the best for one condition and among the worst for another. Improvements 'are quite hard to spread from one ward to the next, never mind from one hospital to another . . .'[8]

We need to deploy *much more powerful incentives* by which to significantly improve health and social care, lower costs, increase productivity in terms of quality outcomes and not only volume, improve value for money and offer genuine incentives for self-responsible lifestyles. And for staff to wash their hands! This last not because we want the state to be our nanny, but because we care about our fellows. And because the medical evidence shows how much better lives can be if we do take more care of our own selves.

At present, however, what Mr Blair called 'the forces of conservatism' remain in command on the bridge. Providers control cultures, limit competition and hold the maps in their hands. Those leading to economic reform are carefully folded away. Purchasing by PCTs, in particular, is failing to alter our course. Nor is the answer 'a new framework', a charter, or a constitution. That is, if this means a 'settlement' and thus a system which can avoid trial and error, evade market discovery and cut us all off from the full benefits of evolutionary, market-based change. It is this which, instead, can prompt new investment, further discovery, innovation, recombination and change. It is right to call for 'an economic constitution' for the NHS. This best makes sense, however, if it means placing all purchasing and all provision in a market where real economic rules lead us forward, with all the benefits both of improvement and surprise. Here, books by economists like Arthur Seldon[9], cultural critics like Virginia Postrel[10] and Jane Jacobs,[11] and consumer-focused analysts and commentators like Regina Herzlinger[12] should be required reading for all NHS staffs, all new NHS entrants, and for those politicians who offer us their statist formulae by contrast with the necessity of trial-and-error adaptation and economic incentives as the only democratic basis for future improvements.

Meanwhile, as Professor Bosanquet has said,

> The current system is a provider dominated one in which the pattern of output reflects the interests and concerns of the providers. The providers also set the costs and the method by which the service is delivered. The NHS can only begin to deliver real value if it uses the forces of competition and choice, rather than fighting them.[13]

NHS Foundation Trusts (albeit, with their competitive prospects much limited by the diluted legislation which set them up) were drawn from the most ambitious and better managed NHS hospitals. But, unsurprisingly, even these are not achieving sustained improvements in performance.[14]

The chief policy requirement is not to continue to ratchet up the levels of spending. Instead, the need is to restructure funding, to make purchasing competitive and to rely on the role of direct incentives. In this way we can construct the conditions for financially empowered individual choice. Here, the effective guardians of competition should be the government as light regulator, and the market itself. This, rather than hoping to rely on PCTs and cumbersome, bureaucratic strategic health authorities, or to hope for disinterested behaviour on the part of vested interests.

The changes I propose more directly address the significant deficits of the NHS, of social care, and the great difficulties of funding long-term elderly care.[15] They meet full on the failures of current NHS purchasing and provision. Current reforms are not providing sufficient incentives to change structures and thus cultures, improve self-responsible preventive care, change local purchasing, increase pluralist competition, or integrate services to the benefit of patients and the enhancement of value for money. Outcomes – including how many people survive treatable diseases rather than die unnecessarily – remain poor by comparison with other advanced countries. The performance of the NHS has recently again been identified as lagging significantly behind other comparable countries over the entire lifespan, what Professor Bosanquet calls the 'cradle-to-grave gap'.[16] The key choice in dealing with these deficits is between dynamism and statism.[17]

We should also ask how we have got into a situation where 'experts' try to make judgements for us, and who claim to know our interests better than we know them for ourselves.[18] These 'experts' continue to seek to intrude their own concepts of 'normality' and 'health' – what Illich called 'medical imperialism', what Skrabanek calls 'lifestylism' – upon our entire 'physical, mental, and social well-being'.[19]

This history suggests, too, that in the two chief left-of-centre strands of British thought about the future of the working class at the beginning of the 20th century grievous errors were made in abandoning active working-class mutualism for central controls.[20] Alas, quite unnecessarily, there is already a lot of wasted sand in the glass.

Notes

1 Nick Bosanquet, Andrew Haldenby and Helen Rainbow, *NHS Reform: national mantra, not local reality* (London, Reform, February 2008). For example, on payment by results. See DoH, *NHS Plan: a plan for investment; a plan for reform* (London, HMSO, July 2000). On the opportunity cost of recent investment in the NHS and welfare see Reform, *Reform Bulletin*, 10 March 2008.

2 See *'Choose & Book': patients' choice of hospital and booked appointment policy framework for choice and booking at the point of referral* (London, DoH, 2004). The DoH reported that in July 2007 only 43% of patients remembered being offered a choice of hospital for their first appointment there, a fall from 48% in March that year. Department of Health, *Report on the National Patient Choice Survey – July 2007 England* (London, DoH, 2007). In February 2008 *Pulse* magazine said hospitals across England were stopping patients from booking advance appointments in attempts to meet government targets of 18 weeks between GP referral and hospital treatment. The DoH also admitted that hospitals rig waiting lists by making it difficult for GPs to make bookings for patients. John Carvel, 'Hospitals do rig waiting lists to hit targets, ministers admit', *The Guardian*, 27 February 2008, p. 9. King's Fund Chief Economist John Appleby reported that only a third of patients seem to have been offered choice, and a similar proportion only were aware of the policy in the first place. In terms of patients' memories of being offered choice there were variations by sex, age and ethnic group. The King's Fund showed in January 2007 that GPs did not offer choice unless a patient asked for this. Rebecca Rosen, Dominique Florin and Ruth Hutt, *An Anatomy of GP Referral Decisions: a qualitative study of GP's views on their role in supporting patient choice* (London King's Fund, 2007).

3 Bosanquet *et al.*, op. cit., p. 44; Health Management Specialist Library www.nhs.library.nhs.uk; SMF Health Commission, *Choice and Contestability in Primary Care* (London, Social Market Foundation, February 2005); Rossiter, *Future*, op. cit., pp. 18–21; DoH, *Practice Based Commissioning: engaging practices in commissioning* (London, DoH, 2004).

4 See DoH, *The NHS in England: operating framework for 2007–08* (London, DoH, 11 December 2006), and *The NHS in England: the operating framework for 2008-09* (London, DoH, 13 December 2007). See also Ann Rossiter, *The Future of Healthcare*. Introduction (London, Social Market Foundation, May 2007). For studies offering contrary perspectives see C Bojke, H Gravelle and D Wilkin, 'Is bigger better for primary care groups and trusts?', *British Medical Journal*, 10 March 2001, 322, pp. 599–602; Robert Town, 'The welfare impact of HMP mergers', *Journal of Health Economics*, 2001, 20(6), pp. 967–90; W Anderson, D Florin, S Gillam and L Mountford, *Every Voice Counts: primary care organisations and public involvement* (London, King's Fund, 2002). Healthcare Commission, *Annual Health Check* (London, Healthcare Commission, 2007).

5 Simon Heffer, 'At last! David Cameron says something I can agree with', *Daily Telegraph*, 13 March 2008, p. 22. But read the '*but*' here, too. Mr Cameron's proposals for reform led by the professionals in health and education were wisely critiqued by Tim Hames. Hames pointed out that Mr Blair, 'like Mr Cameron, kept it vague and adopted positions that had the widest appeal and offended nobody. He, too, sought the votes on the professionals in health and education by promising to scrap Tory measures. And he bitterly regretted it. If you could provide Mr Blair with a swift trip in the Tardis he would trade a smaller majority in the 1997 election for a more substantial programme, rooted in a truly new Labour approach to reform. The principal tragedy of his premiership is that he was not a Blairite at the outset.' Tim Hames, 'A whopping big majority is pointless, Dave', *The Times*, 12 May 2008, p. 19. See also, Ian Martin, 'Unconvincing and unhappy Brown has run out of road', *Daily Telegraph*, 1 May 2008, p. 20, on the caution of 'the Cameroons'; Peter Riddell, 'Mind the gap between Tory plans and reality', *The Times*, 20 May 2008, p. 28.

6 Commission for Health Improvement, *What CHI has found in: primary care trusts* (London, CHI, 2004); Audit Commission, *Transforming Primary Care: the role of primary care trusts in shaping and supporting general practice* (London, Audit Commission, 2004); Audit Commission, *Putting Commissioning into Practice: implementing practice based commissioning through good financial management* (London, Audit Commission, 2007); DoH, *Practice Based Commissioning, GP Practice Survey: Wave 1* (London, DoH, June 2007).

7 Bosanquet *et al.*, op. cit., pp. 31, 34.
8 Jennifer Taylor, 'Driven to sustain improvement', *The Times*, public agenda section, 27 May 2008, p. 5.
9 Colin Robinson (ed.), *The Collected Works of Arthur Seldon* (Indianopolis, Ind., Liberty Fund, 2004–05), 7 volumes: *The Virtues of Capitalism*; *The State is Rolling Back*; *Everyman's Dictionary of Economics*; *Introducing Market Forces into 'Public' Services*; *Government Failure and Over-Government*; *The Welfare State: pensions, health, and education*; *The IEA, the LSE, and the Influence of Ideas* (includes an index to the series).
10 Virginia Postrel, *The Future and Its Enemies: the growing conflict over creativity, enterprise, and progress* (New York, The Free Press, 1998), and *Substance*, ibid.; see also www.dynamist.com.
11 Jane Jacobs, *Cities and the Wealth of Nations* (1984; Harmondsworth, Penguin Books, 1986); *The Death and Life of Great American Cities* (1961; New York, Random House, 2002); *The Economy of Cities* (New York, Random House, 1969).
12 See note 5, in Chapter 3 here on 'Language, and smuggled goods'.
13 Bosanquet *et al.*, op. cit., p. 51.
14 See my article, 'We are arguing about the wrong NHS solutions', *The Independent*, 8 May 2003; Monitor reports at www.monitor-nhsft.gov.uk. On the subsequent weak governance of NHS Foundation Trusts, see *Developing the Role of NHS Foundation Trust Governors* (London, Monitor, June 2008), at www.monitor-nhsft.gov.uk; Patrick Butler, 'NHS governors need a new role model', *The Guardian*, society section, 4 June 2008, p. 4.
15 These deficits include the limits set on flexible change; for example, by targets from the centre and also by inflexible labour markets, national pay scales and central manpower planning. Subsidised public pensions alter costs in favour of public providers, which is an issue to be addressed. These factors all intrude upon the potentials for viable, changing, responsive markets.
16 Bosanquet *et al.*, op. cit.
17 For an extended discussion of dynamism and statism see Postrel, *The Future*, op. cit.; my *Patients, Power and Responsibility*, and also my chapter 'What you believe if you are a dynamist; what you believe if you are a statist', in my *'Coming, Ready or Not!' The Realities, the Politics, and the Future of the NHS: nine studies in change* (Brighton, Edward Everett Root, Publishers, 2008). Also, my essay 'Why does Gissing matter?', in John Spiers (ed.), *Gissing and the City: cultural crisis and the making of books in late Victorian England* (Houndsmills, Hants., Palgrave Macmillan, 2006).
18 See my introduction to *Patients, Power and Responsibility*, ibid., and my chapter 'Sidney Webb, "self-deadness", & the NHS' in my *'Coming, Ready or Not!'*, op. cit. Also, Ferdinand Mount, *Mind the Gap: the new class divide in Britain* (London, Short Books, 2004); PHJH Gosden, *Self Help: voluntary associations in nineteenth century Britain* (London, Batsford, 1973); David G Green, *Working Class Patients and The Medical Establishment: self-help in Britain from the mid-19th century to 1948* (London, Maurice Temple Smith, 1985); WD Reekie, *Government in Health Care: lessons from the UK* (Hayward, Calif., Smith Centre for Private Enterprise Studies, 1995). Pat Thane, *Foundations of the Welfare State* (London, Longman, second edition, 1996).
19 I Illich, *Medical Nemesis: the expropriation of health* (London, Marion Boyars, 1976), revised as *Limits to Medicine* (London, Marion Boyars, 1995); P Skrabanek, *The Death of Humane Medicine* (London, Social Affairs Unit, 1994).
20 Commission for Health Improvement, *What CHI has found in: primary care trusts* (London, CHI, 2004); Paul Corrigan, *Registering Choice: how primary care should change to meet patients needs* (London Social Market Foundation, 2006); Bosanquet *et al.*, op. cit. Also OECD, *Health at a Glance: OECD indicators* (Paris, OECD, 2007).

7

Compare and contrast: performance, probable or actual?

'[Policy] madness, which has been defined as doing the same thing over and over and expecting different results.'

— RICHARD PIPES

'Medicine's real triumphs lie in improving the quality of life for everyone not in death-defying heroics that benefit or torment a few.'

— NEW YORK TIMES

How can we achieve competitive purchasing, to enable every patient to have reliable access to good care?

The answers highlight revealing challenges concerning consumer control, 'personalisation', the coordination of care, and appropriate provider responsiveness. These concern a general theory of mutual and individual obligation and personal responsibility. They also concern practical actions, including providers sorting out their quality, responsiveness, prices and scheduling to attract business. They pose challenging questions about the character of our institutions. In the endeavour to deliver 'world class commissioning' my proposal is for the mutual, voluntary, cooperative patient guaranteed care association, which seeks willing revenues. And which requires providers to genuinely personalise services.

The PGCA will be the consumer's champion, the expert facilitator. It will guide its members to relevant, effective, integrated care. Preferably, to specialists working in disease-specific areas. Professor Herzlinger has called these 'focused factories',[1] in settings which are designed specifically to support the required treatment regime. The PGCA will also expect to tackle unexplained variations in medical practice and the variability of outcomes. To focus on coordinated and integrated care. And to increase the rewards for well-managed providers. The incentive for the insurer/purchaser will be to keep the member healthy. The incentive for the customer will be better, well integrated, thoughtfully coordinated, and almost certainly cheaper and more reliably competent care.

Unexplained variations in practice remain a major issue. In a healthcare system which relies on good intentions (many of which are genuine, of course), we may still be too trusting, too unreflective. There remains a powerful structure of defensive clinical professional guilds, and much secrecy. Dr William Pickering's courage in drawing our attention to inappropriate and unexplained variations in clinical practice, and the prevalence of much uninvestigated variable quality of care, is of sterling value. So, too, are his proposals for different kinds of scrutiny, including an independent medical inspectorate. His approach is more relevant than existing schemes.

The systemic overall answer is for the purchaser and the patient to be on the same team, and with a shared objective: to get good quality services and value for money in a competitive market. A key test is the availability of information, in plain English, and on the issues that matter to the customer. In the NHS, more information is a threat to the stability of institutions. Yet if local people really know that St Hilda's on the Hill has startlingly good or distressingly poor results – if more people die unexpectedly from cardiac disease than at St Wilfrid's Royal Hospital – few will want to go to St Hilda's for heart care. The local media will shine its spotlight on the differences. Even fewer will join the 'Save St Hilda's' marches. Information challenges clinical practice. It is a nuisance to a rationed system. It queries a secretive one. In my market model, information will be an advantage to the patient, to the purchaser, and to the better provider.

A powerful example of the potential for purchasing by a competitive PGCA would be the potentials of 'focused factories' – healthcare facilities which provide highly efficient specialised care. These focused factories can do much to eliminate undesirable but otherwise prevalent variability in quality of care, cost and outcomes.[2] Other examples are facilities which could be increasingly provided in or adjacent to major drive-in retail outlets, where people live their ordinary lives. This is the concept of 'the medical village'.

The PGCA will seek patient satisfactions. It will want to work with all possible quality measures. It will ask such questions on its report cards as would the patient want to go back to that facility, that physician, that reception? Would they recommend the service to others? Were they treated as an individual? Were people kind, or rude, tactful and welcoming, 'too busy' and dismissive? What was the physical environment like? How long did they have to wait? Was the wait unexpected? Were explanations offered? Were their views asked for in a consultation? Did they feel they were involved in shared decision making? Were they given clear information? And emotional support? Did people listen? Was confidentiality respected? Were they given guidance on when to take medicines, and why, and on what to eat and drink? Was the care plan clear, explained to them, and did they understand the explanation? Were they given a recording of guidance and literature to take home, and which they could discuss with their loved ones and friends?

The PGCA will publish aggregated data on the patients' experiences. Separately, its own doctors in management will audit medical records, assess the appropriateness of treatments, their efficacy, the necessity of tests, costs, and the monitoring of recovery and of care.

The NHS has proposed 'world class commissioning'. But the performance of local monopoly PCTs as 'lean, mean commissioning machines' has been the subject of much anxiety concerning their capabilities and expertise. These have not seemed fit for purpose. The Health Commission's Annual Health Check in 2007 reported PCTs as the worst performers 'on the things that matter most'.[3] And so it is not sufficient to call for 'improved' local purchasing – no doubt, to be driven by more central direction. We know, too, that trends towards even greater local monopoly make this improvement much less likely. To achieve effective (and reflective) purchasing it is essential that the conditions for a market to grow and to thrive are set in place. Instead of the present limited reforms, we should introduce a structure of *competitive* purchasers and informed financially empowered choices. The situation that would arise in an open market of competitive purchasers can be seen by comparison with what PCTs (and many GP practices) are currently doing on some key elements in care. They are, indeed, a critical barrier to effective change.

PGCAs vs. PCTs

These points are best clarified by experience and example. Let's compare what the competing PGCAs could do and what the now monopoly PCTs do or do not do.

Coordinated care

This is a crucial objective, for all users of NHS services. The competing PGCA would exert all its management and leadership skills to achieve coordinated provision and care. Its lack is at the root of much failure in the NHS, notably in cancer care. The predominant users of the NHS are long-term chronic sufferers, who need coordinated care and who have to re-negotiate their care regularly. Many have co-morbidities. Two critics of NHS reforms, Professor Bob Sang and Professor Chris Ham, have both questioned whether the current reforms will support the development of integrated care, or reduce the use of hospital services. They question, too, the project to increase the diversity of provision (which evidence suggests PCTs are, in any case, deliberately reducing now) to support patient choice. PGCAs, however, would combine choice and an insistence on buying coordinated care – just as they would combine negotiating personal care for chronic long-term sufferers with choice to make such negotiations effective. Advocacy and negotiation, coordination and choice are all one of a piece. They are *not* alternatives.[4]

Competition

PGCAs would compete with other purchasers for members joining with willing revenues. PCTs do not. They are local monopolies. They disable the development of a market. They supervise the setting of the concrete. It is essential to the evolution of a market that NHS institutions accept that their share of work will very likely reduce, that new providers are encouraged to invest, and that a critical mass of independent provision is created, with all services and all managements contestable. The most essential lever will be competitive purchasing organisations, who press at every boundary for change, just as new providers will make new offers to consumers. The most recent government suggestions for failing NHS hospitals to be placed under private sector management again evades the real issue – which is that improvements will only come from the aggregate decision making of purchasers representing willing members, and with competitors coming into the market as providers.[5]

Information

There is no prospect of achieving the much vaunted 'World Class Commissioning' in the NHS, for without good information there is no possibility of making informed comparisons. The competing PGCA would ensure that good information was made available through conventional market pressures. They as well as purchasers would have to invest in it. Indeed, the providers and purchasers most likely to succeed would compete in part on the basis of the information they offer: 'Come to us. We have the best doctors in management and we buy the best outcomes. Look at the figures.' As I show, below, at present PCT purchasing managements *actively* resist such ideas, as do consultants within provider institutions. They do all they can to limit choices, as do GPs.[6]

Prices

We would get away from bundled tariffs, block budgets and national prices. PGCAs would negotiate prices locally. They would buy quality, access, timing and cost. PCTs are restricted by national tariffs. Here, the Reform proposal by Professor Bosanquet *et al.* for an independent authority to set tariffs in the short-term is not a market approach. Avoid![7]

Payment by results

As PGCAs will monitor provider performance against customer-defined expectations as well as by standard clinical audit, this will be the basis of negotiated payments, and the timing of cash flows, between the PGCA and any provider offering services. The present national tariff structure does not facilitate such negotiation.

Budgets

No PGCA could survive unless it had full knowledge of budgets and financial flows with appropriate management controls. Many PCTs do not yet have these in place. Why? Because under the present reforms it does not matter.

Patient choice

The PGCA would market its services directly to potential members who were in control of their own health savings account as a mobile fund. Such a mutual organisation would understand this as an essential of a democratic, open, competitive structure. And that choice and thus risk to their income is a condition of markets and of potential successes as well as losses if they failed to meet the wishes of their members. PCTs do not have to do any such things. They do not have to improve in response to the wishes of members who can otherwise go elsewhere. They have no such risks because 'consumers' have no such choices. The increasingly monopolistic local situation protects them. Even the prospect of very limited patient choice is seen as a risk to their planning. Professor Bosanquet reported that 'In private conversations, one independent sector hospital provider reported being told by a PCT that a particular ISTC [Independent Sector Treatment Centre] would be taken off the choice menu if it proved too popular.'[8]

Contestability of services

The success of a PGCA in attracting willing members would in part turn on the access and improved services they can achieve from competing providers. PCTs are too cosy with traditional providers, who also predominate in terms of financial surpluses, and management skills. They also have cultural clout in that consultants have great political influence through the Royal Colleges and also with the media.

Employment of GPs

Currently, GPs employ themselves. Some also buy services from providers which they own. The PGCA would not directly employ any doctors, save in the management of its business. It would buy services from competing GP practices. It would negotiate access, weekend services, the hours to be covered and by whom. Alan Johnson's long (and costly) struggle with the GPs and the BMA would be a thing of the past. Markets would decide. The competitive PGCA would set out the conditions of its proposed purchase of services from GPs. Those who did not wish to offer weekend cover, longer hours, or times of opening convenient to patients who were members of a competitively managed PGCA would attract very little business. As with GP contracts, or the controversial new polyclinics – recommended by Lord Darzi – let the market decide.[9]

Independent sector provision

The open market, which PCTs deliberately restrict, would follow from willing revenues taken to a PGCA which would then buy advantageously on behalf of its members and from any suitable supplier.

Employment of staff

Competing purchasers would set their own contracts with staff. The advent of competition would establish market levels of pay and conditions, and end inflexible national structures. Some incomes would rise, others fall. Good performance would also be properly rewarded. PCTs, NHS hospitals and other public providers do not have these freedoms.

Entry and exit

Necessarily, some existing providers would lose support; others would gain this from willing purchasers. Some strategic oversight would be necessary, and this remains to be debated. However, the protection of the inadequate provider and the poor purchaser would cease. The incentives would be to improve, retrain, retool or remove. Clearly, big hospitals remain in an advantageous position since this is where the specialists are employed. They are protected, too, by the presence of A&E where just over half of NHS hospital work is done. Similarly, large providers are protected by Royal College controls over the approval of doctor training. Even with some services being moved into the community, this powerful structure will remain considerable. The contestability of management is an important issue of public policy even as improved purchasing will continue to shift work and roles from traditional settings.

Patient-reported outcomes

The Liberal Democrat spring 2008 conference policy paper *Empowerment, Fairness and Quality in Health Care* rightly proposed piloting patient-reported outcome measures which would measure real patient experiences and address and assess whether the treatment has actually benefited their physical and mental health.[10] However, we do not need another unaccountable and costly quangocracy to do this. The PGCA would do this as a matter of routine in a market, and would negotiate payments based on outcomes as reported by patients.

An example: closures

Local hospital closures would happen or not happen depending on the decisions of purchasers. There would have to be some strategic negotiation nationally and locally, and the relationships between this and the impact of an open market need to be very carefully debated. A complex problem is where A&E is located, and the contestability of its management. This process of discussion, and of relationships between a market and national strategic questions, is not helped, however, by politicians declaring – in 'vote-buying' – that they will protect local hospitals. This is a matter primarily for purchasers locally.[11]

An example: relocated services

Well-led PGCAs would have encouraged many GPs to set up surgeries in places where people live their normal lives. Heywood, Middleton and Rochdale PCT gave a lead here in March 2008, setting up the first GP surgery located in a Sainsbury's supermarket. But it has taken an age for such an innovation to occur anywhere. Similarly, there should be GPs in A&E, with consequent savings.[12]

An example: lack of Customer power

The NHS has disproportionately benefited the middle classes to the detriment of poorer people, the elderly, and other fragile users of services such as the mentally ill. It has been persistently 'ageist'. One of the most striking recent examples has been the case of Mr James Tagg, the 88-year-old Second World War bomber pilot from Torquay in Devon who suffers from wet age-related macular degeneration (AMD), which attacks central vision. As we age, there are many physical changes to be faced and endured. The debilitating effects of impaired vision caused by this condition shouldn't be one of them. Unfortunately, this progressive sight disorder is the leading cause of impaired vision in people aged over 65. It is a prime threat to continuing independent living. The first telltale signs of AMD are loss of fine vision and colour at the centre of the eye. Sharp vision in this part of the eye is essential for reading, driving, writing, watching television, recognising people and performing tasks around the home. Mr Tagg experienced this eye condition but he was refused treatment by Torbay PCT. Apparently, he would have to go blind in one eye before the PCT would agree to fund the injections that could save his sight. Is such a situation conceivable if Mr Tagg was in control of his own health savings account, which he could take to a preferred purchaser of his choice? Could he, as an older person who has paid his dues to his country, be then denied service, marginalised and disenfranchised? Mr Tagg fought the case. He used media exposure and achieved the funding for his treatment. Well-wishers, including doctors, sent him cheques amounting to £1000 which he presented at No. 10 Downing Street, to pay for his treatment. The PCT relented, on a technicality – as some NHS Trusts now appear to be doing in June 2008 in seeking to free themselves from the obloquy of denying people the opportunity to pay for cancer drugs that the NHS does not supply. Elsewhere in the South West of England the treatment denied to Mr Tagg was available from other PCTs, so the argument that it does not work falls. Mr Tagg was tenacious, and went public. But in a system where individuals were financially empowered the structure would give choices to the silent, too.[13]

An example: more lack of customer power

The case of Cora Slade, the retired NHS nurse suffering from wet age-related macular degeneration is a second recent example of the same denial of services. Mrs Slade is 74. Her local PCT (Devon Primary Care Trust) refused to pay for treatment. She paid for her own care, which is another example of a willingness to pay which is a case both of self-responsibility but also of being cheated by a 'service' for which the individual believed she had already paid in taxes. Her husband Don has Parkinson's disease, and Mrs Slade is his carer. In different parts of the country the service Mrs Slade sought is either provided or denied. Each time the media take up such a case some technicality is discovered by which local criteria are 'adjusted'. What a perfect example we have here of unjoined-up-thinking. Instead, we need to do all we can to endorse the informal carer, the family member and the friend, as I examine in my later focus on long-term elderly care. What power there would be if individuals held mobile money and if this was gathered together by a PGCA, purchasing on their behalf. In the draft Queen's Speech of May 2008 Gordon Brown warned that hospitals which fail to treat patients well will have their funding cut. Why not enable PGCAs to make such decisions about which providers to fund, and allow them to move funds to those who offer the best services? Mr Brown has said that people will have more personal budgets. The logic then is to permit real empowered choice. We wait to see the details.[14]

Notes

1 For Herzlinger's most recent comments on this see *Who Killed Health Care?*, op. cit., pp. 78–9, 168–72, 220; Stuart Lovett, 'Chronic problems: innovative solutions: paving the way to the focused factory', in Herzlinger, *Consumer-Driven Health Care*, op. cit., pp. 635–42.

2 See JC Goodman, op. cit., p. 235.

3 Healthcare Commission, *Annual Health Check* (London, Healthcare Commission, 2007).

4 See Bob Sang, 'Don't let's forget, we're in it for the long-term', *British Journal of Healthcare Management*, 2007, 13(4), pp. 122–5 and 13(5), pp. 160–1; Chris Ham, 'The reforms need reform', *The Guardian*, 26 February 2007. Prof. Sang is Professor of Patient and Public Involvement, South Bank University. Prof. Ham was Director of Strategy, Department of Health, 2001–04 and is Director of the Health Services Management Centre, University of Birmingham. See also Alastair Mant, 'The triumph of big-business think', *International Journal of Leadership of Public Services*, 3(1), April 2007, pp. 37–46.

5 John Carvel, 'Failing hospitals to get private sector bosses', *The Guardian*, 4 June 2008, p. 2.

6 Nick Bosanquet, Andrew Haldenby and Helen Rainbow, *NHS Reform: national mantra, not local reality* (London, Reform, February 2008), p. 52.

7 Ibid., p. 36.

8 Ibid.

9 See John Carvel, 'Angry GPs reluctantly accept plan for weekend and evening surgeries', *The Guardian*, 7 March 2008, p. 7; National Audit Office, *NHS Pay Modernisation: new contracts for general practice services in England* (London Stationery Office, 27 February 2008); Nigel Hawkes, 'Contract was a windfall for GPs but "not a good deal for patients"', *The Times*, 28 February 2008, p. 4. Also, James Gubb, *Why the NHS is the sick man of Europe* (London, Civitas, 2008). Many practices are rigid and inflexible in their hours, have inflexible appointment booking arrangements, and have restricted services. The costs of this lack of flexibility to the British economy have recently been estimated at £1 billion, and at the loss of 3.5 million working days a year. Confederation of British Industry, *Just What the Doctor Ordered: better GP services* (London, CBI, September 2007). Unlike continental Europe, too, patients cannot go direct to a specialist. On his appointment Mr Johnson made improving primary care access a national priority, emphasising the importance of competition. Victoria Vaughan, 'Johnson wants competition to prop up poor GP access', *Health Service Journal*, 26 July 2007, p. 5. David Rose, 'GPs face penalty if patients need out-of-hours care at hospital', *The Times*, 15 November 2007, p. 24. See also Alan Johnson, speech on improving primary care to NHS Confederation Primary Care Network, 6 March 2008. But the government's view is that 150 centres of primary care are required, and must be opened. It also proposes a new central agency to support innovation. In fact, innovations best arise from an open market, as Virginia Postrel's books illustrate for the modern period and earlier. See Kate Devlin, 'Polyclinics "will mean longer trips to see your GP"', *Daily Telegraph*, 9 June 2008, p. 1; Keith Hopcroft, 'A nasty case of clinical detachment', *The Times*, 12 June 2008, p. 28.

10 Liberal Democrats, *Empowerment, Fairness and Quality in Health Care*, Policy paper for Spring conference (London, Liberal Democrats, 22 January 2008).

11 David Cameron, speech to the Conservative Party annual conference, 3 October 2007. Labour politicians are said to have sought to protect hospitals from closure in marginal seats. Nigel Hawkes, 'Labour ploy to protect hospitals in marginals', *The Times*, 15 September 2006.

12 Daily Telegraph reporter, 'GP's surgery opens in supermarket', *Daily Telegraph*, 4 March 2008, p. 14.

13 Laura Clout, 'Veteran wins fight for NHS sight treatment', *Daily Telegraph*, 29 February 2008. Max Pemberton, 'Finger on the button', *Daily Telegraph*, 3 March 2008, p. 23. For background on top-up payments, see Paul Charlson, Christoph Lees and Karol Sikora, *Free at the Point of Delivery – Reality or Political Mirage? Case studies of top-up payments in UK healthcare* (London, Doctors for Reform, April 2007); Sarah-Kate Templeton, 'Cancer pair win fight for top-up drugs', *Sunday Times*, news section, 22 June 2008, p. 7. See also Age Concern, *The Age Agenda 2008: public policy and older people* (London, Age Concern, 26 February 2008) and N Seddon, *Quite Like Heaven: options for the NHS in a consumer age* (London, Civitas, 2007). See also www.caredirections.co.uk and www.stanthonys.org.uk/AMD_treatment.html.

14 Daily Telegraph reporter, 'Nurse refused NHS funding to save sight', *Daily Telegraph*, 7 March 2008, p. 14. On propensity to make top-up payments, one in four pounds of UK healthcare spending is now spent privately. *Reform Bulletin*, 22 February 2008, at www.reform.co.uk. See Andrew Porter, 'Cash threat to hospitals where patients suffer', *Daily Telegraph*, 15 May 2008, p. 4. Junior Health Minister Mr Ben Bradshaw MP has also said that the government's proposals for changes in the provision of GP services are 'an open procurement process so that any prospective provider – a group of GPs, a voluntary organisation, a cooperative or an independent provider – can put forward proposals. . . . In practice the contracts will be based on local decisions about which option provides the best quality and value for money.' But who will make these contract decisions? See B Bradshaw, 'Our proposals are about improving the NHS, not privatising it', *The Guardian*, 14 May 2008, p. 31.

8

What are politicians *for*?

'. . . *whether we do little or much we are sure to discontent everybody . . . and we had better satisfy our consciences by doing what is just and right between the contending parties.*'

– LORD CLARENDON

'*I give you bitter pills in sugar coating. The pills are harmless, the poison is in the sugar.*'

– STANISLAW LEE

'*Controlled democracy is an oxymoron. Democracy in voting, like democracy in media, is about risk, or it is about nothing.*'

– SUSAN BUCK-MORSS

Clearly, no politician can do anything very much until elected. But to be elected we expect them to have a purpose. To be elected politicians surely pose and answer the question of 'what is a political party *for*?' And 'Why do we want power?' There are fundamental issues about the funding, provision and consumption of health and social care which will engage them at the coming general election. These do need political action – significantly, indeed, by politicians standing aside. These issues need urgent and bold attention. They are about values and principles as well as provision. Indeed, those who seek radical solutions have not abandoned morality. They insist upon it, which is why they want radical change. However, the reform picture that UK politicians offer us is very muted. We have seen that Mr Alan Milburn continues to push for change. From his general statements about the kind of society we would like to live in Mr David Cameron, too, has encouraged the hope that he can move us towards consumer control. We need to remind leaders in all three main parties that the evolution of personal budgets has genuinely positive and revolutionary potential.

The emphasis on choice offers the opportunity of much greater self-responsibility, a commitment to the consequences of our actions, and significant improvements in preventive care. The key is to empower every individual by specific control over funds. Every other instrument – such as the 'public value' idea and an NHS constitution promoted by Mr Gordon Brown and Mr David Cameron – is, however, blunt and rusty.

Some politicians, out of sheer frustration, have, however, actually made a huge difference. I take the view that Mr Tony Blair and Mr Milburn offered clear, thoughtful and vigorous leadership in difficult circumstances. They moved the NHS and social care to an agenda of 'choice'. As Anthony Seldon described this in July 2001:

> Blair was in bullish form, dismissing anyone who urged caution on reform: When someone suggested 'preference' might be an easier sell to the unions and the party, he replied simply: 'Choice is choice'. At one point in the discussions Mr Blair added: 'It's going to be hell for a large part of the time we're doing this . . . I don't see any point in being Prime Minister unless we take risks.'[1]

And in August 2002: '"Don't worry," he used to say, "whether you think this is deliverable for the party or the government. Tell me what you think is right and let's work out how we can do it."'[2] This is much more unusual than many give credit.

By contrast, much Conservative Party thinking on health and social care was for a long time left in a dangerous statist vacuum, in part because of the work of its own 'Health Commission' on which provider interests exerted very considerable influence. It said very little about choice or empowerment. It was not dynamist. During more than a decade in opposition, too, the Conservative Party accepted the arguments of the liberal intelligentsia in favour of the state controlled NHS. This, despite its very well recorded deficits in every key area including many poor outcomes – for example, in cancer care which eventually affects virtually every family in the country.

However, under a section headed 'Full Engagement', its Health Commission stated on 'Accountability' that 'The NHS of the future must be accountable to patients not bureaucrats. Patients must understand why they are receiving a particular care package; they must be able to effect change if appropriate.'[3]

The language here was not helpful. Patients *must* understand? They are *receiving*, not choosing? They must be able to effect change *if appropriate*? The document said that engagement needs to be based on the principle of informed choice. *Informed?* On the basis of whose *values* and *preferences*? Who makes which *trade-offs*? May we not make our own informed – and even uninformed – choices? Who says which is which? Who decides which is relevant information? When would our choices *not* be appropriate? How do we make sure the apparent choices are real? That we can secure what we want, and for which – as the document notes – we have paid already in taxes? Who *decides* who decides?

Fortunately, the Institute of Economic Affairs, Progressive Vision, The Adam Smith Institute, Politiea, Reform and Civitas in the UK; The Cascade Institute, The Cato Institute and others in the USA and elsewhere continue to consider the endemic and systemic problems of state controlled and predominantly state provided health and social care. They have offered detailed and carefully researched free market solutions, too; for example, the many writings of Arthur Seldon and the two publications by Professor Phillip Booth on the funding of long-term elderly care.[4]

Some Liberal Democrats have also given serious thought to these issues, notably David Laws MP who has clearly influenced the 2008 policy paper *Empowerment, Fairness and Quality in Health Care*. This is radical in that it urges 'Expanding direct payments and individual budgets in the provision of social services and introducing the concept into specific areas within the NHS', although it then limits ideas of choice to increased local control in a framework of 'the new localism'. However, the party leader Nick Clegg made a speech in mid-June which took his party well beyond its most recent position as the advocate of increasing the powers of local government, and of voter influence over this. He proposed a 'patient premium' for the poor. This could be part of the weighting of an HSA. More radically he also advocated the extension of individual budgets to the NHS. He still spoke in term of the party's argot of local government, and in 'new localist' language. But there was more: 'The pruning back of the central state; the devolution of power to local communities; *and the empowerment of individual service users* [my italics].'[5]

'The party of the NHS'

Mr Cameron has headlined his party as 'The party of the NHS'. The suggestion that it is better management that will get the job done is, I suggest, insufficient. Certainly, good management is necessary. But the issue is what do we mean by better management, and of what? And then on which basis can it be specified, and by which incentives and structures can it be measured and achieved? The Party's Green Paper of June 2008 addressed these issues on important topics, but as yet there is no commitment to financial power to make individual choice effective.

The operational and intellectual deficits are indeed formidable. Clearly, the information deficits as we have seen, on outcomes and the experiences of patients. But also on basic financial matters, too. Here, and at the current level of spending of £100 billion, the NHS does not know in detail how the money is being spent because its financial controls are so poor.[6] Nor is additional spending a proper measure of improvement. The required difference is in management, coordinated care, the benefits of choice and competition including much more coordinated care and measurable outcomes. Meanwhile, in the UK the unprecedented levels of NHS investment have been introduced but with no advance in productivity. We still lack quality measures. The public sector, too, finds any measure save volume elusive. There is no guarantee of any kind that increased spending will achieve the high quality services, prompt and integrated access, competition and consumer choice which other differently managed health systems have consistently achieved. Without directly linking funding to root-and-branch reforms those ambitions remain beyond our reach.

International evidence and authoritative national audit shows that the UK performs poorly on many major and modern care challenges. There is thus much unnecessary suffering, and avoidable early death. The catalogue of difficulty is truly forbidding. I suggest that improving the management of the NHS will not be sufficient. As we have seen, many of the problems are summarised and commented upon in the think-tank Reform's fourth annual report on the NHS. It finds that there is inadequate diagnosis, insufficient specialisation, inadequate treatments, little outcome data, too little coordination of care, poor management, and often not even basic financial controls. Corporate failures and cost over-runs are constant, as the recent Cabinet Office review noted. In terms of modernisation and innovation (found in competitive systems) the NHS does not meet many of the best requirements for treatments. For example, it does not provide the latest Down's syndrome screening. There are no seamless prescription or booking systems, and too little care integration. There is a failure to innovate or to adopt promptly those improvements shown to be effective overseas; for example, in cancer care, stroke care, chronic care, mental health, fracture care, dementia care, end-of-life care, maternity services. In infant mortality the UK rate of 5.12 deaths per 1000 is worse than most European countries including the Czech Republic. There is the systematic mismanagement of patients' records, too, as cited by Health Commission Chief Executive Anne Walker.[7]

In 2007–08 junior health minister and surgeon Lord Darzi conducted a national consultation to review the fundamentals of clinical care, patient dignity and safety, integrated services, patient control, choice and local accountability – all of which were listed as challenges which one would have thought would long ago have been sorted, with the NHS in its sixtieth year. Absurdly, too, it was said that the consultation would help ministers set priorities in a national blueprint (and then 10 regional ones) not for the next three, four, or even five years but *for the next 60 years*. This is a ludicrous old Soviet-style idea in a fluid, fast changing, adaptive society where only a very few years ago no one had even thought of the Internet or even heard of AIDS! However, it shows how hard the concrete has set. Lord Darzi, it seems, is unfortunately both a-historical and uninformed about the past. He might re-educate himself helpfully, perhaps beginning with Eric Hobsbawm's David Glass Memorial Lecture, 'Looking Forward: History and the Future' in Hobsbawm's *On History*.[8]

Meanwhile, many will have been surprised to learn that average life expectancy in the UK is less than in other developed countries, such as France or Australia. There are also wide regional variations within the UK.[9] Such a fundamental service as neonatal care does not meet national guideline standards, is poorly provided and under-staffed, and offers 'a lack of clear data on outcomes'.[10] Accident and Emergency services fail to meet necessary standards in key respects. For example, in the care of patients involved in severe traumas where some 60% of patients were found to receive care that was less than good practice required.[11] Waiting times – such as for psychotherapy and counselling for mental healthcare patients, which is up to three years – remain shocking. Waiting times which were not put under intense pressure by targets remain longer than in Europe. NHS hospital standards of cleanliness remain a scandal, too.[12]

The facts about NHS realities challenge the positive myths of the service. They disturb what has become fantastical propaganda about 'the best service in the world'. To insist on more of the same is to set aside experience, to fail to make sense of experience, and to substitute for experience attitudes which evade the realities of the world. In particular, this harms the interests of the weak. Monocultures are not adaptive. They are dangerous. Indeed, Bob Ricketts, the Department of Health system management and new enterprise director, said in November 2007 that 'The worst of the NHS is a disgrace'.[13]

Living detail

Here are 14 recent examples of this living detail – by contrast with politicised genera-lisations – with references. Each of these underlines that consumers are not customers. They have no power. If they had economic power, how many of the following problems would be tolerated? These examples might be viewed as what ecologists call 'an indicator species'. Or messages about the underlying soil, the culture, context and disempowering realities. The list could be much longer, if space allowed. Better management by politicians seems unlikely to be sufficient for necessary change. And, as Sir Gerry Robinson showed in his enquiry into the NHS, to announce a policy is not necessarily to fix a problem.[14]

1 Despite referrals by her GP and midwife for her to see a consultant obstetrician, no appointment was made for a 22-year-old woman with a family history of brain haemorrhage, and who then died during childbirth. The need for her to receive specialist care was overlooked by midwives and doctors on up to *six* further occasions.[15]

2 Patients are being allowed to starve on NHS wards, particularly the elderly, according to Department of Health figures.[16]

3 Frail and elderly people in care homes are often mistreated or intimidated, despite very expensive government inspection and regulation.[17]

4 Hospital staff at Tameside General Hospital in Manchester were 'simply too busy' to care properly for an 11-year-old girl with suspected meningitis, a Coroner was told in January 2008.[18]

5 Children's bodies are being taken many miles from families due to a shortage of pathologists.[19]

6 Despite the NHS commitment to dignity, hospitals continue to fail to treat people with respect. Complaints to the Healthcare Commission revealed patients were left unwashed, in soiled bedding and in other humiliating conditions. In April 2008 the Commission said that the number of complaints had soared, and a growing number were upheld. There were falling nursing standards, rushed GP appointments, and failings in basic care such as clean bedding.[20]

7 One in 10 hospitals did not reach agreed standards of patient privacy and confidentiality.[21]

8 Mixed wards persist, despite promises to do away with them. Labour scrapped its manifesto pledge in 1997 – repeated in 2001. These remain a bitter source of complaints, but in an insufficiently funded system with no incentives to self-care and increasing demands NHS managers have no option but to use mixed wards to meet the volume of demand. Large 'Nightingale' wards, virtually unknown around the developed world, remain a similar concern.[22]

9 The NHS abandons many dementia patients and their families, according to the House of Commons Public Accounts Committee.[23]

10 NHS maternity care is 'crumbling', with a shortage of midwives. The sum of £828 million has been spent on settling clinical negligence claims in childbirth cases since 1995. The lives of newborn babies are at risk due to underfunded/ overstretched neo-natal units.[24]

11 The first ever survey of radiological tests showed that there were 329 cases of patients being given the wrong doses of radiation between November 2006 and December 2007. A third involved staff sending the wrong patient to be X-rayed or scanned. Others had the wrong body part scanned, or got the wrong dose of radiation, or had the wrong radioactive substance injected. The Commission said 77 NHS hospital trusts had reported no mistakes. 'This may indicate high levels of safety or a poor reporting culture.' The Health Commission said the errors highlighted 'a systems failure that has much broader implications'.[25]

12 A doctor made 'barn-door sized errors' in reading breast cancer scans, with women suffering delays in being diagnosed and receiving treatment. The errors were uncovered by colleagues who reviewed his notes. Dr William Pickering has proposed for many years now that an *independent* inspectorate should have access to all notes, and examine these on a random basis, to reveal the level of error and to encourage higher standards. This proposal has been ignored although changes in the scrutiny of medical practice still do not meet Dr Pickering's valid criticisms.[26]

13 Despite the successful investment in IT systems by individual NHS trusts and by GPs, and the enormous potential for improvements in clinical practice, on the largest scale, NHS IT is still chaotic. The project for electronic patient records is a major example. The DoH also recently missed the deadline to deliver a turnaround plan.[27]

14 Only one in 10 women with breast cancer are getting access to reconstruction surgery at the time of their treatment, despite recommendations from NICE in 2002 that this should be available to all. The entire picture of cancer care is of the greatest concern.[28]

Local managers themselves report that they have low aspirations and fear failure. According to one well-known and thoughtfully sensitive NHS manager, they were only shaken up when targets and benchmarking to improve services were introduced. 'This revealed for the first time the true extent of variation in service delivery and outcomes and provided a basis for local performance management. This would never have been attained by allowing us to establish our local targets – our low aspirations and fear of failure would have limited ambition.'[29] This is a reminder that even with a 'new localism', little will change without much intensified competition and choice.

The so-called policy of 'free choice' in elective care – being able to choose from among a list of providers – is a hint of promising possibilities. But it has not been made a priority for PCTs to implement. As the review from Reform put this:

> The current drift of policy ignores the very clear international evidence about the gains to choice and competition. Strong use of incentives and pluralism have practically eliminated waiting times in a range of developed countries including Denmark, Belgium, Spain and Australia, and have achieved as good or better outcomes and better access than in England. England has seen significant reductions in waiting but these have been bought at a huge cost. They could have been achieved much more quickly by use of competition and pluralism with a more limited and targeted increase in funding.[30]

There is another point here for politicians. Milton and Rose Friedman wisely showed in the 1980s that once elected there is only a short honeymoon enjoyed by any politician. Therefore, they advised: prepare carefully with detailed policies when in opposition, and enact them during the honeymoon before the self-protective system closes ranks again. For special interests threatened by any changes will mount noisy and costly media campaigns to prevent the removal of sinecures and privileges created by government. Mr Blair wished he had been more radical sooner. He found, like predecessors, that the moment to make radical changes is earlier rather than later. Even after six months or so in office further change is much more difficult. Counter-attacks develop against changes. Those who are affected by the changes mobilise. The typical media campaign in these circumstances is not intended to inform. It is intended to assure that the majority are not well informed.

The emphasis for an intending radical national leader then is necessarily to focus on several elements. First, get elected without frightening people, but with a purpose. Second, *have* a purpose. Third, implement quickly those detailed policies worked out carefully in opposition. The Friedmans stressed: do not wait until in government to consider the detailed actions required to implement a general policy position. Do the work now. Indeed, work with the ideas of those who have already done the work – like the Institute of Economic Affairs. Third, be aware that once in government, the reality of the 'iron triangle' of vested interests, bureaucracies and political self-interest will embrace you, too. I say more on the 'iron triangle' in a moment.[31]

Competing answers

Historically, there have been three chief answers to healthcare reform competing for our attention. First adaptive, evolutionary shifts in society set in open markets for which philosophers like Friedrich von Hayek, economists like Arthur Seldon and Ludwig von Mises and cultural critics like Michael Oakeshott, Robert Nozick and Virginia Postrel have argued.[32] Second, centralist state-run services, managed ('rationed') on our behalf and for our own good. Third, the shining vision of an allegedly predictable socialist revolution, always begun in violent upheaval and then to be followed (we are promised) by a society with no problems of production or distribution. The choice between 'real-land' and 'dream-land', or between 'day-mare' and 'night-mare'. The British post-war welfare state with its monopoly services has been an uncomfortable and always uneasy compromise between the two.

Yet in the global aftermath of failed communism the popular pressures to open up to adaptive change are considerable. These pressures raise fundamental questions for politicians about social cohesion, legitimacy, solidarity, coherence, equity, access and autonomy. All of the questions and credible answers converge on active 'choice' and self-determination. They ask us to be clear how the user of a service is to have genuinely enforceable power. The answers pivot on who has power over themselves and over others. *Especially, who has power to command the services, the time and the consideration of others.* They concern, too, how much society values the self-esteem of the individual, and how this is a key link to self-development and self-responsibility.

The institutional answers concern mutuality and self-organisation. They offer to combine individualism and collective action, not to contrast them. They stand in a long tradition of mobility, of choice, and of self-respect – rather than in a tradition of 'arithmetical equality of social status'. Indeed, as Christopher Fry says in *Venus Observed* (1950), 'Equality is a mortuary word'. Instead, we echo a tradition which would have been recognised by John Ball and Gerald Winstanley, and by William Beveridge.[33] Democratic means of accountability are important, too. But, as I suggest below, they are too limited and too generalised. They work best when the state does less, with the individual responsible for more. Crucially, occasional voting does not ensure that the individual user of services can secure a necessarily intimate, individual, separable, timely and effective service. As they seek our suffrage, politicians need to know this, even if they do not openly admit it.

Economics and democracy

We know that democracy is a limited means for such decision making. The economists Anthony Downs and Duncan Black first offered an analysis of the 'economic theory of democracy', which suggested that the self-interest of politicians prompted a market exchange between votes and benefits in the political process.[34] This viewed politicians as 'entrepreneurs', who pursue policies to attract the most votes in competition with other parties.

This theory predicts that in a two- or three-party democracy the competitors converge. They seek the centre ground, relying on the idea that those on the extreme wings of their parties have nowhere else to go. The incentive is for ambiguity in policies, to capture as wide a range of support as possible. Politicians 'buy' votes, too, and they use the taxpayers' own money with which to bribe them with policies.

The theory describes British politics very clearly since 1990. We know, too, how ineffective an individual vote can be. Elections offer voters policies on all manner of things, however vaguely expressed. One vote in the political marketplace is of small account, unless it happens to be in the swim of the majority. Most British governments are elected with minority support. And since both parties – for example, on health and social care – often offer virtually identical policies there is little or no choice on key issues. In addition, it is difficult to show that a majority vote for one party indicates decisive support for any one line in a manifesto.

As Arthur Seldon has argued, too, in political elections 'producer interests normally prevail over consumer interests. Producer interests are concentrated, they are more easily crystallized, and their beneficiaries are identifiable (they can also generally charge their costs against income tax)'.[35]

If we do not now opt to decide for ourselves in the marketplace we have no one to blame but ourselves. We cannot look to 'politics' for lifeboats. We must look to ourselves. We must encourage open and democratic markets. We must, too, accept that life is risky. As I recall David Lloyd George to have once said, 'We cannot build navies against nightmares.' But we can build lifeboats against the state.

My own Westminster conversations and professional observations as a National Commissioner persuade me that one of the great strengths of the former Secretary of State for Health, Alan Milburn, was that he fully understood these issues and sought to act upon them. The most promising developments in policy are now following on from his initiatives, especially the introduction of personal budgets in social care. The fundamental challenges which these make explicit are also helping to reveal how to increase incentives to save for the long term and how to fund the present gulf in elderly care. I address these problems in detail in later chapters.

Robert Browning wrote:

> Which was it of the links
> Snapt first, from out the chain which used to bind
> Our earth to heaven . . .?

And TH Huxley:

> It is certain that there is an immense amount of remediable misery among us; that in addition to the poverty, disease and degradation, which are the consequences of causes beyond human control, there is a vast, probably a very much larger, quantity of misery which is the result of individual ignorance, or misconduct, and of faulty social arrangements.

One of the shrewdest contemporary observers and formerly one of the most senior advisers to Mr Blair at No. 10, Geoff Mulgan, said in his important study *Good and Bad Power* that 'Governments can't help but see people as problems to be managed, and they can't help preferring passive gratitude to active scepticism.' Like him, 'I argue that the best way to understand government both within nations and globally is through the lens of service.'[36]

Geoff Mulgan also very wisely observes:

> What makes the difference? For any one of us the prospects of happiness will depend on such things as our genetic endowment, our character and relationships and where and in what circumstances we were born, as well as sheer luck. But for the larger populations of cities or nations what matters most to human happiness is not the climate or the landscape, genes or national characters but rather the quality of government in its widest sense, and the extent to which people can govern their own actions. People blessed with peace, order, equity and rights, and governed by benign rulers, stand a far better chance of living a good life, whatever their personal qualities. People living under dictators, without rights, laws or honest officials, risk misery and suffering.[37]

Conventionally, even in a benign democracy, politicians 'buy' votes. Special interests, too, have achieved extraordinary 'provider capture' in the NHS, and on a large scale. It is very striking, for example, that in May 2008 29 of the top 30 posts in the Department of Health were occupied by people who had come up through the NHS, the one exception being the Permanent Secretary. Provider capture indeed![38]

But if we hope for better services in a dynamic, evolving structure which can meet the empowered wishes of consumers, politicians must step aside and provider interests must be disciplined by the open market. Politicians should put as few obstacles as possible in the way of an evolving market – which is our only means and method by which we can solve 'the problem of knowledge'. They should, too, in the wise words of Sir Alfred Sherman, 'stop trying to bribe people with their own money'.[39]

Meanwhile, the task of radical politicians is to protect innovation, competition and the market for better care. The cry is for major reform to cultures, purchasing, provision and funding. And, as President Woodrow Wilson said, 'Freedom exists only where people take care of the government.'

Notes

1 Blair comments in July 2001: Anthony Seldon, with Peter Snowdon and Daniel Collings, *Blair Unbound* (London, Simon & Schuster, 2007), op. cit., p. 44; also especially pp. 33, 68–72, 114–16, 240–7, 298, 333. See also Alastair Campbell, *The Blair Years: extracts from the Alastair Campbell Diaries* (London, Hutchinson, 2007), edited by Alastair Campbell and Richard Stott; Andrew Rawnsley, *Servants of the People: the inside story of New Labour* (London, Hamish Hamilton, 2000; London, Penguin Books revised edition, 2001).

2 Seldon, *Blair Unbound*, ibid., p. 114.

3 Conservative Party, *The National Health Service – Delivering Our Commitment. Submission to the Shadow Cabinet Public Services Improvement Policy Group*. Published June 2007. Chaired by Stephen Dorrell MP and Baroness Perry. Document written by Dr Andrew Jones, policy adviser to Mr Dorrell. Neither Mr Cameron nor Mr Lansley has said very much about patient choice or empowerment, save in very general terms. Individual financial control has not been proposed. Nor competitive purchasing. This remains the case, even with the Green Paper, *Delivering Some of the Best Health in Europe*, op. cit., and Mr Cameron's speech to the Royal College of Surgeons, 24 June 2008. See also David Cameron, speech 'The Conservative approach to improving public services', *The Guardian* public services summit, 26 January 2007; Cameron, speech 'The NHS at 60', after visit to Trafford General Hospital, Manchester [where Aneurin Bevan launched the NHS in 1948], 2 January 2008; Andrew Lansley interview: Francis Elliott and Sam Coates, 'Tories seek to set the pace on NHS spending', *The Times*, 28 February 2008, p. 1; Francis Elliott and Sam Coates, 'We still have some way to go to win the electorate's trust, top reformer admits', *The Times*, 28 February 2008, p. 3. Jonathan Morgan AM, Welsh Assembly Member for Cardiff North and Shadow Minister for Health & Social Services in the Assembly, made a speech on 1 March 2008 in Cardiff which favoured the NHS structure but said it would be better managed in self-governance. He announced the Welsh Conservative Party Health Commission, headed by Professor John Fairclough, orthopaedic surgeon, and dominated by provider interests. See www.conservatives.com. See also Andrew Lansley speech to BMA Staff and Associates Specialists annual conference, 8 June 2006, www.andrewlansley.co.uk, and his comment 'Why is the government so afraid of choice?' on EU proposals for access in Europe for patients on waiting lists, 19 December 2007, www.conservatives.com. Hayek's *Socialism: the road to serfdom* (London, Routledge, 1944), was dedicated to 'The socialists of all parties', the planners.

Mr Cameron told his party conference on 3 October 2007 that top-down targets must be scrapped, and professionals trusted, while emphasising outcomes. 'What we have got to do is make the NHS and doctors answerable to the patients and not the politicians.' But how? Francis Elliott, '"Unscripted" Cameron delivers a textbook speech to the faithful', *The Times*, 4 October 2007, pp. 6–9. On Cameron see Kieron O'Hara, *After Blair: David Cameron and the Conservative tradition* (Thriplow, Cambridge, Icon Books, revised edition 2007). Plato, in his *Republic*, gave us due warning of politicians.

In November 2007 Mr David Cameron unveiled the Conservative Co-operative Movement. This is chaired by Jesse Norman, a Senior Fellow and formerly Executive Director of the think-tank Policy Exchange and Conservative candidate for Hereford and South Herefordshire. He is the co-author of a pamphlet on co-ops and social responsibility which urged a radical programme of change away from the centralised state and towards the individual and constitutional reform. Alas, Norman urges those old panaceas 'devolving more power from Whitehall to local government and a delocalisation of public services' without reference to individual financial empowerment. However, he says he wants new life to be breathed into cooperative organisations, and promises that he and his colleagues 'will be looking at how shared ownership can be extended into the public services, in key areas such as education, social services and the welfare system which rely so much on personal engagement and the human touch'. In February 2008 Jesse Norman said that 'We ... will be looking at schools, housing, healthcare and other public services.' We shall see. Will the Conservatives apply these ideas to healthcare and to education? Or will New Labour do so, prompted by Alan Milburn? If so, the Tories will be too late. See Jesse Norman, 'Buy into Cameron's co-op', *Sunday Times*, 11 November 2007, p. 23; Jesse Norman, Kitty Ussher MP [Economic Secretary to The Treasury] and Danny Alexander MP [Liberal Democrat Shadow Secretary of State for Work and Pensions], *From Here to Fraternity: perspectives on social responsibility* (London, CentreForum, 2007); Jesse Norman, 'Co-ops are not left-wing', *The Guardian*, 21 February 2008, p. 32; Amy Coyle, *Nuts and Bolts – Or, How to Start a Food Co-op* (Conservative Co-operative Movement, 2007); David Cameron launched this book when he spoke to the National Farmer's Union on 24 January 2008.

4 Robinson (ed.), *The Collected Works of Arthur Seldon*, 7 vols., ibid. See Philip Booth, *The Long-Term View: financing care for the elderly* (London, Politiea, 1996), and Philip Booth, *Caring for the Long Term: financing provision for the elderly* (London, Politiea, 2000). Also Tom Sorrell (ed.), *Health Care, Ethics and Insurance* (London, Routledge, 1998), with contributions by Philip Booth and Gerry Dickinson among others; P. Booth, 'The transition from social insecurity', *Economic Affairs*, 18(1), March 1998, pp. 2–12; *The Geneva Papers on Risk and Insurance* [series], at www.ideas.repec.org/s/bla/geneva.html, and The Geneva Association Information Newsletter at www.genevaassociation.org. See also E Bramley-Harker and T Booer, *Mind the Gap: sustaining improvements in the NHS beyond 2008* (London, BUPA, 2006), and Rossiter, *The Future*, ibid.

5 Paul Marshall and David Laws (eds.), *The Orange Book Reclaiming Liberalism* (London, Profile Books, 2004), especially Introduction by Paul Marshall, Chapter 1 'UK Health Services: a Liberal agenda for reform' by David Laws, Chapter 2 'Liberalism and localism' by Edward Davey, and Chapter 5, 'Liberal Economics and social justice' by Vince Cable, and Chapter 7 'UK health services: a Liberal agenda for reform and renewal' by David Laws. See also Julian Astle, David Laws, Paul Marshall and Alasdair Murray, *Britain After Blair. a Liberal agenda* (London, Profile Books, 2006), especially Chapter 6, 'Welfare reform: from dependency to opportunity' by David Laws. Also, Duncan Brack, Richard S Grayson and David Howarth (eds.), *Reinventing the State: social liberalism in the 21st century* (London, Politico's, 2007) especially Chapter 17, 'Reforming the NHS: a local and democratic voice' by Richard S Grayson; Liberal Democrats, *Empowerment, Fairness and Quality in Health Care*, ibid; Nick Clegg, speech, 'Nick Clegg on the NHS: a liberal vision for the future', 10 June 2008, to King's Fund health group; Nicholas Watt, 'Lib Dem leader warns against imposition of polyclinics', *The Guardian*, 11 June 2008, p. 17.

6 Monitor, *Guide to Implementing Service-Line Management* (2007); Bosanquet *et al.*, *NHS Reform*, op. cit., p. 52.

7 'Walker claims admissions of failure show assessment works', *Health Service Journal*, 21 June 2007, p. 7. 'Safe crackers', *Health Service Journal*, 26 July 2007, pp. 23–9.

8 EJ Hobsbawm, *On History* (London,Weidenfeld & Nicolson, 1997), pp. 37–55.

9 Helen Mooney, 'Making your mind up on the NHS's next step', *Health Service Journal*, 27 September 2007, pp. 14–15

10 Healthcare Commission, *State of Healthcare 2007: improvements and challenges in services in England and Wales* (London, Healthcare Commission, 2007); OECD, *Health At a Glance 2007: OECD indicators* (Paris, 2007); LJ Gray, N Sprigg, PMW Bath *et al.*, 'Significant variation in mortality and functional outcome after schematic stroke between Western countries: data from tinzaparin in acute ischaemic stroke trial (TAIST)', *Journal of Neurology, Neurosurgery, and Psychiatry*, 2006, 77, pp. 327–33; Hugh Markus, 'Improving the outcome of stroke' *British Medical Journal*, 25 August 2007, 335(7616), pp. 359–60; Royal College of Physicians, *National Report: clinical audit of falls and bone health in older people* (London, Royal College of Physicians, 2007); National Audit Office, *Improving Services and Support for People With Dementia* (London, NAO, 2007); Healthcare Commission, *Maternity Service Review* (London, Healthcare Commission, 2008); Confidential Enquiry Into Maternal and Child Health, Saving Mother's Lives: *Reviewing Maternal Deaths to Make Motherhood Safer 2003–2005* (London, NCE, 2007); National Audit Office, *Caring for Vulnerable Babies: the reorganisation of neonatal services in England* (London, NAO, 2007); Unicef, *Report card 7, Child Poverty in Perspective: an overview of child well-being in rich countries* (Geneva, Unicef, 2007); OECD, *Health at a Glance: OECD indicators* (Paris, OECD, 2007).

11 National Confidential Enquiry into Patient Outcome and Death, *Trauma: who cares?* (NCEPOD, London, 2007).

12 See, for example, Healthcare Commission, *Investigation into Clostridium Difficile at Maidstone and Tunbridge Wells NHS Trust* (London, Healthcare Commission, 2007); Nick Clegg, speech to *The Guardian* public services summit, 8 February 2008.

13 *Health Service Journal*, 29 November 2007.

14 Other recent reports said that heart patients are dying due to poor hospital care; hundreds of thousands of patients are seen every year without the clinician having their medical notes; that there are large numbers of unreported adverse 'patient incidents' in the NHS every year; that infection control still receives less attention than is necessary; that almost half of nurses who report serious concerns about patient safety say that the matter was ignored, covered up or not addressed by managers. 'Sorry record on patient notes', *The Times*, public agenda, 27 May 2008, p. 4; Sarah Boseley, 'Heart patients dying due to poor hospital care, says report', *The Guardian*, 4 June 2008, p. 5. On politicians announcing policies but this does not mean anything is then actually done locally, see Sir Gerry Robinson, the 'management guru', in his programmes based on Rotherham General Hospital, in South Yorkshire. *Can Gerry Robinson Fix the NHS?*, a fully funded Open University project, broadcast on BBC2 on three consecutive nights, 8–10 January 2006, and *Can Gerry Robinson Fix the NHS? One Year On*, broadcast on BBC2, 12 December 2008.

15 Lucy Cocksfoot, 'Expectant mother was third in her family to die aged 22', *Daily Telegraph*, 9 January 2008, p. 11.

16 Rosa Prince, 'Thousands of patients are being allowed to starve on NHS wards', *Daily Telegraph*, 5 January 2008, p. 10.

17 Commission for Social Care Inspection, *Rights, Risks and Restraints: an exploration into the use of restraint in the care of older people* (London, CSCI, 2007).

18 Daily Telegraph Reporter, 'Hospital staff too busy to care for meningitis baby', *Daily Telegraph*, 11 January 2008, p. 11.

19 David Rose, 'Children's bodies taken miles from families over shortage of pathologists', *The Times*, 4 January 2008, p. 11.

20 Healthcare Commission, *State of Healthcare 2007* (London, Healthcare Commission, 2007); Healthcare Commission, *Spotlight on Complaints: a report on second-stage complaints about the NHS in England* (London, Healthcare Commission, 2008); Kate Devlin, 'Number of complaints against the NHS soars: soiled bedding and rude nurses among lapses in care', *Daily Telegraph*, 7 April 2008, p. 12.

21 Healthcare Commission, *State of Healthcare 2007*, ibid.; Rebecca Smith, 'NHS patients face humiliating treatment and filthy bedding', *Daily Telegraph*, 5 December 2007, p. 5.

22 Lord Darzi, House of Lords, *Hansard*, 28 January 2008, cols. 440–1. There remain wide performance gaps between hospitals, shown in a survey of 76,000 patients at 165 NHS trusts. More than 3 million people are still being treated in mixed-sex wards. Health Commission, *National Survey of Adult Inpatients 2007* (London, Health Commission, 14 May 2008); John Carvel, 'Survey of patients shows big NHS performance gaps', *The Guardian*, 14 May 2008, p. 10; Rebecca Smith, 'Mixed-sex wards for 3m patients', *Daily Telegraph*, 14 May 2008, p. 1; Nigel Hawkes, 'The hospitals that still aren't getting a clean bill of health from patients', *The Times*, 14 May 2008, p. 31.

23 House of Commons, Public Accounts Committee, *Improving Services and Support for People with Dementia*, report 24 January 2008), HC 22; National Audit Office, *Improving Services and Support for People with Dementia*, Report by the Comptroller and Auditor General, 2006–07, HC 604, 4 July 2007; Nigel Hawkes, 'NHS abandons many dementia patients and their families', *The Times*, 24 January 2008, p. 22.

24 Evidence from a recent series of very critical reports on the NHS based on patient experiences. See Healthcare Commission, *Review of Maternity Services* (London, Healthcare Commission, January 2007); Rebecca Smith, 'Mothers failed by NHS, says watchdog', *Daily Telegraph*, 25 January 2008, p. 1. See also Sophie Borland, 'UK fertility treatment "among the least safe in Europe"', *Daily Telegraph*, 7 April 2008, p. 12; House of Commons, Public Accounts Committee, *Caring for Vulnerable Babies: the reorganisation of neo-natal services in England*, 26th report of session 2007–8, HC, 390, 17 June 2008.

25 Health Commission, *Ionising Radiation (Medical Exposure) Regulations 2000: a report on regulation activity from 1 November 2006 to 31 December 2007* (London, Health Commission, 14 March 2008). John Carvel, 'Patients put at risk by being sent for x-ray by mistake', *The Guardian*, 14 March 2008, p. 7.

26 Gary Cleland, 'Doctor told 17 women with cancer they were in good health', *Daily Telegraph*, 14 March 2008, p. 11. William G Pickering, 'An Independent Medical Inspectorate', in *Regulating Doctors* (London, Institute for the Study of Civil Society, 2000).

27 Roger Evans, 'DoH misses deadline as it fails to deliver own turnaround plan', *Health Service Journal*, 2 August 2007, p. 5; Simon Bowers, 'Fresh trouble for NHS IT system', *The Guardian*, technology section, 5 June 2008, p. 1.

28 Royal College of Surgeons of England, *Mastectomy and Breast Reconstruction: a national audit of provision and outcomes of mastectomy and breast reconstruction surgery for women in England and Wales* (London, RCS/NHS Information Centre, on behalf of Health Commission, 10 March 2008); *Improving Outcomes in Breast Cancer* (London, NICE, 2002); Franco Berrino, Roberta De Angelis and Milena Sant *et al.*, and the EUROCARE Working Group, *Survival for Eight Major Cancers and All Cancers Combined for European Adults Diagnosed 1995–1999: results of the EUROCARE-4 Study* (Paris, EUROCARE, 2007); Mike Richards, 'Eurocare Studies-4 bring new data on cancer survival', *The Lancet*, 8(9), September 2007, pp. 752–3; K Sikora, M Slevin, and N Bosanquet, *Cancer Care in the NHS* (London, Reform, 2005); N Bosanquet and K Sikora, *The Economics of Cancer Care* (Cambridge, Cambridge University Press, 2006); Michael Coleman, Delia-Martine Alexe, Tit Albrecht, and Martin McKee (eds.), *Responding to the Challenge of Cancer in Europe* (Brussels, European Observatory on Health Systems and Policies, 4 February 2008); National Audit Office, *Tackling Cancer in England: saving more lives* (London, National Audit Office, 19 March 2004) HC288; *The NHS Cancer Plan and the New NHS. providing a patient-centred service* (London, Department of Health, 2004); *Implementing the NHS Cancer Plan* (London, DoH, 8 February 2007); *Cancer Reform Strategy* (London, DoH, 3 December 2007); Professor Mike Richards [National Cancer Director], *Cancer 2012 Visions*, Open letter, 3 December 2007, at www.dh.gov.uk. See also Cancerbackup facts sheets at www.cancerbackup.org.uk. And Olivia Timbs and Karol Sikora, 'Cancer in the Year 2025', *Cancer World*, September–October 2004. This report is based on a meeting in 2003 of 50 contributors to a two-day study, of which I was one. The NHS has now developed National Service Frameworks in cancer care, coronary heart disease, paediatric intensive care, mental health, and older people's services. See also 'Does the UK really have an effective cancer plan?', Editorial, *The Lancet Oncology*, 8(9), September 2007, p. 747. There remains a regional lottery. For example, men with prostate cancer are two and a half times as likely to die in some areas as in others. Nic Fleming, 'Prostate cancer postcode lottery exposed', *Daily Telegraph*, 11 March 2008, p. 10.

29 Sophia Christie, 'On the power of targets', *Health Service Journal*, 12 July 2007, p. 12.

30 Bosanquet *et al.*, op. cit., p. 50.

31 Milton and Rose Friedman, *Tyranny of the Status Quo* (San Diego, Calif., Harcourt Brace, 1983; London, Martin Secker & Warburg, 1984; Harmondsworth, Penguin Books, revised edition 1985), pp. 43, 46.

32 F Von Hayek: The University of Chicago Press has in progress a superlative 19 vol. *Collected Edition* of Hayek's works, general editor Bruce Caldwell. The original editions of his works include *Individualism and Economic Order* (Chicago, Chicago University Press, 1948); *The Constitution of Liberty* (Chicago, Chicago University Press, 1960); *Studies in Philosophy, Politics and Economics* (London, Routledge, 1967), and *New Studies in Politics, Economics and the History of Ideas* (London, Routledge, 1978); *Law, Legislation and Liberty: a New Statement of the Liberal Principles of Justice and Political Economy* (London, Routledge & Kegan Paul, 1973–82). Arthur Seldon: Colin Robinson (ed.), *The Collected Works of Arthur Seldon* (Indianapolis, Ind., Liberty Fund, 2004–05), seven volumes. Ludwig Von Mises: *The Theory of Money and Credit* (1934); *Human Action* (1948); *Theory and History* (1957); *Epistemological Problems of Economics* (1960), and *The Ultimate Foundation of Economic Science: an essay on method* (Indianapolis, Ind., Liberty Fund, 2006), edited by Bettina Bien Greaves. Michael Oakeshott: *On Human Conduct* (Oxford, Clarendon Press, 1975); *The Politics of Faith* (New Haven, Conn., Yale University Press, 1996); *Rationalism in Politics and Other Essays*, new expanded edition, Timothy Fuller (ed.) (Indianapolis, Ind. Liberty Fund, 1990); Also, Jesse Norman (ed.), *The Achievement of Michael Oakeshott* (London, Duckworth, 1992); Paul Franco, *Michael Oakeshott: an introduction* (New Haven, Conn., Yale University Press, 2004); Stuart Isaacs, *The Politics and Philosophy of Michael Oakeshott* (London, Routledge, 2006). Website: www.michael-oakeshott-association-org; Robert Nozick: *Anarchy, State and Utopia* (Oxford, Basil Blackwell, 1974). Virginia Postrel: *The Future and Its Enemies: the growing conflict over creativity, enterprise, and progress* (New York, The Free Press, 1998), and *The Substance of Style: how the rise of aesthetic value is remaking commerce, culture, and consciousness* (New York, HarperCollins, 2003; Harper Perennial edition, 2004). Website: www.dynamist.com.

33 William Beveridge, *Voluntary Action: a report on methods of social advance* (London, George Allen & Unwin, 1948).

34 I am indebted to the discussion in Arthur Seldon and FG Pennance, *Everyman's Dictionary of Economics* (1965; revised, 1975), reprinted in *The Collected Works of Arthur Seldon*, vol. 3 (Indianapolis, Ind., Liberty Fund, 2005), pp. 173–4. Also, Anthony Downs, *An Economic Theory of Democracy* (New York, Harper & Row, 1957) and Duncan Black, *The Theory of Committees and Elections* (Cambridge, Cambridge University Press, 1958).

35 Robinson (ed.), *Collected Works of Arthur Seldon*, 7 vols, op. cit.

36 Mulgan, *Good and Bad Power*, op. cit., pp. 1–2.

37 Ibid., pp. 5–6.

38 Private information, May 2008.

39 Private conversation JS/AS at the Centre for Policy Studies, London, 1994. See also Alfred Sherman, *Paradoxes of Power: reflections on the Thatcher interlude* (Exeter, Imprint Academic, 2005).

9

Cancer and 'the efficiency myth'

'It was not the Carthaginian army which crossed the Alps: it was Hannibal.'
– HUGH ROSS WILLIAMSON

'Efficiency ... should possess a sweeping gesture – even if that gesture may at moments sweep the ornaments off the mantelpiece.'
– HAROLD NICOLSON

The 'efficiency myth' is an absolutely key issue. The NHS is *not* the best system in the world, as key OECD indicators on clinical outcomes show. No other country has ever copied it. Huge new investment has been made but productivity has not risen. Indeed, leading respected authorities suggest that it has actually declined. Productivity has fallen by 20% since 1997, according to the Prime Minister's own Strategy Unit, and the OECD. The Atkinson Review for the Office of National Statistics puts this fall at a lower level, but still at 1% per annum between 1997 and 2004. As Dr John Meadowcroft has said, 'The belief that more money will lead to better outcomes is intuitively appealing, but it ignores the political realities that face a nationalised health service where producer interests inevitably become all-pervasive. Here, in terms of productivity, efficiency and value for money, more really can mean less.'[1] Niall Dickson, Director of the King's Fund – in reviewing healthcare change – has pointed out that despite NHS reforms the system is still 'relatively inefficient, reactive without being responsive, and still too dominated by provider interests.'[2]

It is no surprise that without the stimulus of competition, innovation, productivity and service quality is static or worse. It is crucial that there is a clearer understanding of why these deeply embedded problems persist, if we are to have any chance of making major changes.

Perhaps the most glaring example of continued failure concerns cancer care. Cancer care is both a particularly urgent area for action, in terms of diagnosis, treatment and outcomes. It is an example of what the NHS has signally failed to do to achieve reliably competent patient care. It is, too, a key arena where so much more can be done, notably by proper coordination of care. Yet today – and despite the new NHS Cancer Framework and the Herculean efforts of cancer director Professor Mike Richards – Britain has some of the lowest survival rates of countries with *similar* health spending. For most cancers the UK performs less well than the European average. Many suffer unnecessary pain and many still die earlier than they need. Professor Richards recently said that patients are dying because doctors are failing to detect cancers, and that incorrect diagnosis has become 'a significant concern'. And: 'Ultimately, it can mean that the cancer has progressed to a stage where it can't be cured.'

Late diagnosis is a major reason why Britain lags behind other European countries in terms of cancer survival rates. This is partly due to failures of people to go to the doctor in time. But it is also an issue of professional competence and of the uncoordinated systems of the NHS itself. An unpublished joint study by the Department of Health and the National Patient Safety Agency found that from January 2004 to November 2006 more than 1900 patients suffered a missed or late diagnosis.[3] In addition, there are thousands of mistakes in treating cancer. In 2007 more than 500 cases were missed by doctors, according to official figures. The scale of the problem was disclosed when the NHS in England and Wales was shown to have paid out £47 million in negligence claims related to cancer since 1995. The government has a further £50 million of claims outstanding.[4]

The annual number of new diagnoses of cancer in Europe is expected to rise by 20% by 2020. The number of cancer sufferers in Britain is expected to rise from 1.3 million now to 3 million by then. Meanwhile, regional imbalances in spending and in UK care persist. Some of our survival rates are equivalent to the lowest in Europe. Cancer Partners UK in February 2008 found that there were marked differences in care across Europe leading to inequalities in survival. The UK has lower all-cancer survival rates than countries spending similar sums on healthcare. We are far less successful than the Nordic countries (which encourage choice and competition), and we do no better than some recently communist eastern European countries which spend less than a third of our UK per capita healthcare budgets.

Grin and bear it? Key aspects of this situation have long been – and remain – quite unnecessary. Had there been competition and an open market then we should have had much better performance produced by more specialisation in care. Many necessary skills are there, but they are not well organised or coordinated. Where rare cancers are dealt with by specialist care we do much better. But the poor integration of services – on which competing purchasers could *insist* – means that many common cancers are not dealt with well.[5]

Professor Karol Sikora, the leading cancer specialist, has recently said that the UK cannot afford new cancer treatments without changing funding mechanisms. New, more effective but more costly treatments are emerging. Yet ethical dilemmas remain. We cannot guarantee that a cancer sufferer will see a cancer specialist, or that they'll see a doctor who has ever seen their condition before. New cancer drugs are not available on the NHS due to their cost and to local funding policies. These include Avastin and Erbitux (for treatment of colorectal cancer), Tarceva (for lung cancer), and Herceptin (for other cancers). People are not free to pay themselves for drugs known to be effective when these are not made available because of local funding policies. New drugs which inhibit cancer growth and affect the blood vessels around cancer sites will make the issue more pressing. If individuals owned their own fund they could provide for these drugs. So, too, could MS patients seeking beta interferon, which has been denied to them on the advice of the government's own rationing body, the cumbersome and slow-moving NICE. Similarly, those 400,000 people in Britain suffering from rheumatoid arthritis – 10% of them with a severe form – who are now denied access to the drug Abatacept (Orencia) by NICE. These would negotiate with their PGCA about its provision.

Own goals

We worsen the situation quite unnecessarily by our insistence that no one should pay for cancer care which cannot be provided for everyone, even though such individual co-payments could transform many lives. These would, too, be exactly an expression of the self-responsibility we otherwise seek to endorse and engage. The case of Colette Mills, 58, the former nurse who was a patient, highlighted the issue in 2007–08 when she was denied cancer drugs for which she was prepared to pay.[6] This is culturally authorised suffering. If she had held an HSA, Colette Mills could be alive today.

So, too, Mrs Linda O'Boyle. The case of this patient has once again challenged the legitimacy of the system. Mrs O'Boyle (a retired healthcare worker from Billericay, Essex), died aged 64 in May 2008. She, too, fought for the right to top up NHS treatment with privately purchased cancer medicine that the NHS refused to provide. She was denied a drug – Cetuximab, also known as Erbitux – which offered her the chance of living at least six months longer. Instead, she paid for this with her own savings of £11,000. She was then told by Southend University Hospital NHS Trust that she could choose between continuing with the treatment for her bowel cancer available under the NHS, or opt to go privately for a different treatment regime. She could either have treatment under the NHS (to whose costs she had contributed as a taxpayer), or privately. But she could not have both in parallel. She could not continue with NHS treatment and, in addition, pay for the drug which is not routinely funded by the NHS. The campaigning group Doctors for Reform has now raised £35,000 to fund a legal challenge. Six other patients are taking legal action, too, against the NHS as their own treatment was cut off because they, too, wished to pay for life-prolonging drugs, although they denied no one else treatment by paying for these themselves. No one would be worse off since they were adding resources, not taking these away from anyone. The policy of refusal denies both the opportunity to have the drug and the rhetoric of patients having more say in their treatment. The *Daily Mail* columnist Melanie Phillips described the decision of Mr Alan Johnson, Secretary of State for Health, to refuse patients the right to pay for additional medicines as 'the equality of the graveyard, and inimical to a free society'. My PGCA model would allow the integration of tax-based funds and additional personal co-payments. These could also be tax deductible.

Meanwhile, Britain has among the worst cancer survival rates in Europe, to which this policy of denial contributes. The NHS now spends roughly the same on cancer per patient as the rest of Europe, but there are 10 new drugs 'routinely available in Boulogne but not in Brighton', as Professor Karol Sikora recently said. These new cancer drugs can make a significant contribution to extending lives, often with good quality of life. According to an ICM poll for Doctors for Reform only 7% of the public support the policy of denying NHS care to patients who choose to pay for extra drugs. In addition, 65% of people said they would pay extra towards their treatment if diagnosed with a life-threatening condition.

There is thus in progress a rapid and enormous revolution in cancer drugs. Some 20 new drugs for a range of cancers will be launched in the next two years. There is the prospect of a whole set of promising follow-ons. The really fundamental issue here is structural: how to ensure that every patient can secure modern and effective treatment. It is time that all politicians faced this. The challenge is not to avoid commenting on such a case as Mrs O'Boyle's for fear of being thought to favour the middle class which might afford treatment. It is, instead, to show how all in every class can properly secure the necessary drugs and preferred treatment. In response to the fuss about the denial of drugs Mr Cameron said he was 'minded' to support co-payments. But we need a commitment on the basis of principle.

This is my argument for health savings accounts and individual financial empowerment. The alternatives, as Professor Sikora has pointed out, are unethically to hide innovations from patients. Or to provide opportunities for patients to contribute more to costs. Or to oblige patients to go completely private, having been taxpayers all their lives. Or to allow a dangerous underground market in top-up drugs. Or to radically change financial structures, as I have proposed.[7] Present policy seeks to iron out diversity to produce a flat system. Yet Professor Baroness Finlay, President of the Royal Society of Medicine, has stressed that we already have a multi-tier system of care, different definitions of an 'episode of care' in different parts of the country, and even provision for the NHS to charge patients or insurers when people are treated initially privately but who then come into A&E through complications.[8]

American systems are often abused by British politicians. We are often warned not to be like America in healthcare, as if this was the only option or alternative to the present failing structure of the NHS. Indeed, adopting the American approach is not what is required or proposed. However, *en passant* we might note that in America there are twice as many cancer specialists available to patients and twice as many obstetricians and gynaecologists per 100,000 of population. There are, too, three times as many cardiologists. For some cancer survival rates, where in the UK only 5% of patients with stomach cancer survive for more than five years, over 40% do so in the USA. In any language this is a startling difference. And it is achieved despite intrusive interference and over-regulation by Washington and by the individual states. One of the authors of the study which gave these figures has said that the quality of care and the friendliness and responsiveness of nurses was very much better than in the NHS. Again, what we would expect in a market. Dr Richard Smith, then editor of the *British Medical Journal*, said that the study 'exploded' the myth that the NHS was 'remarkably efficient'.[9]

Cancer care – including who survives and who dies – is but one mirror of a class society. The NHS has significantly functioned as the mirror of a class society over 60 years. Inequities in access and treatment remain significantly class-based, and with major regional variation. Many of the disadvantaged in this and in other areas of care – such as the disabled, one of the most neglected and institutionalised groups – remain marginalised. The NHS has never been a universal service, nor has it made the hoped-for contribution to inequities in access or health outcomes between social groups. As Nick Edwards, Editor of the *Health Service Journal*, wrote in April 2007, 'The fact that the best hospital trust is twice as good as the worst trust in terms of its standardised mortality rate is an indictment that strikes at the core of the NHS's values and gives the lie to its first initial.'[10]

Questions: it all depends . . .

But the British love the NHS, don't they? Opinion polls in favour of the NHS but with no costs attached to decisions tell you very little. It is easy to demand more when you can pass the bills to someone else. Markets with real costs tell you what people really value. We would know much more clearly what the British public really feel about the NHS if they had financially empowered individual choices. This is *the* only true and verifiable test of success. It is also important to appreciate that the answers you get depend on the questions you frame. If people are asked, 'Do you want the NHS privatised?' you may get one kind of answer – although this is changing. If they are asked, 'Do you want billions more spent?' you get a predictable answer. It's always someone else's money. But if you ask, 'If we give you control of an individual fund, would you like to spend it with the doctor of your choice, the treatment of your choice, and the hospital of your choice? And we will give you lots of information, advice and help' you will get another kind of answer. If the individual can spend the money in a free market you get, cumulatively, the answers which test every service in the real world. Meanwhile, by 2010 annual spending by the state will have doubled since 1997, to £674 billion. Cumulative public spending since 1997 stands at £4500 billion. Mr Andrew Lansley, Conservative Shadow Secretary of State for Health, proposed to increase this spending. Yet services continue to be run on behalf of the producer, not the consumer. However, this orthodoxy seems to be challenged by recent opinion polls, which suggests that people are sceptical about the value that they get from taxation. We need to base evolutionary change not on opinion but on the surprises which the market unveils as we discover distributed knowledge and as it influences services.[11]

We know that cancer care in the UK is unsatisfactory, even despite the fact that otherwise much of the outcomes data in the NHS remains poor. But we are not entirely in the dark concerning overall NHS performance. Indeed, on the available information we rank poorly compared with most other comparable systems. It is then a surprise perhaps that the US research organisation the Commonwealth Fund has ranked the NHS the best in the English-speaking world in terms of value for money. But a cheap or 'value for money' service is not necessarily the same as a good service. It is certainly not an optimal service.[12] The healthcare press and daily media regularly cites such deficits as poor cancer care; very unpopular and widely resisted hospital closures; one in five patients leaving hospital malnourished; financially enhanced doctor and dentist contracts but continued failures in services including inadequate out-of-hours cover; lengthy hospital waiting times; inadequate public health outcomes; desperate delays for mental health patients; disabled children especially marginalised; filthy facilities despite costly management; MRSA and hospital-acquired infections/avoidable deaths; patients with hearing and balance disorders waiting *years* to be seen by an appropriate specialist; muddles in medical training and employment; enormous waste; the prevalence of mixed sex wards in contradiction to promises of change; IT failure in a system costing £12 billion to centralise data unsafely, instead of each patient holding an electronic record of their own; and so on.[13]

Is even more spending the answer?

The new funding announcement by Mr Lansley – which follows the 'fast-track' funding recommendation of Gordon Brown's former adviser Sir Derek Wanless – came on the very day when the National Audit Office reported that the new GP contract had cost the NHS £1.76 billion more than NHS management had predicted in its first three years. There had been no improvements in productivity. Incompetent DoH planning and management was blamed. GP practices were earning 58% more for 5% less work. The new consultants' contract has also led to a fall in activity, with consultants working fewer hours. Activity per consultant had reduced, according to the House of Commons Public Accounts Committee. There is also the prospect now of government closing some 5000 hospital beds as part of its reorganisation of cancer treatments.[14]

The NHS has also recruited 40,000 additional administrative staff, including 30,296 senior managers. But we do not yet have any further outcomes data to see the effect on people's health. Nor do not yet know the results of the Quality and Outcomes Framework by which GPs now target patients at risk of heart attack, strokes and other serious health consequence – although this work is an important part of the new deal. So far the measurement of productivity merely deals with volume, and not yet with outcomes. In addition, evidence obtained under the Freedom of Information Act suggested that the continuity of care which was a proud boast of the system has been seriously compromised.[15]

The public policy issue is *not* how much more to spend on the NHS, despite the increasing demands of an ageing population. It is to spend the existing budgets efficiently, to achieve better outcomes. It is also to empower the individual in command of self-responsible personal choice. It is vitally necessary to increase funding for elderly care by introducing more powerful incentives for savings. The financial base for health and social care needs to be broadened, too, rather than to rely on tax increases. A savings account model is a very attractive route.

We need *dramatic* improvements in the management, in the explicit coordination and in the diagnosis and treatment quality in British cancer care services. Who will unfold the new map?

Notes

1 Cabinet Office, *Department of Health Capability Review* (London, Cabinet Office, 2007) and the response, Department of Health, *Department of Health Development Plan: planning our future together: developing together: feeling the difference* (London, DoH, 2007). See also National Audit Office, *NHS Pay Modernisation: new contracts for general practice services in England* (London Stationery Office, 27 February 2008); Nigel Hawkes, 'Contract was a windfall for GPs but "not a good deal for patients"', *The Times*, 28 February 2008, p. 4; John Meadowcroft, 'In the NHS, more can mean less', *Economic Affairs*, 26(3), September 2006, p. 81. See also Office of National Statistics, Public Service Productivity, *Healthcare*, January 2008.

2 Niall Dickson, '1997 and all that: Blair remembered', *Health Service Journal*, 10 May 1997, p. 17.

3 Gary Cleland, 'GPs' failure to spot cancer is pushing up death rates', *Daily Telegraph*, 14 April 1008, p. 8. OECD, *Health at a Glance: OECD indicators* (Paris, OECD, 2007); *OECD Health Data 1998: a comparative analysis of 29 countries*, and *OECD Health Data 2001: a comparative analysis of 30 countries* (Paris, OECD, 2001); Cancer Research UK, *Trends in Mortality Statistics* (London, Cancer Research UK, 2007); North Ireland Cancer Registry, *Cancer Incidence and Mortality*, 2006 data, Belfast, NICR, online, accessed 2 June 2008; Welsh Cancer Intelligence and Surveillance Unit, *Cancer Incidence in Wales 2000–2004. WCISU Annual Publication No. SA6/01* (WCISU, 19 April 2006); ISD Online, *Cancer Survival (1980–2004)* (Information and Statistics Division, Scotland, 18 December 2007); Anna Dixon and Sarah Thomson, 'Choices in healthcare: the European experience', *Journal of Health Services Research and Policy*, 11(3), July 2006, pp. 167–71; David Marsland, *Welfare or Welfare State Contradictions and Dilemmas in Social Policy* (London, Macmillan Press, 1996); E Jabubowski, *Health Care Systems in the EU, A Comparative Study. European Parliament Working Paper*, SACO 101/revised. Brussels, European Parliament, 1998; World Health Organization, *World Health Report 2000* (Geneva, WHO, 2000); David G Green and Benedict Irvine, *Health Care in France and Germany: lessons for the UK* (London, Civitas, December 2001); James Gubb, *Just how well are we? A glance at trends in avoidable immortality from cancer and circulatory disease in England and Wales* (London, Civitas, 2007).

4 Sarah-Kate Templeton, 'Cancer woman runs out of time in NHS battle', *Sunday Times* news section, 27 January 2008, p. 1. See also B Jonsson and N Wilking, *A Pan-European Comparison Regarding Patient Access to Cancer Drugs* (Stockholm, Karolinska Institute and Department of Economics, Stockholm University, 2005). Janet Daley, 'Forget fair trade – only free trade can lift people out of poverty', *Daily Telegraph*, 25 February 2008, p. 20, makes important points. See also Sikora, Slevin, and Bosanquet, *Cancer Care*, ibid; N Bosanquet and K Sikora, *The Economics of Cancer*, ibid; Michael Coleman, Delia-Martine Alexe, Tit Albrecht, and Martin McKee (eds.), *Responding to the Challenge of Cancer in Europe* (Brussels, European Observatory on Health Systems and Policies, 4 February 2008); Kate Devlin, 'Thousands of mistakes in cancer treatment', *Daily Telegraph*, 11 March 2008, p. 6. Scotland's NHS clinical negligence bill in 2005–06 was £5.4 million.

5 Richard GA Feechem, NG Sekhri, KL White, 'Getting more for their dollar: a comparison of the NHS with California's Kaiser Permanente [with commentaries by J Dixon, DM Berwick, and AM Enthoven], *British Medical Journal*, 19 January 2002, 324, pp. 135–43; Chris Ham, Nick York, Steven Sutch, and Rob Shaw, 'Hospital bed utilisation in the English NHS: Kaiser Permanente and the US medicare programme', *British Medical Journal*, 29 November 2003, 327, pp. 1257–60; Jonathan Shapiro, 'Lessons for the NHS from Kaiser Permanente', *British Medical Journal*, 29 November 2003, 327, 7426, p. 1241; Richard Smith,' The NHS experiment', *British Medical Journal*, 327, 29 November 2003; Les Zeddle, 'An innovative approach to population health. Kaiser Permanente Southern California', in Herzlinger, *Consumer-Driven Health Care*, op. cit., pp. 661–8; Also Herzlinger, *Who Killed Health Care?*, op. cit., pp. 41–9. See also correspondence on Kaiser over a lengthy period at www.bmj.com.

6 'Patients forced to provide their own food', *Daily Telegraph*, letters, 18 December 2007; 'Hospitals patients provide their own food but are banned from paying for drugs', *Daily Telegraph*, Comment, 18 December 2007; Sophie Borland, 'NHS may deny care to woman over Avastin', *Daily Telegraph*, 17 December 2007; Sarah-Kate Templeton, 'Cancer woman runs out of time in NHS battle', *The Times*, 27 January 2008.

7 Sarah-Kate Templeton, 'NHS scandal: dying cancer victim was forced to pay', 'Cancer patients "betrayed" by NHS", and 'Voters call for end to ban on cancer drugs', *Sunday Times*, 1 June 2008, pp. 1, 7; Melanie Phillips, 'Labour's playing medical poker – and the stakes are patients' lives', *Daily Mail*, 2 June 2008, p. 12; Andrew Levy, 'This cancer victim had the temerity to buy her own drugs. The result: an NHS bill as she lay dying', *Daily Mail*, 2 June 2008, p. 8; Richard Alleyne, 'Cancer patient dies after NHS ends care', *Daily Telegraph*, 2 June 2008, p. 8; Karol Sikora, 'A patient must be allowed to top up their treatment', *Daily Telegraph*, 2 June 2008, p. 8; Sarah-Kate Templeton, '"We've paid into the system all our lives. Why has the NHS turned on us?"', *Sunday Times*, 8 June 2008, comment section, p. 12, and 'Doctors anger at cruelty to patients', *Sunday Times*, 8 June 2008, news section, p. 1. For an apparently contrary view see Allyson Pollock, 'Operating profits, *The Guardian*, 11 June 2008, p. 232. The authentic voice of the statist past.

8 Ilora Finlay, 'Trust me, top-up care is fair', *Sunday Times*, comment section, 8 June 2008, p. 19.

9 See references in note 1 of this chapter.

10 Nick Edwards, 'Variation in quality: the figures are standardised, but the care certainly is not', editorial, *Health Service Journal*, 26 April 2007, p. 3.

11 Philip Johnson, 'This waste of our money is just madness', *Daily Telegraph*, 17 March 2008, p. 21, commenting on John Seddon, *Systems Thinking in the Public Sector: the failure of the reform regime* (Axminster, Triarchy Press, 2008); ICM Poll, March 2008, see Rosa Prince, 'Tories mired in confusion over policy on tax cuts', *Daily Telegraph*, 17 March 2008, p. 10.

12 Karen Davis, Cathy Schoen, Stephen C Schoenbaum *et al.*, *Mirror, Mirror on the Wall: an international update on the comparative performance of American healthcare* (New York, Commonwealth Fund, May 2007). 'UK healthcare ranked best value for money', *Health Service Journal*, 24 May 2007, p. 8.

13 The Health Commission recently found that the top five overall issues in patient complaints were safety; poor communication; ineffective procedures; poor complaints handling; and dignity and respect. See www.healthcarecommission.org.uk. The NHS has a standing committee on malnutrition. See Malnutrition Study Group, *The 'Must Report': nutritional screening for adults – a multidisciplinary approach* (London, MAG, 11 November 2003).

14 See also Helen Nugent, 'Foreign GPs flown in for one in ten areas', *The Times*, 1 March 2008, p. 29.

15 National Audit Office, *NHS Pay Modernisation: new contracts for general practice services in England* (London Stationery Office, 27 February 2008); Nigel Hawkes, 'Contract was a windfall for GPs but "not a good deal for patients"', *The Times*, 28 February 2008, p. 4. This article discussed many of the complexities and reports the case put by doctors, too. DoH, *Quality and Outcomes Framework in Revised General Medical Practices Contract*, April 2004. [Wanless Report], *Securing Our Future Health: taking a long-term view. Interim Report.* (Health Trends Team, London, HM Treasury, 2001); *Securing Good Health for The Whole Population* (Health Trends Team, London, HM Treasury, 2004) Subsequently, Wanless also wrote *Securing Good Care for Older People: taking a long-term view*, commissioned and published by the King's Fund in March 2006. See also interview with John Carvel, *The Guardian*, 12 September 2007, and DoH, *On the State of Public Health, Annual Report of the Chief Medical Officer* (London, DoH, 17 July 2006). On IT see Tony Collins, 'Secret Downing Street papers reveal Tony Blair rushed NHS IT', *Computer Weekly*, 18 February 2008. House of Commons Committee of Public Accounts, *Pay Modernisation: a new contract for NHS consultants in England* (London, House of Commons, 10 October 2007) 59th report of session 2006–07, HC 506. See also Andrew Spooner, *Quality in the new GP Contract: understanding, designing, planning, achieving* (Oxford, Radcliffe Publishing, 2004). For a contrary view to the government's see Gordon Monbiot, 'Making GPs more accessible is just a disguised concession to big business', *The Guardian*, 11 March 2008, p. 37. On closure of beds, see Sarah-Kate Templeton, 'Up to 5,000 beds facing axe in cancer shake-up', *Sunday Times*, 11 May 2008, p. 8.

10

The 'choice agenda' and the problem of knowledge

'There is no absolute knowledge. Those who claim it . . . open the door to tragedy. All information is imperfect. We have to treat it with humility.'

– JACOB BRONOWSKI

'All genuine knowledge originates in direct experience.'

– MAO TSE-TUNG

'. . .the decision maker's efforts to become informed are often complicated by the fact that those who possess the relevant information have no incentive to reveal it truthfully.'

– ROBERT H FRANK

The 'choice' agenda engages us all in 'the problem of knowledge', or of how we can know what other people want and how anyone in advance can know what we want or are likely to want and be prepared to pay for. The credible answer, as Richard Rorty argued, is one where we must each reach our own conclusions about life and where we should respect the differences between us.[1]

The realisation of changes relies, too, on practical steps to address inevitable vulnerabilities and to support different kinds of authenticity. My emphasis is on authenticity defined by the user of services. On authenticity as self-expression and self-responsibility. On authenticity as identity. On authenticity as truth 'from within'.[2] And on ideas of mutuality.[3] There are many fruitful ways to cooperate which need not be imposed on us by collectivist theory. We can have collective action without collectivism.

Each of these questions asks us to consider how we understand cultural change, and how we permit it. They ask us to take a view of how and why organisations change, how they gain knowledge, how they sustain themselves, what motivates staffs, how organisations learn and innovate, what culture is and how it changes. These issues ask us to consider how organisations remain effective, how they remain competitive, and the importance of decentralised, competitive, open systems. They ask us to take a view about how entire societies evolve, and what it is that constitutes creative order.[4]

'Choice' is now being given many tasks. It is, as we have seen, the only way to gather knowledge of what services people want and will pay for – either by taxes or by other payments. It is democratic. It encourages self-responsibility. It endorses the development of the unexpected, in trial-and-error evolution. It helps remove poor attitudes, poor practice, poor outcomes. Indeed, it will make up for the many disappointments of many years of almost continuous NHS reform. Thus, we can address the long-term failures in equity, as well as other issues of efficiency, responsiveness and competence, along with the recent failures to sustain – let alone improve – productivity, despite unprecedented new investment.[5] The continuing lack of good outcomes data. The convenient (?) 'ignorance' of consumers. The deficits of information of all kinds which make it very difficult for patients to make comparisons between services and practitioners. The prevalence of vested interests which have long achieved 'provider capture'. The privileges granted by governments to the medical Royal Colleges, to trade unions such as the British Medical Association and the Royal College of Nursing, and to undemocratic quangos like the General Medical Council. The deficits are significant, and they are due to failures of the state to work properly with knowledge derived from customers.

All these interests obstruct necessary market change and open access in markets to services. They have successfully limited professional accountability. The embedded inertias in the existing culture – much of which is the direct result of powers granted by governments – have long included the very slow uptake of new technologies, of new drugs and of new procedures. These have been more successfully and rapidly introduced in open markets. Working patterns and practices of professionals have, too, long been beyond the control of local management.

A genuine 'choice agenda' can prompt much more patient control. But if – and only if – service-users control the money and express their self-knowledge. This will encourage initiative and self-responsibility. It will increase investment and the transfer of successful technologies from other areas of the economy. It will widen access, lower costs and increase offers from new providers. These changes, too, will help professionals to fulfil themselves. In this important sense choice is conciliatory. As my colleague at the think-tank Reform, Professor Bosanquet, has written,

> Clients need to have access to services within days or weeks. They deserve to have a choice of services. Health professionals will be able to build new kinds of partnership between patients and professionals. The abilities and talents of health professionals should be used to the full so patients can benefit from effective long-term programmes, which maximise support in a community setting.[6]

The proponents of 'voice' instead of empowered 'choice' do, though, continue to put their case. However, this requires the user of services to be politicised. And to be limited to 'involvement' and 'consultation'. This is the concept of the activist patient. One prominent advocate of this case is Professor Bob Sang, who opposes 'demand management thinking', as he does centralised 'protocol-driven' and 'pathway obsessed' care. He calls instead for 'Holistic commissioning of integrated service systems, building on current local government and patient and public involvement reforms.' Thus, 'A shift in the healthcare narrative, away from consumerism and tariffs, towards citizenship, stewardship and co-production . . . with patients as active, effective partners in the transformation of health and social care.'[7]

Professor Sang is right to insist that chronic sufferers are not marginal, but core to the NHS business. However, it is precisely economic power and consumer pressure and thus effective choice which can make a reality of people being able to successfully negotiate continuing and coordinated care. And so I seek to offer a critical corrective to Professor Sang's arguments against demand-management, and in favour of genuinely empowered knowledge and choice in a pluralist age. I believe that empowered choice is the means to achieve his objectives, of personal, adaptive, real controls in people's lives. The case for choice is both moral and instrumental. Economics is the science of choice. This can make a reality of 'shared decision making' with clinicians. We need to examine economic ideas. We need to address how to change cultures, too. To see how and why particular ideas are at the root of specific attitudes, including the cultural and political rejection of choice by many in the NHS and in social care. There are, alas, essential ideas which many in the NHS and in social care ignore or do not fully appreciate.

In terms of what the NHS said it was intending to achieve, to help the poor and disadvantaged, the fragile and helpless, we need to rediscover how those who are not by any means the greatest beneficiaries of any economic system – those accommodated in 'steerage' – can be given *personal* power to get the things they want. And thus to ensure that they have an equal claim on the resources which the wider risk taking and dynamic economy generates for health and social care spending.

This asks us to acknowledge that power and knowledge is dynamic. It is not easily removed from society, not even by the temporary power of centralised terror. We have to do what we can to distribute it without undermining dynamism and while recognising that it will always creatively prompt new possibilities to which we again have to readjust, until the next time.

The arguments emphasise that we need a well-rewarded, welcoming and committed workforce. We and they need, too, a changed cultural ethos which gives permission for local initiatives and welcomes them. We need a structure which is responsive to individual consumers. One which welcomes enterprise and innovation. One which pivots on pluralism and choice as the keys in the doors. These approaches can finally achieve justice in access, and a new balance between the individual and the state. This cannot be achieved by centralised controls or by even more expenditure.

Personal budgets demonstrate what can be achieved, and by which means. Even so – and despite their success – government still seeks other ways to achieve necessary reforms, and without the full realisation of the lessons of its own actions. It still fails the test of the problem of knowledge. But, it seems, sometimes almost any method will do, provided it does not give people control over money. Thus in March 2008 Hazel Blears MP, the Communities Secretary, unveiled proposals for a white paper on 'empowerment'. This is promising to extend community rights to information, accountability and sometimes redress from a gamut of public services, including neighbourhood policing and PCTs. 'Ministers are also looking at the idea of extending the concept of community kitties by giving local areas, potentially the size of three council wards, access to £1m annual budgets to spend on priorities selected by local bodies.' Money to be an incentive to action – yes. But *on priorities selected by local bodies?* We have seen that this cannot deliver a personal, timely, intimate service to an individual. If this is what we want, we should follow the concept of the money working by creating health savings accounts and patient guaranteed care associations. Why take the tortuous, cumbersome, costly, bureaucratic quango-ised local government route, when the market will do it better, and which bureaucracies cannot do at all?[8]

We need to distinguish clearly between the objectives of good health and social care and the means and policies chosen to achieve these. As we do, too, between the ideologies or theories by which both the objectives and the means have been and are to be justified. Especially, if we are to move the stone.

Notes

1 Richard Rorty, *Philosophy and the Mirror of Nature* (Princeton, Princeton University Press, 1979); *Contingency, Irony and Solidarity* (Cambridge, Cambridge University Press, 1989); *Objectivity, Relativism and Truth: philosophical papers* (Cambridge, Cambridge University Press, 2001). For a recent American perspective on planning and the problem of knowledge see Randal O'Toole, 'Why government planning always fails', *Cato Newsletter*, The Cato Institute Washington, DC, 6(1), Winter 2008, pp. 1–5, and O'Toole's *The Best-Laid Plans: how government planning harms your life, your pocket-book and your future* (Washington, DC, Cato Institute, 2007). It was planners, too, who destroyed Britain's steam railway heritage and much of our best Victorian architecture.

2 A fascinating and difficult concept. See discussion in Virginia Postrel, *The Substance of Style: how the rise of aesthetic value is remaking commerce, culture, and consciousness* (New York, HarperCollins, 2003; Harper Perennial edition, 2004), pp. 110–17.

3 See Mount, op. cit. Also, my discussion of social enterprises, and the limits on empowerment in my chapter 'Only half way to paradise? Social enterprise initiatives: the opportunity, the challenge, and the deficits of individual empowerment', in my book *'Coming, Ready or Not'*, op. cit.

4 See the valuable modern discussion in Postrel, *The Future and Its Enemies*, op. cit.

5 National Audit Office, *NHS Pay Modernisation: new contracts for general practice services in England* (London Stationery Office, 27 February 2008); Nigel Hawkes, 'Contract was a windfall for GPs but "not a good deal for patients"', *The Times*, 28 February 2008, p. 4.

6 Nicholas Bosanquet, *A Healthy Future for Scotland* (Edinburgh Policy Institute, 2003), p. 9.

7 Bob Sang, 'Don't let's forget, we're in it for the long-term', *British Journal of Healthcare Management*, 2007, 13(4), pp. 122–5 and 13(5), pp. 160–1.

8 Hazel Blears, speech 'Putting communities in control', to regeneration conference, London, 5 March 2008; 'Unlocking the talents of our communities – an overview', www.communities.gov.uk. Also, Patrick Wintour, 'Blears wants police, NHS and councils more locally accountable', *The Guardian*, 5 March 2008, p. 5.

11

'When the axe came into the forest . . .'

'In the Carboniferous Epoch we were promised
abundance for all
By robbing selected Peter to pay for collective Paul . . .
And that after this is accomplished,
and the brave new world begins
When all men are paid for existing,
and no man pays for his sins.'

– RUDYARD KIPLING

'The pragmatist knows that doubt is an art which has
to be acquired with difficulty.'

– CHARLES SANDERS PIERCE

As the old Turkish proverb has it, 'When the axe came into the Forest, the trees said "The handle is one of us".' But are the NHS reforms really 'ours'? Can we 'be the change', as Mahatma Gandhi urged? My concern is with *enabling*, not imposing, change. And with how a successful transition to an improved structure of health and social care can evolve in a free society.

I have stressed the necessity of moving to a structure of individual financial empowerment, and then of *competing* purchasers. This would come about through passing individual control of funds to individual customers, who then choose with which purchasing body to spend their funds. We hear much of the necessity of pluralism in supply. But many in the NHS reject the idea that health service-users should even be conceived as customers at all. Even when they seem to accept the possible yields of some market mechanisms they reject the necessary context and culture. Yet it is pluralism in purchasing led by customer decisions about who should spend their money for them which is the essential lever of change. Then alternative offers by providers can be considered in the market, and endorsed or rejected by customers and their purchasing bodies. Innovation, new experiments, new technologies can then be adopted by purchasers on behalf of their willing members and by prospective providers who want to stay in business. It is the free market which has delivered most improvements in healthcare, and the NHS which has obstructed change. Professor Nicholas Bosanquet and Dr Jim Attridge remind us that cataract surgery was developed against strong professional opposition, and that the NHS has been very slow to adopt improvements. It opposed the early hospices, and was laggardly in using hip replacement surgery which was much more used in the USA. There is evidence of persistent differences of diffusion rates for medicines between countries, slow UK take-up and avoidable failures in equity. We are very late adopters, even of our own inventions. We need much more push, and pull. This approach would be a genuine test of a market society. Its results would be a welcome corrective to the typical bias against market society on which much NHS and much associated British University writing or 'commentary' is founded. Too many British University commentators make a living by staying one raindrop ahead of the current wave and describing the weather. Here Professor Bosanquet and Dr Attridge are among the happy exceptions.[1]

Do we mean it?

The adoption of bold change would show that we mean it. This is a vital cultural point in all this, if we are to expect the staff in health and social care to truly commit themselves to change. Especially when so many have been through the reform mill several times before, and with results that have hardly impressed many. NHS reforms are like buses. There is the widespread idea that you do not really need to change. Of reforms people say, 'There will be another one along in a minute.' The move to individual financial empowerment and to a new structure of competing purchasers would be the clearest possible statement that *we mean it*. That change is not an illusion. That it is not to be one step forward, and two quick steps back. That the stone will be moved. That we will not allow it to roll back upon us. That new purchasers and new providers will be an unavailing feature of developing markets to improve British health and social care. That vested interests will not be allowed to derail the train. That regulation itself will be light, inexpensive and focus on protecting competition so as to armour the consumer rather than the producer. That this will lower prices, too.

Here we need to be grown up about profit or operating surpluses. For without these, no new purchaser or provider will invest. There will be no service differentiation in existing or new locations. No consumer-led improvement will come about. Those who really know how to serve the customer will not come into the services. Without convincing people of the certainty of change and the predicted results we will not be able to reach out to the continuous innovation which can create customer-value, and which will be shared between all service-users. Innovation, too, will inevitably prompt imitation, and thus new experiments, further recombinations, and more new innovation. If we truly want this we have to be persuasive about the conditions for its success and permit the risks.

Priced services are an important element in any possible transition which can then be politically irreversible because it will produce results which people will insist on retaining. What is hidden must be revealed. The patient and the payer must become one. This must be so, even though inevitably but helpfully payers will come together voluntarily in mutual, cooperative purchasing bodies. Then the financially empowered individual will choose between priced alternatives. These will be alternatives offered both by purchasing bodies – 'Join us!' – and providers. Then the benefits will be many – including a decline in administrative costs associated with accompanying state bureaucracies. These costs, indeed, are invariably excessive when compared with the competing costs of private provision. There is also enormous and well documented public-sector waste.[2]

Incentives are critical: incentives to save, to prepare for the future and to be self-responsible. These appreciably increase personal freedom and choice. They enhance justice and social contentment. They increase the dignity of the users of services. The equal right of every individual can truly be expressed only with individual control over the necessary funds. The argument is that markets work in the public and the private interest. They enable people to build choice and spontaneity into their lives. They allow an expansive view of opportunity. And an equality of decisions about personally and often diversely preferred outcomes. Always provided, that is, that the individual is financially empowered by a health savings account. Emphasis: essential here is economic power.[3] Emphasis: beware diversionary tactics to evade these truths. Emphasis: beware mistaking what we are told we must have for what we need to discover for ourselves, in our own authentic experience. Beware mistaking what *is* for what our own subjective experience tells us is truly authentic, and which differs from the official account. Beware the risk of misleading ourselves that what we now have is 'inevitable' and serves us best. Recall, too, that the opportunity costs of failing state services has been the services which could have evolved under free if regulated markets. History exposes untaken roads, and the opportunity costs, the lost achievement and the other realisations denied by the introduction of the NHS.

'When I speak of cultures . . .'

Structural changes are essential to cultural change. And so we need to consider cultures carefully. The content of 'culture' is neatly summarised by Sir Douglas Hague (formerly Chairman of the Economic and Social Research Council):

> . . . when I speak of cultures, I mean nothing more sophisticated than those sets of beliefs and behaviours, aspirations, expectations, values, senses of duty and right, those ways of evaluating what is prudent and legitimate and so forth, that inform the decisions of politicians, bureaucrats, organisations, the users of services or the public at large.[4]

Stewart Brand, in *How Buildings Learn*, offers a parallel analysis. Buildings contain six nested systems: Site, Structure (the foundation and load-bearing elements), Skin (the exterior), Services (wiring, plumbing, heating, etc.), Space (plan; the layout), and Stuff. As he says, 'the lethargic slow parts are in charge, not the dazzling rapid ones. Site dominates Structure, which dominates the Skin, which dominates the Services, which dominate the Space plan, which dominates the Stuff. . . . The quick processes provide originality and challenge, the slow provide continuity and constraint.'[5] We need to sort out what is Site and what is Stuff. We need to ensure that a well-designed structure is adaptable, and respects the different speeds and functions of these nested layers, allowing evolutionary change without disrupting the necessarily permanent systems – the plumbing and the load-bearing beams.

The possible advance of healthcare especially concerns how to encourage a willing acceptance of many roles being redefined. I say more on this in my final chapter, 'How many fingers make five?' It asks for sometimes painful processes of adjustment, among staff whose perceptions of themselves and of the public often encourage them to resist change. It focuses particularly on those economic instruments which can be persuasive. It does so from an awareness that other incentives and persuasions have been much less effective. Reform is particularly concerned with practical steps to effect favourable and irresistible democratic change. It emphasises social solidarity and coherence, equity of access and good outcomes. It outlines the social and economic approaches which do most to ensure these. It seeks to empower the individual to decide about them for themselves. It appeals particularly to the legitimacy of British feelings of fairness.

This surely means equal access to the use of care services. It does not mean an imposed 'equality' of outcomes, which is impossible to achieve. But it should not mean levelling down. Or all joining hands together to cross the finishing line joint last but together. Indeed, it is divergence and not convergence which creates new opportunities for all. 'Fairness', too, should be about equal opportunities for self-responsibility and self-determination in a vibrant and free economy, where, inevitably, too, there will be disparities of wealth which reflect many factors including the different energies and abilities of us all. 'Fairness' means the justice and basic decency of equity or equal access among people who are otherwise inevitably unequal in their genes, parentage, talents, opportunities and efforts in life. It does not, however, require an imposed politicised equality.

This does not mean we cannot seek a structure which properly serves the poor as well as the better-off. Indeed, the opposite is the case. This again emphasises the power of positive incentives to encourage people out of poverty and to help those who remain disadvantaged through no fault of their own. Incentives have a key role in enabling choice, achieving stable funding, promoting fruitful investment, generating savings, preferring pluralism in provision, and both improving and endorsing good professional performance. Such a structure needs to recognise, too, that life *is* risk. And that we should accept the responsibility for our own actions.

This contrasts these endeavours with those luminous, synoptic visions and transcendent answers where experts know our interests best; indeed, claim to know our interests better than we know them themselves. This aspect engages us all in 'the problem of knowledge'.[6] The realisation of changes relies on practical steps to address inevitable vulnerabilities and to support different kinds of authenticity. On authenticity as identity. On authenticity as truth 'from within'.[7] There are many fruitful ways to cooperate but which are not imposed by theory.

When all these fundamentals are addressed by real markets the results for staff as well as for consumers can be positive, although obviously there will be some losses of privileged controls. There can, however, be more flexibility at work for many staff, freedom from politicised supervision, and a stimulating and creative environment. This can include the immediate satisfaction of knowing that you have satisfied the customer's wishes, and the prestige which that will bring. The 'naturalisation' of choice can, indeed, transform the theories and practices of public sector management, for the benefit both of staff and consumers. It can so transform the allocation of resources that the poor will no longer receive much less attention and much less spending on their care than the middle classes within the state system. Financially empowered choice can quite literally re-make organisations in ways which other reforms have failed to achieve. It will certainly do so on the big issues: with regard to behaviour and relationships, policy making, resource allocation, consumption, planning, organisation, investment and management. And, most notably, with regard to culture in which the privileges granted by government to professionals, coercive local controls and central targets will be replaced by the cumulative decisions of consumers in the ever-evolving market. The structure will be reorganised in favour of the consumer. A vital issue, too, is whether clinicians will be allies for change. I argue that a rapprochement between clinicians and markets has many values, not least to them. Adaptive professionals will surely prefer to answer to informed patients and their local purchasers, rather than to more distant bureaucracies or to Whitehall. They will surely wish to collaborate more closely with cost-conscious, more risk-aware patients, and their skilled advisers. The necessity of cultural change is not merely decorative. Here, local permission to effect change is crucial. We need to open many closed doors, and to see what lies behind them. For example, every doctor knows (if I may say this, without offending) to whom they would not send their daughter. They know the identity of 'Dr Up-to-date' and of 'Dr Deadwood'. This is, however, not public information. Nor have doctors been rewarded for what happens to their patients, or on the basis of outcomes. But, after all, doctors striving for good outcomes came in good part into medicine, and underwent its onerous training, to tailor their skills for best care to the specific individual. They should and could be rewarded for best care. Similarly, we – and they– should know who is the best at what they do. In the US a firm called Best Doctors has built up a database on US and international physicians which helps here. This informs customers, and encourages proper rewards. The 'best doctors' are those which have been selected by their peers. This move gives credibility and authority to the project. The firm uses this detailed material, and supplements it by surveys. The project helps the 'outsider' identify the right doctor for a particular health problem. The US Department of Health and Human Services has, too, launched a pilot project to provide physicians with incentives to use health IT. They are investing $50 million immediately. The two largest Massachusetts health insurers – Tufts Health Plan System, and Harvard Pilgrim Health Care – recently expanded their use of physician ranking systems and tied these more closely to co-payment discounts. This despite clinical opposition. Those members who seek care from top-rated or top-tiered physicians have lower co-payments.

It is important, too, that customers hold a full electronic record of their history. This will benefit care and also enhance their potential to move to another purchaser if they so wish. In the US, Kaiser Permanente and Microsoft in June 2008 launched a personal health records pilot of this kind. These initiatives are intended to help customers make informed decisions and to help clinicians to benefit both from peer review and from market choices being more effective. We need such initiatives in the UK, with medical technology personalised in this way.[8]

There are questions of decision making of two kinds. The first concerns enabling individuals to ask which service do I want and can or will pay for, either by a health savings account or by optional insurance and cash top-ups. The second concerns the issue of those services for which government must make *strategic decisions* and which the market will not necessarily make if left entirely free and open. This question asks us to consider situations where the cumulative consequences of policy must be considered, and which for various reasons markets may not produce an entirely satisfactory answer. The outstanding example in healthcare is thought to concern A&E services which have been thought to be beyond the reach of competitive provision. Here we need to consider how local A&E management can be contestable. As we know, market failures are self-correcting. Government failures are much harder to influence. Yet A&E – where, in 2007, waiting times rose *again* by more than half – is another significant local monopoly where we require real levers for improvements.[9]

Ignorance of information

But consumers are ignorant, aren't they? It is no accident that information is poor. It has been a requirement of a rationed system which, in the words of Professor Nicholas Bosanquet and Stephen Pollard, 'has universalised the inadequate'.[10] Clearly, poor information hinders the test of predictability, of the user being able to find out about the likely effects of the service in advance. This matters even if we accept the distinction between 'search goods' (which can be tested before purchase, like cars) and 'experience goods' (such as holidays, or medical treatments, on which a judgement about satisfaction is often necessarily retrospective, but which can be guided by the experiences of others if fully reported. For we do want to know what happened to other patients 'like me'. And which doctors did best; who does the procedure most often; what do other patients say about their experiences and results; who lived and who died; who lived on well, who is still in chronic pain? Why? Here, fortunately, many user groups are expert patients who have gathered much valuable information on experiences, performance and outcomes. For example, those with long-term, chronic illnesses offer much information to one another about treatments, outcomes, risks and benefits. They have developed detailed knowledge which they can use to consider alternatives, challenge medical judgements, choose interventions which they know from experience produced effective outcomes, at least for them. We then have to try to make relevant comparisons for ourselves. User groups also help people to form good and informed mutually constructive relationships with providers. Such mutual negotiations will be more balanced and more fruitful if the user of a service is informed in these complex and shifting processes.

A special issue of *Economic Affairs* was concerned with pharmaceuticals and government policy. This recently demonstrated that restrictions in information and services contradict the rhetoric of the NHS about access and equality. Indeed, the denial of information is an integral part of the rationing process. It remains a persistent feature.[11] In addition, there is a concern about special interests including user groups. When government confers benefits on a special interest, the recipients are a relatively small group in society. They are better informed. But since the costs of such benefits are spread widely, thinly, and over the population as a whole, one result is that a few have a powerful incentive to lobby intensively, but the many usually do not bother to inform themselves about it, or to take any actions. This is, curiously, one of the reasons for consumer ignorance in public services, for which the consumer is usually falsely blamed.

The 'iron triangle'

We should remind ourselves of the 'iron triangle' which Milton and Rose Friedman enunciated. Government, vested interests and the bureaucracy would recognise the handle and the axe as the blunted partners which they too often are. For these special interests form the iron triangle in which politicians, vested interests and bureaucracies run things together and in their own interests even when proclaiming the general interest. They have the longest tenures, too, and outlast prime ministers. As the Friedmans have argued, good people with intentions are not sufficient. And governmental employees, no less than those of private businesses, will put their own interests above the interests of others. 'Calling them public servants does not alter that fact.'[12]

There is a fundamental issue here about economics, politics, and how democracies actually work. This concerns what the Friedmans called 'the tyranny of the status quo'. It is also an important element in the relative ignorance of consumers about choices. As the Friedmans put it,

> Any measure that affects a *concentrated* group significantly – either favourably or unfavourably – tends to have effects on individual members of that group that are substantial, occur promptly, and are highly visible. The effects of the same measure on the individual members of a *diffused* group – again whether favourable or unfavourable – tend to be trivial, longer delayed, and less visible. Quick, concentrated reaction is the major source of the strength of special interest groups in a democracy – or for that matter any other kind of government. It motivates politicians to make grandiose

promises to such special interests before an election – and to postpone any measures adversely affecting special interest groups until after an election.[13]

In the British context, such interests include such trade unions as the British Medical Society, the Royal College of Nurses, and Unison in healthcare, the various teaching unions in education, and so on. These commonly seek to show the immediate and direct effects of any proposed changes, which they show as visibly disruptive. Those seeking changes have to argue for longer term and often delayed benefits. It is the contrast between the dramatic and the gradual. And between a balance of costs and benefits which special interests usually express as 'the general interest' but which usually mainly concerns a special interest of their own. These are usually presented as 'the national interest'.

When government confers benefits on a special interest, the recipients are a relatively small group in society. But the costs are spread widely, thinly and over the population as a whole. One result is that a few have a powerful incentive to lobby intensively, but the many usually do not bother to inform themselves about it, or to take any actions. As the Friedmans say, 'When we are among the few to benefit, it pays us to keep track of the vote. When we are among the many who bear the cost, it does not pay us even to read about it.'[14] This is one of the chief reasons for consumer ignorance in public services, for which the consumer is usually falsely blamed. The problem is worsened, too, by recent developments in the nature of the political class, and the professionalisation of politics, which Peter Oborne has vigorously analysed. Here there is further convergence against the interests of the wider public.[15]

Protecting competition

Government meanwhile will not vanish, but its role should be limited to protecting competition so that markets protect consumers. Government should verify standards and deal with a limited number of externalities (such as clean water). The relationships between government and markets are complementary. Every market is embedded in social structures and networks, including regulation. But the balance should not be such that government overwhelms the creative forces.

Competition innovates, teaches, experiments and improves. It evolves, as we did biologically, by trial and error, in a complex, responsive, experimental process of change. It has solved many manufacturing problems, lowered costs, made goods and services widely available to an unpredicted extent, offered multiple improvements, and given better lives, pleasure and fulfilment to billions. It has liberated people from politics and in their personalities and personal lives. In the wider economy competition has improved productivity and pushed quality so high and prices so low that many manufacturers have to find ways to distinguish themselves besides price and perform ance. Thus, they emphasise aesthetic qualities and appeals to taste. The characteristic of mass markets is now mass customisation to support as many different personal styles as possible, as the cultural critic Virginia Postrel shows in detail in *The Substance of Style: how the rise of aesthetic value is remaking commerce, culture, and consciousness.*[16]

As Postrel makes clear, this is not merely a business strategy. It is a major ideological shift. In the modern economy we have enjoyed the benefits of standardisation, convenience, mass distribution, predictable minimum quality and also personalisation. They are not mutually exclusive. But what has happened in 'public services', sheltered from competition, busy in their rigid, mandatory 'services', overseen by hierarchies which are out of the reach of the market? Businesses which have to seek willing revenues and welcome clients focus on comfort, friendliness and reassurance. 'Services' which wait for money to fall from above, in politically managed bundles, and whose 'clients' have no choices, are very different. They represent an elite imprimatur which is averse to personalised services. 'Radical' sociologists study 'material culture', but from a Marxist perspective. They do not appreciate sufficiently that it is 'material culture which makes culture material' – that the expressions of lifestyle are more than mere reflections. They are in some cases its substance. And in all cases they give it substance.[17]

The NHS is still systematically disconnected from the modern world where competition has driven up standards, reduced costs, enlarged expectations, believed in demand and enhanced choice so that all our lives have changed for the better. What was once extraordinary is now ordinary. What was once reserved for the rich is now enjoyed by the poor. What was once only for the middle class is now class-less. What was once beyond the reach of any working person's dreams is now the conventional reality, and unnoticed as it is so ordinary. There are five fundamentals in our life: sex (for pleasure and reproduction), food, shelter, healthcare, and education. Yet the last two remain exempt from all the improving forces which have changed everything else. This makes no sense. It is literally *none* sense.

It is only real competition which can entirely change the daily operational necessities. Only this can really bring 'public services' to the tipping point, where a different perspective offers 'critical mass' for change. In the wider economy it prompts managers to think many things creatively and consciously: 'The sky's the limit.' 'Dream your dreams.' 'We do it because our customers demand it.' 'People *like* that.' 'Let's make it special.' 'Every working day *is* special.' 'Everything here is the best of its class'. 'We do it as well as anyone anywhere in the world.'

Hand on heart, how many of us have *ever* heard *anyone* in *any* public services *ever* say *any* such things?

Notes

1 But Ruth McDonald, Sudeh Cheraghi-sohi, Peter Bower, Diane Whalley and Martin Roland, 'Governing the ethical consumer: identity, choice and the primary care medical encounter', *Sociology of Health and Illness*, April 2007, 29(3), pp. 430–56 make the case for the relevance of the concept in improving our understanding of the ways in which individuals manage their health and service use. See also Nicholas Bosanquet, 'The long-term economic gain from new models of healthcare provision: the opportunities for pharmaceutical companies', *Economic Affairs*, 26(3), September 2006, pp. 10–16. See Jim Attridge, 'Equity of access to innovative medicines: mission impossible?', *Economic Affairs*, 26(3), September 2006, pp. 17–23.

2 See, for example, National Audit Office, *Prescribing Costs in Primary Care* (London, Stationery Office, 18 May 2007), HC 454 2006–2007.

3 I rely on the arguments of Ludwig von Mises, Arthur Seldon and others, cited elsewhere. The statistician Carol Propper and colleagues have sceptically reviewed several interlocking aspects of current choice policy including competition between hospitals, responsiveness of patients to greater choice, provision of information, and fixed prices, and the impact of competition on improved outcomes. Carol Propper, Deborah Wilson, and Simon Burgess, 'Extending choice in English healthcare: the implications of the economic evidence', *Journal of Social Policy*, 35(4), October 2006, pp. 537–57. See also Simon Burgess, Carol Propper and Deborah Wilson, *Will More Choice Improve Outcomes in Education and Health Care? The evidence from economic research* (Bristol, Centre for Market and Public Organisation, University of Bristol, 2005); Carol Propper and Katherine Green, 'A larger role for the private sector in financing UK healthcare: the arguments and the evidence', *Journal of Social Policy*, 30(4), October 2001, pp. 685–704.

4 Douglas Hague, 'Transforming the dinosaurs', in Geoff Mulgan (ed.), *Life After Politics: new thinking for the twenty-first century* (London, Fontana Press, 1997), note 1, p. 424. Hague's study originally published as *Transforming the Dinosaurs: how organisations learn* (London, Demos, 26 July 1993).

5 Stewart Brand, *How Buildings Learn: what happens after they're built* (New York, Penguin Books, 1994), pp. 12–23. I owe the reference to Postrel, *Substance*, op. cit., p. 154. See also the works of economist Jane Jacobs on the necessity of trial-and-error adaptation as the only democratic basis for future improvements. Jane Jacobs,

Cities and the Wealth of Nations (1984; Harmondsworth, Penguin Books, 1986); *The Death and Life of Great American Cities* (1961; New York, Random House, 2002); *The Economy of Cities* (New York, Random House, 1969).

6 Richard Rorty, *Philosophy and the Mirror of Nature* (Princeton, Princeton University Press, 1979); *Contingency, Irony and Solidarity* (Cambridge, Cambridge University Press, 1989); *Objectivity, Relativism and Truth: philosophical papers* (Cambridge, Cambridge University Press, 2001).

7 Virginia Postrel, *The Substance of Style: how the rise of aesthetic value is remaking commerce, culture, and consciousness* (New York, HarperCollins, 2003; Harper Perennial edition, 2004), pp. 108–9.

8 There are, of course, many good doctors – although we do not have the information we need to know quite who is who. However, consider the dramatic and very public case of the highly skilled international footballer, Eduardo da Silva of The Arsenal – who suffered a compound fibula fracture to his left leg and a dislocated ankle with medial ligament damage in February 2008 when brutally mis-tackled in the away game at Birmingham City. The quick thinking and the medical skills of The Arsenal medical staff, the long-serving Arsenal and England physiotherapist Gary Lewin, and the doctors at Selly Oak Hospital saved his leg and his career and livelihood. They deserve our admiration and gratitude. Birmingham City was relegated at the end of the season. Quite right. Martin Samuel, 'The tackle that broke a leg and divided a nation', *The Times*, 28 February 2008, pp. 92–3, and Tom Dart, 'Arsenal staff credited for quick action with Eduardo', *The Times*, 28 February 2008, p. 92. On US information, Steven W Naifeh, and Gregory White Smith, 'Providing the most wanted information when most needed: best doctors', in Herzlinger, *Consumer-Driven Health Care*, ibid., pp. 458–66; www.news-medical.net, 11 June 2008, and www.kaisernetwork.org.

9 'A&E waiting times rise by 52 per cent', *Daily Telegraph*, 16 February 2008, p. 1. See www.dh.gov.uk for figures published on 15 February 2008.

10 Nicholas Bosanquet and Stephen Pollard, *Ready for Treatment: popular expectations and the future of health care* (London, Social Market Foundation, 1997), p. 1.

11 Jim Attridge, 'Equity of access to innovative medicines: mission impossible?', *Economic Affairs*, 26(3), September 2006, p. 21. Mike Dent, 'Patient choice and medicine in healthcare: responsibilization, governance and proto-professionalisation', *Public Management Review*, 8(2), June 2006, pp. 273–96 offers – despite its dreadfully ugly jargonised title – a useful review of some changing processes.

12 Milton and Rose Friedman, *Tyranny of the Status Quo* (San Diego, Calif., Harcourt Brace, 1983; London, Martin Secker & Warburg, 1984; Harmondsworth, Penguin Books, revised edition 1985), pp. 43, 46.

13 M and R Friedman, *Status Quo*, ibid., pp. 14–15.

14 Ibid., p. 56.

15 Peter Oborne, *The Triumph of the Political Class* (London, Simon & Schuster, 2007). See also Anthony Sampson, *Who Runs This Place? The anatomy of Britain in the 21st century* (London, John Murray, 2005).

16 Postrel, *Substance*, op. cit., p. 108, passim; Grant McCracken, in *Plenitude*, 2.0, beta version, at www.cultureby.com, p. 26, cited in Postrel, *Substance of Style*, op. cit., p. 31. See also Postrel, *The Future*, op. cit.

17 The ideas, too, reflect a mistaken Marxist idea that producers simply manipulate consumers and decree what they will buy. Managers who read novels and consider aesthetics, who imagine new services, who believe in the empowered consumer have not much flourished in the NHS. The man who should have been appointed to succeed Sir Duncan Nicoll in the 1990s was Chris West (then Chief Executive of the Portsmouth Hospitals Trust). He was an outstanding, cultured and patient-focused NHS manager, but he died too young. There were many others with imagination in the 'third-in-line mafia' – in the main, women – but they were not valued in the culture, and few played golf.

12

Will 'a new localism' answer?

> 'The English think they are free but they are quite wrong; they are only free when
> parliamentary elections come round; once the members have been elected they are
> slaves and things of naught.'
>
> – JEAN JACQUES ROUSSEAU

> 'The people who have been running the system are not bad people; they are usually
> very good people. But it's a bit like male drivers – you can head down that road,
> won't take directions, and won't turn back admitting you have gone down the
> wrong road.'
>
> – STEPHEN DUFFY

The chief alternative offered to direct control over money by the users of services is
'the new localism'. Will it answer?

The Liberal Democrat Edward Davey MP has written with delicious understatement
that 'the public's experience of local government is not uniquely positive'.[1]

Direct elections may strengthen local government, including the election of local
mayors. But they will not secure a specific service for a particular individual. Localism
is not local enough. In addition, most of those lower-income people who the NHS was
intended to help most take no part in democratic processes. One in three low-income
voters do not vote; do not urge others to vote; do not present their views to local coun-
cillors; do not join pressure groups; do not write to MPs or to the media, and do not
take any part in political campaigns.[2]

Elections, too, see politicians devising offers to maximise votes, but voters cannot
express themselves by voting in such a way as to be sure of a personal and individual
timely service. Nor is the evidence from voting in national or local elections a good
guide to attitudes to specific issues, since elections are determined by a variety of
pressures and issues. Participation, too, is slipping. General election turnout has
fallen from 77.7% in 1992 (in what was a rather different Britain), to 71.4% in 1997
and 59.7% in 2001 – the lowest since the introduction of universal adult suffrage. In
2005 it rallied to 61.3%, but there was much postal ballot fraud. In addition, membership of political parties has halved in the last 25 years, whereas by contrast public
involvement in civil society (or alternative forms of activity such as volunteering and
protesting at 'hospital reconfiguration') is increasing. Despite proposed stunts such
as offering a lottery prize for voting in local council elections, there seems to be an
appreciation that voting does not deliver individual services, which are controlled

by bureaucracies, but that two other things do help change systems: markets, and media protest.[3]

When still Chancellor, Gordon Brown told Labour's 2006 annual conference that 'I want a radical shift of power away from the centre'. This speech chiefly concerned giving NHS bodies more local freedom, rather than empowering individual users of services.[4] Alan Milburn had made some limited and constrained progress here with foundation trusts. The hope of more local voting has not, however, changed the world. At the moment the government's Appointments Commission selects non-executive directors to PCTs and to other NHS trust boards. Local accountability is said to exist via local council health scrutiny committees. PCTs, too, use consultations, as do regional health boards, to 'embrace patients in decision making'. However, national experience is 'patchy ... with far too few examples of it being embedded in culture and practice' (according to the *Health Service Journal*). And in any case this is only about a 'voice' not a 'choice'.[5] Further, Health Minister Ben Bradshaw has said that there is a 'problem' with the accountability of PCTs to patients, who have found it difficult to influence decisions and to make their voices heard. We have already seen why in our discussion of the true sources of elusive knowledge.[6]

Two other innovations are proposed by some: more delegation of central powers to localities and more voting for such people as the management boards of hospitals. Mr Milburn is one who has advocated this.[7] The Liberal Democrats have also proposed that PCTs be replaced by elected local health boards, or alternatively that their work be transferred to local government to improve accountability. They also favour a local income tax. They argue for decentralisation as a source of greater freedom to experiment, and 'to embrace the choice agenda, so crucial to the reform of public services'. They talk of institutions which are to be 'as democratically accountable *as possible*'. David Laws MP has written of 'power being exercised either by individuals themselves, or as "close" to them *as possible*' (my italics). But this idea does not show how this would empower the individual to secure a preferred, individual service. The rationing of social care by local government, too, is a decision taken as close as possible to the individual concerned. This does not help when service is denied – as Ivan Lewis MP has appreciated, with his current work on a Green Paper on elderly care. Vince Cable MP is more favourably disposed to vouchers in further and vocational education, but not in mainstream health or education. Here, he lags behind Mr Milburn's current thinking. David Laws is more radical than his colleagues – and much more radical than his Conservative Party counterparts. He dislikes the dilution of traditional liberal beliefs in the benefits of markets, choice, the private sector and competition. He wishes to step back from statist solutions. He advocates a national health insurance scheme where the individual could choose either the NHS or an alternative insurance provider. These funds would be mobile, with a choice of health providers.

Even so, his colleague, Edward Davey MP, writing on 'Liberalism and localism', shows that the new localism continues the existing system of central–local relations, and that it,

> can appear to mean anything to anyone at any time – all within the current constitutional centralism. The Treasury's vague talk of managerial decentralisation completely avoids democracy. Concepts such as 'earned autonomy' reveal that no power shift is envisaged. An agenda of 'freedoms and flexibilities' is set in terms of Whitehall's own targets, inspections and judgements.

He urges that there must be mechanisms for checking state power, and promoting quality and choice by the individual. The division of powers, the localisation of actions and the restraint of the centre is attractive if genuinely radical steps follow. Some European examples have, indeed, been very radical. Sweden, for example, 30 years ago allowed local areas to opt out of parts of the welfare state and declare themselves as free communes, running their own services. Nothing like as radical an idea is now offered by our three main political parties, but a 'new localism' is on their common agenda. Yet this suffers from the many known contradictions, ambiguities and dilemmas of all democratic devices. It highlights the many illusions about the identity between the 'people', their 'will' and how democracy actually operates. However, as this book went to press Nick Clegg, Liberal leader, suggested that individual financial empowerment should be extended. We await details.[8]

Politics and priorities

Even in an active democracy we face the realities that for much of the time, as Geoff Mulgan notes, the political world is a specialised domain sufficient to itself, governed by professional politicians, scrutinised by media professionals in arguments constructed by paid lobbyists, with the voters left outside as consumers who can only choose at regular intervals between (apparently) contending alternatives.[9]

'Self-rule', or rule by popular opinion, does not guarantee that minorities will be taken seriously, that the powerless will have any power, or even that the majority will be able to exercise any command over services between elections. 'Rights' clash. Politics ultimately determines 'priorities'. Even if the official policy is to redirect resources for the health and education of the poorer majority it remains very difficult for people to see how to ensure that the state either locally or nationally is the vehicle by which their individual wishes are made real. Many of these wishes, too, in a multi-cultural and multi-racial society, will inevitably clash.

We agree and accept democratic compromises in order to keep our swords in their sheaths. But in terms of healthcare most of us do not want the vague promises of some theoretical over-arching thing called 'power' in terms of this politician or that. We want *a service*. We want it now. We want it free at the point of demand. We usually want it locally. We want it to work. We want it safe. We want it clean. We want to be able to live with the consequences, if at all possible. We want to choose between outcomes, if there are real choices to be made. We want to be treated fairly, and we want the same for others. Yet by voting we cannot be sure of *any* of this.

A 'new localism' may do little or nothing to change these realities. Indeed, it can further solidify existing inequalities. Democratic elections and politics are a lot better than dictatorships. Yet when all elections turn on ambiguities – in part, to enable politicians to manage their often fractious parties, in part to get elected at all, in part because more decentralisation (even if it were 'real') would not necessarily improve government – we cannot be sure what gains a new localism might offer. There is, too, the underlying challenge to monocracy itself: that although in theory people are fundamentally to be equal, deep inequalities of wealth and income enable the rich to capture better services than the poor, however they might vote, if they do. If economic equality is a prerequisite of political equality then the 20th century experiments to impose this by communist regimes have not been an encouraging experience. As the poor opt out of participation in elections, the answer is to give them the power they understand best because of its lack in their lives. Money.

The caucus at the beginning of the American primary elections in January 2008 created great excitement, and reminded us of the Athenian model of democracy when public decrees were displayed and debated in the marketplace, and where the majority of citizens were able to read them. This process dramatised many of the ambiguities and dilemmas of democracy. It engaged some of the US public in self-responsibility about power and in robust argument about decisions. Many responded to the opportunity by making the effort to learn about the issues. For a short time each four years the image of ancient Athens arises again in this ferment of ideas and debate, at least in the USA primaries. Here, voting is not necessarily 'rational'. This is not new. As John Vincent showed in his study of the formation of the British Liberal Party, people voted for WE Gladstone as an expression of who they thought they were, as an expression of their self-esteem, and not because Gladstone enacted radical policies to help them. For he did nothing of the kind. He was the symbol, 'the People's William' notwithstanding.[10]

In Iowa in 2008, many felt that an individual vote mattered, although it is quite normal for one vote to make no difference. Such conversations highlighted how we decide, who decides, and the limits of such decision-making processes. They tested individuals, ideas and a system. Yet the Athenian approach in a complex modern society raised – in the context of NHS reform – basic difficulties about the competence of such a model. It involved only some 340,000 Iowans out of 2 million registered voters. This was twice as many as have ever voted in person in the Iowa caucus before. But, still, not many. It involved huge expenditure on modern media, with significant funds raised via the Internet.[11] There was little discussion of specific policies, but there was much emotional eloquence. This event suggested that such a model can perhaps handle only a very general proposition – such as 'Change You Can Believe In'. Like our own local government, it is a blunt instrument, if sometimes personally a bloody one. Unless we are all to meet very often indeed to consider many detailed issues together, trying to control local institutions by a state of permanent consultation looks far from practicable. Or we might elect healthcare managers or boards. But what would this achieve? How has it helped with foundation trusts?

Geoff Mulgan on democracy suggests that 'all states have three characters – that of a servant, that of a captured master, and that of a servant of themselves'.[12] Much of the contemporary state remains pre-democratic. It is still designed around command rather than accountability, with authority directed downwards. Officials and managers are hostile to openness and public activism as 'consultation' on hospital 'reconfiguration':

> This is not a model that encourages or can cope easily with intensive public involvement. In no nation has it come close to Lincoln's idea of government of, by, and for the people. Instead we have government chosen by electorates, respectful of the people, and to varying degrees, committed to their welfare – which is a great advance over what went before but it falls short of full democracy. The command of the state has been transformed but not the state itself. The nineteenth-century French anarchist Proudhon's lifelong denunciation of the perversion of democracy into a mere competition for the '*imperium*' seems vindicated.[13]

The challenge then is to organise democracy or the bureaucratic state, or people's power, differently, to secure a better alignment between rulers and ruled. But how? A 'new localism' offers to do something to break it up. Edmund Burke believed in small platoons. My own proposals with regard to healthcare concern shifting financial power so that people can exercise their personal freedoms within collective provision, amid competitive pluralist options. In our democracy the theory is that ultimate power rests with the voters. But in national and local elections we are powerful on one day only very occasionally. Between elections the vocal and the organised pressure groups as clients of government win the tug of war over resources. The gap between those in power and those outside remains huge. After the election we cannot reliably secure that for which we voted. And we are likely to be in a minority in any case. There is no known voting mechanism which can add every voter's preference together to form a coherent whole. This is, of course, the problem of knowledge which markets solve but which is beyond the reach of 'experts'. People do not, in any case, necessarily vote for what they want. They often vote strategically, to help achieve an outcome they want ('anyone but the Tories', as in 1997). We can evict governments together, of course, but do we thus gain a choice? If we do it is only of a very general nature. The process as a whole legitimises government, and leadership. Here, Mr Blair, for example, demanded more of people than before, and challenged the nation to change by supporting major NHS reform. This was not what a vocal minority at least had wanted. Further, neither voting nor ministerial leadership can enable us to reliably command a local, personal, intimate and timely healthcare intervention unless we control the money.

In addition, minority governments often rule, by default. The mathematics of elections shows that governments are usually returned by minorities, with a divided majority voting for other parties and leaders who are not then returned to office. Even aside from the usual practices of deals of various kinds between politicians – usually within their own party where conflicting perspectives coexist uncomfortably – the otherwise unorganised voter cannot insist on getting what he or she thought they voted for. And they will be elbowed aside by the vocal 'inside-track' pressure group or the 'client' interest – doctors, in healthcare, farmers in agriculture and so on, in often quiet and private symbiotic bids for resources and policies in their intended capture of the state machinery.

The low level of participation in local government is another disabling factor, but even a high level of voting would not secure an individual service. The issue for the 'ordinary' patient is how to secure a service when they want it, not to spend their life in agitation, in strategic debate, in being 'consulted'. The same is true of proposed reforms via electronic voting and other instant consultation.[14] It is worth noting, too, that even general elections can only offer voters leverage sometimes. Gordon Brown became leader of his party and Prime Minister without being submitted to a popular electorate, as did John Major – although he subsequently won the 1992 general election.

Ken Livingstone's autobiography was called *If Voting Changed Anything, They'd Abolish It*.[15] It is quite a thought.

Notes

1 Edward Davey, p. 45, 'Liberalism and localism', in Paul Marshall and David Laws (eds.), *The Orange Book Reclaiming Liberalism* (London, Profile Books, 2004). See also Alan Milburn, 'Empowering citizens: the future politics', Speech to the Global Foundation, Sydney, 2 May 2006. Simon Jenkins has argued for more elected mayors. See Simon Jenkins, 'Ken is a squandering, crony-ridden mayor – but look on the bright side', *Sunday Times*, comment, 27 January 2008, p. 18.

2 Robert Winnett, 'Vote for your council and win a lottery prize', *Daily Telegraph*, 10 December 2007, p. 14. Leading article, 'Making voting easier won't make it popular', *Daily Telegraph*, 12 January 2008, p. 31.

3 'Scepticism greets plans to take politics out of NHS', *Health Service Journal*, 28 September 2006, p. 4. On the rationality or otherwise of voting (and costs/benefits) see Levitt and Dubner, op. cit., 'Why Vote?', pp. 222–6, originally published in the *New York Times Magazine*.

4 Editorial, 'Accountability: patient involvement can help siphon control from the centre', *Health Service Journal*, 13 September 2007, p. 3.

5 On the then Chancellor's reservations, Gordon Brown, in offering these changes, has been sceptical of 'marketisation'. See Gordon Brown, 'A Modern Agenda for Prosperity and Social Reform', speech to the Social Market Foundation at Cass Business School, London, 3 February 2003. On the return on the investment see Ruth Lea, *The NHS Since 1997: modest improvement at immoderate cost* (London, Centre for Policy Studies, 2005).

6 Roger Evans, 'Bradshaw calls for action to fix primary care democratic deficit', *Health Service Journal*, 13 September 2007, p. 5.

7 'Milburn calls for PCT elections', *Health Service Journal*, 28 September 2006, p. 7.

8 See note 5, in the chapter 'What are politicians *for*?', above. Also, Rebecca Evans, 'Lib Dems: time to scrap PCTs', *Health Service Journal*, 20 September 2007, p. 9. On central/local relations and funding see Simon Jenkins, 'Politicians are too terrified to devolve power to the people', *The Guardian*, 14 November 2007, p. 33. Mr Nick Clegg, Liberal leader, favours local income tax and radical centralisation and choice expressed by more voting for local boards. But he has also now urged extending personal budgets. See Rosie Millard, 'The big dreams of a genial waffler', *Sunday Times*, 23 December 2007, news review, p. 4; Nick Clegg, speech, 'Nick Clegg on the NHS: a liberal vision for the future', 10 June 2008, to King's Fund health group;

9 Geoff Mulgan, *Good and Bad Power*, op. cit., p. 228.

10 JR Vincent, *The Formation of the Liberal Party, 1857–68* (London, Constable, 1966; second edition Brighton, The Harvester Press, 1980).

11 Figures from politics futures trading at realclearpolitics.com; Michael Barone, 'A good starter – but where's the meat?', *The Times*, 5 January 2008, p. 23; Tim Reid, 'Stunning win lifts Obama's bid to become first black president', *The Times*, 5 January 2008, pp. 6–7.

12 Mulgan, *Good and Bad Power*, op. cit., p. 319.

13 Ibid., p. 245. The novels of CP Snow are, of course, an insight into how democracy in academe has often 'worked'. So, too, Noel Annan's discussion of life at Oxbridge. See *The Dons*, op. cit., esp. Chapter 13, 'The Don as Administrator'.

14 It isn't worthwhile for people to find out more. See Harford, *The Logic of Life*, op. cit., pp. 29–30, pp. 194–214; Bryan Caplan, *The Myth of the Rational Voter* (Princeton, NJ, Princeton University Press, 2006). For other theoretical and practical problems see Kenneth Arrow, *Social Choice and Individual Values* (New York, John Wiley & Sons, 1963).

15 Ken Livingstone, *If Voting Changed Anything, They'd Abolish It* (1987, London, Fontana, 1988). See also Steven E Landsburg, *The Armchair Economist: economics and everyday life* (1993; New York, The Free Press, 1995), p. 18.

13

Will giving power back to the doctors answer?

'The idea that powerful elites like to share power voluntarily is a comfortable myth that helps societies recover from conflict, but it bears scant relation to the truth.'

– GEOFF MULGAN

'People should be compelled to be freer and more individualistic than they naturally desire to be.'

– WYNDHAM LEWIS

'If we want things to stay as they are, things will have to change.'

– GIUSEPPE TOMASI DI LAMPEDUSA

As Adam Smith famously said in *The Wealth of Nations*, professionals do not necessarily meet together only for 'merriment and diversion', but often in conspiracy in pursuit of their own interests. Experts often use their information to serve their own agenda.

We are concerned with the basic ethical claim that the system, which is maintained at the public expense, should serve the user of services rather than the interests of the provider. And that much more explicit audit is required – including measures cast in terms of the patient's own wishes and preferred outcomes. It is this claim to which we look to politicians to make paramount. It is they who must find the common ground and negotiate a new settlement with professionals. As I have suggested, the best means is by a non-political free market.

Professionals are often accused of regarding themselves with marked self-satisfaction. Certainly, experience suggests that they will not normally vote for change if this threatens something of substance which they hold to be valuable. They have often been an intransigent, high-status minority living in a protected environment ('The Secret Garden') within the wider structure.

Yet Mr David Cameron has proposed giving power back to the front-line, to doctors. He also wants NHS budgets to be handed to GPs.[1] These two demands take insufficient account of two very important factors. First, the writings of public-choice economists such as James Buchanan, Gordon Tullock, and Arthur Seldon which explain the processes by which the capture of services by producer interests occurs, to the detriment of consumers.[2] Second, the actual recent results within the NHS of these actions. Dr John Meadowcroft (Lecturer in Public Policy at King's College, London) has summarised these developments. Since 1999 NHS funding has increased by 9% per annum, rising from £40 billion in 1999 to more than £80 billion. Yet services remain in a perilous state, many even more so than before. By 2010 the NHS will face an annual shortfall of some £7 billion. Unprecedented new funding has produced only minor benefits in terms of outcomes. Instead, systemic failings persist: many waiting times have increased, hygiene remains dangerously poor, the elderly are persistently neglected. And the key point is that much of the additional money has been garnered into their barns by producer interests, instead of being spent on improving care. Mr Cameron should appreciate that, even in retreat, 'experts' can be self-serving.

A large proportion of the additional funding – some estimates put it at 40% of the total – has been transferred to NHS staff in year-on-year above-inflation pay increases. GP's have received staggering new contracts since 2003, giving the average GP a salary of £100,000 per annum. More, for doing less. Producers have captured the budgetary process, and allocated themselves large sums of new money. Staff numbers have grown, too. Producers have thus taken control of the expansion of their own organisations. But with what results in terms of patient care? We still have little or no information on outcomes or quality. However, productivity has fallen by 20% since 1997, as we have already seen.[3]

Quasi-markets

On the demand side, what Mr Cameron has proposed is to revive the GP Fundholder or 'quasi-market' of the Thatcher years. This initiative in the 1990s was positive, although it was widely resisted within the service on the basis of 'equity'. But this does not go nearly far enough in the new context. And, indeed, the Conservative governments of Mrs Thatcher and Mr Major did not ultimately benefit in terms of votes from drawing back from the logic of this reform. The political lesson is that you should go for it, if you believe it. Of course, the necessity is to go beyond the by-now old model of GP fund-holding to what I have called patient fund-holding, or what are now known as personal budgets. For the GP fund-holding model does not hand financial power to the patient. 'Quasi-markets' are operated by proxies on the user's behalf, not by consumers. And even if users have information on services and local performance they are not in a position to insist on a choice. In addition, 'strategic' priorities about the allocation of resources or the legitimacy of provision which are beyond the control of the quasi-market may determine whether or not services exist locally in the first place.

A&E services have always been paid for centrally, and remain outside the quasi-market. Consumers may be offered only choices at the margins. Many may be forced if they can afford it to exit to alternatives. Many will have no such choice. In addition, there is no competition between PCTs for the NHS tax-based funds. No consumer has control of 'their' money. Block contracts prevail. In these circumstances, where is there any individual empowerment? For example, if none of the available options described by the GP Fundholder is considered by the individual (in an increasingly multi-cultural society) to be capable of delivering the outcomes sought by the user, being able to consult about them with a GP Fundholder/PCT and even being able to 'have a say' (even 'a greater say') in choosing between them will not be empowering.

Confusingly, too, Mr Cameron speaks of patients and professionals being 'properly in charge'. It is not clear what this means. How can both patient and professional be in charge? Indeed, what can 'a patient-led NHS' mean? In January 2008 Mr Cameron said that NHS patients would be able to choose their own GP and hospital consultant, which would help drive up standards in an age when 'doctor no longer knew best'. He applauded the market, but said that his party would be 'the party of the NHS', as 'an honour to be earned'.[4] Mr Cameron told the *Health Service Journal* in June 2007 that

'The big nature of the change we are arguing for is to empower GPs and clinicians and what you have then is decision making in the NHS being led by what patients and GPs choose to do with their budgets.' Does this mean patient fund-holding, and a shift towards a health savings account or a voucher? It seems not. Greater clarity may emerge if the Conservatives return to government, and then find a new language which means markets but does not actually say so. But at present what is being said is unclear. Meanwhile, Mr Cameron's White Paper proposes yet another quango – Health Watch – as a national body for patient voice. So this is not individual budget holding; it is voice instead of choice.[5]

On the basis of recent NHS evidence alone it is a risky proposition which asserts that the interests of the consumer are necessarily best served by giving more power to the providers or to vested interests. For the primary task of professionals has always been to save themselves from being called to account, as Geoff Mulgan has stressed. They, too, have been in control of the definitions of 'quality' based on producer autonomy. They have resisted control from above, and exerted control on those below. They have long avoided pressures from the bureaucracy of NHS management and from the market. But definitions are necessarily changing. Chiefly due to cultural change rather than political pressures – as quality is much more evidently a vital aspect of an economy which depends on price, on empowered demands, on opportunity costs, and on rewards for those who best serve their clients.

Professionals typically want to regulate themselves, to set strict limits to the risks of being held responsible by the outside world. As Geoff Mulgan put this as long ago as 1974, 'Any serious programme for spreading responsibility would have to start not with those at the bottom of society, those out of work and on welfare, but rather with the most powerful.'[6] By contrast, more power to the medical professionals in the 'front-line' is one of Mr Cameron's chief offers. This may have electoral attractions, as it sounds as if services must inevitably improve as a result. But it is a moral trap – as, indeed, is the pursuit of efficiency as an end rather than as a means.

We might remind ourselves that it is the people for whom the service exists and who make the jobs for those delivering the services, not the other way around. It is the recipients who should be deciding on the necessary trade-offs and the required outcomes. It is politicians who should protect the terms of service and delivery, notably of choice, competition and plurality. It is markets, indeed, which should effectively make the rules. Rightly, the market should be lightly regulated by government. It is government and not the providers who should make these rules. The Hippocratic oath may indeed protect the patient, not least from some doctors who may know more technically and scientifically than the patient but who practise doubtfully. The professional structure of self-regulation protects doctors from the scrutiny of others. For all these reasons I take Mr Cameron's view to be a mistaken one, philosophically, morally, politically, and in terms of practical management. Similarly, the think-tank Reform runs a campaign of 'Doctors for Reform', but not one of 'Patients for Reform'. I would still like to see such a parallel campaign, to emphasise recipients rather than to highlight providers, however persuasive they might be to politicians. Mr Cameron's party is offering a really radical reform of welfare. Why not of healthcare, too?[7]

Generational change

Here, Mr Cameron's 'narrative' is, rightly, for a smaller state, and perhaps for the historical British individualist market economy within an assertive democratic culture. David Willetts for one has previously made this case.[8] But in healthcare Mr Cameron has said that he wants his to be 'the party of the NHS'. Thus he seems to distrust markets, and the potential for entrepreneurs – so lacking in the NHS itself – to dramatically improve healthcare provision. There is, though, no prospect of redesigning the system in the customer's interests and achieving productivity gains and a flow of innovations without releasing the control over buying power and giving it the consumer. Meanwhile, Mr Cameron seeks to recover the support of medical staff who were once the natural allies of Conservatism – and who vacillate between the two ancient poles of knowledge as a possession to be exploited and of knowledge to be shared. However, when producer interests predominate over those of service-users, a 'doctor knows best' mentality contradicts the themes of endorsing personal autonomy and self-esteem and choice based on the intimate values of the user of the services. The 'docs know best' idea continues to see consumers as largely passive recipients of services.

This is increasingly a difficult case to make, both in terms of the changing structure of contemporary society and of individual access to the information and the experiences of others. The Internet; YouTube; Facebook; Bebo; MySpace; Last.fm; blogging; e-mail, and online comparisons of services are all integral, in particular, to the way in which young people now present themselves, manage relationships and make decisions. Several of these start-up enterprises are British. Their power was underlined by the sale of Bebo to AOL for $850 million in March 2008. As Libby Brooks has written, 'This is the first generation to grow up beyond the digital divide – now that social networks are available on mobiles and that there is free internet access in schools and libraries, the barrier is no longer about hardware but literacy.'[9]

This is a huge generational change. It is one which is shifting the world more rapidly than anything since the advent of the railways in the 19th century, when WM Thackeray said that the railway embankment was like a wall, dividing past and future. Here, the advent of real-time global connections facilitated by new social software technologies has changed every relationship, between the individual and the state and between the individual and others like them, as well as with professionals. This involves millions in rolling conversations and check-ups on possibilities in a newly borderless and diverse world. It is one factor helping to unfetter services from the state.

Professor Buck-Morss has said that 'There are producers of culture working on another level to open up alternative spaces – on the margins, at boundary crossings, at cultural intersections, within electronic landscapes . . . taking advantages of its electronic infrastructures and technological forms. . . . These technologies are cultural weapons which confront older structures of power that continue to own them and try to contain them.'

The political principle of geographical and intellectual isolation is then a left-over from an earlier age. People now see and experience the world via the global media. They look beyond the view presented to them by national state power. They are interrupting and querying the legitimacy of contexts which deny them control over their own lives. We have seen this in the row over the NHS denying cancer drugs otherwise available in other jurisdictions, and visible to all on the net.

The deficits and denials are then a shock to ideological preconceptions – and which may not have previously been realised by these individuals. The experience of a patient refused cancer drugs, and the option of co-payment, is materially and politically subversive. It challenges those rationalisations offered as reasons, an NHS 'consulting' culture offered as control, and the politics on which these ideas are based. For the patient these are both philosophical and material experiences, and the source of new understandings. These experiences, too, are occurring in the patient's 'own world' and not just in Dr Coulter's and Mr Redding's 'community'. Here, as we see with growing anxieties about care, these experiences are increasingly preoccupying many with how to challenge and change the prevailing cultural and its political preconceptions. They will continue to insist on moving beyond 'involvement' and 'public value' to personal empowerment.

As Susan Buck-Morss has written, new IT is transforming 'the masses' into a variety of publics – 'including a virtual global humanity, a potential "whole world" that watches, listens and speaks, capable of evaluating critically both the culture of others and their own.'[10]

The terms of all politics, and of individual relations to their locality and to others, have changed indelibly. Every marketplace is being reshaped as a result. Everywhere people search for something better, cheaper, more suited to their individuality. They find information at the click of a mouse. They pass it round. They expect more. They demand more. This defining change contributes to a lack of deference towards authority, and an unwillingness to take what you are given. Shoddy public services are rejected. People will not wait for delivery. They are frustrated by bureaucracies, and by incompetence. It is too soon for many in this new generation to have to tussle with the NHS and its bureaucracies. But when they have to they will be much less tolerant and accepting than the baby-boom generation. Few indeed will uncritically accept that they must listen when politicians tell them whom to trust. The world has changed forever. But why do we still seek to make an exception of the two critical areas, health and education? How can this make *any* sense?

Whether or not new technologies will be trusted as a democratic means of voting electronically, it is clear that a market system is now made much more workable by new forms of credit and distribution. The introduction of the credit card was a vital step, which allowed convenient distant purchase, especially when linked to instantaneous electronic connection. Electronic money, credit cards and organisations such as e-bay, Amazon, PayPal, and the websites of individual providers have made more buyers and more sellers who have tailored offers to customers preferences. This is the Hegelian argument revived. That we are only fully formed as free subjects by our experience of working to shape the world, and puzzling over the problematic nature of *actualité*. The electronic revolution has thus made people actually or potentially more knowledgeable. This can increase both moral and actual autonomy. Information, which stressed professional authority, is no longer the perquisite of elites, nor is it any longer under their control. Passive trust – with its 'faith' merits as well as its demerits – is a thing of the past. Trust in medical competence remains important, but it is contingent. Recent evidence of very varied medical performance and disturbing reports – together with the availability of information about actual patient experiences on the web – properly prompts individual questioning about the merits of individual doctors and specific treatments and their outcomes and side-effects. Everyone can look up information about the performance of professionals, and what patients thought of their experiences and outcomes of treatments. They can consider such assessments before making their own trade-offs. This is both a moral and an instrumental shift. There is more mutual dependence to help individuals secure independence.

And, as Geoff Mulgan says:

> Bad power is power that refuses to answer for itself, that hides, that believes itself to be its own justification, and demands accountability of everyone else. Bad power is power that seeks to make its own reality. Good power, by contrast, opens itself to scrutiny and accepts that truth is something to be sought, not asserted. Yet this blurring of the boundaries between the state and society is not quite as automatically good as it at first

seems. The knowledge that is produced at one remove from the state is also produced at one remove from the people it is there to serve. Most intellectual disciplines have a far stronger sense of service to themselves than of service to the people, and most assume that the public are incapable of competently interpreting their own lives . . . it is all too easy for knowledge to become detached from humanity and care. And for professionals to see other people as means not as ends.[11]

And so we need to recombine autonomy, individual control of money, self-knowledge, advisory and support services and professional judgement and advice, with the presumption that the individual should have the final say about their own fate.

All power to the doctors? In terms of professional performance, failures of diagnosis, of sufficiently early referral to specialist treatment, and the varied quality then found by the patient is one set of problems.[12] Many older doctors, too, have not grasped the changing nature of patient attitudes and knowledge in a consumerist society. I review the literature on this in my chapter 'My body, but your decision?' And so this particular proposal by Mr Cameron to privilege producer interests again seems wide of the mark. Especially so since a principal characteristic of a failed NHS monopoly has been the dominance of producer interests. Mr Cameron has also affirmed his commitment to increasing NHS funding, and to the 'NHS ideal'. He has rejected any move towards changes in the basis of funding and its operation – such as an HSA or an insurance-based system. If Mr Cameron comes to power, liberal economists at the Institute of Economic Affairs and elsewhere will seek to persuade him otherwise. We have already considered the successful example of Singapore, and we might note here, for example, that France has a much higher proportion of privately run hospitals and healthcare centres than the UK, with these services integrated within the overall health system. Indeed, it has one of the best healthcare systems in the world. There, in a social insurance system, patients have a choice of private or state-based care, and private clinics provide 40% of healthcare, but account for only 22% of costs. So they are more efficient by a goodly margin than the state providers.[13]

Mr Cameron has also said he wants to free up all hospitals from close state surveillance. We must hope this will mean by the power of customer choice. Meanwhile, the NHS is ranked between number 18 and number 24 in terms of international comparisons of health systems. Mr Cameron has not yet expressed faith in the abilities of 'ordinary' people to make good choices for themselves. He has made no proposals for individual empowerment.[14] It will be a loss to customers of care if he shares the assumptions of academic, statist 'experts'. As mentioned earlier, Lord Anthony Giddens has commented: 'In his speech he used words which even Aneurin Bevan might have blanched at: "I believe that the creation of the NHS is one of the greatest achievements of the twentieth century"'.[15] Lord Giddens also noted that under recent reforms medical pay rises eased shortages, but working practices did not change sufficiently. That productivity has hardly improved. That local managements 'game' the statistics to match government wishes. That over-spends are very significant. He adds: 'These shortcomings will not be remedied by relaxing the pace of reform, or by supposing that one can "return power to the front-line professionals". Increasing patient choice can help stimulate productivity, but so also can more effective and selective incentives for medical staff.'[16]

With this wise advice in hand it hardly seems sensible to decline to consider the effective alternatives which can achieve better coordinated care, higher standards, the significant saving of life and freedom for many from quite unnecessary pain. Why try to sustain provider power as an alternative to individual choice?

Clinicians as allies?

Here a key issue is whether clinicians are to be allies in the achievement of the 'choice agenda'. Several leaders in this kind of change have described in detail the ways and means by which success here can be achieved with clinical leadership and management support. For example, the cultural change-maker Patricia (Pat) E Natale, RN, MSN, Chief Nursing Officer at the Detroit Medical Center. This large cluster of facilities has a total revenue of $3.8 billion. It has 2230 inpatient beds, 66,000 surgeries annually, 3000 physician (700 faculty), and 13,400 full-time employees.

Pat Natale has said, 'It is important to use the ethical imperatives of excellence and patient safety to enable clinicians to tolerate the churn of change and create ownership.' In adopting a system-wide approach to care fully using new information technologies management made it clear that it was committed to success, and that paper was not an option. There was to be one system of care across the entire facility. Clinicians directed the project of change. Patient satisfaction and patient safety drive change, and these were the values which have aligned quality and financial data points. New IT now makes decisions possible more securely and more quickly, and issues are resolved at conversion. IT enables a leveraged approach to developing employees, too. The system can be designed to support outcome reporting. Training is based on workflows. Clinical adoption has been key. It is important, too, that adoption is reproducible, iterative and applicable to all new processes. The expectation that this will be has to be established. At Detroit it was decided that implementation of new IT had to be rapid, thorough and deep, and with expectations carefully managed. Strong and persistent leadership on all levels was and is essential if planned results are actually to happen. The Detroit Medical Center, of course, is 'driven by the need for discriminating difference for the health system is in a very competitive environment'.[17]

Choice distorting priorities?

Some say that more individual choice will distort 'clinical priorities'. What might this mean? We should be careful not to assume that only clinicians can determine appropriate outcomes, aside from the values of the service-user. Clinicians ('scientific experts') respond to incentives. For all people respond to incentives. 'Experts' are people. How any given expert treats you will depend in part on how that expert's incentives are set up. We need to be sure that incentives – which are both economic, moral and social – work in favour of the users of services. Indeed, incentives can be designed to improve the lives *both* of clinicians and service-users. Every doctor already has strong incentives to do the best for his own family. He/she knows where they would send their daughter. We need incentives to work so that we are all in the same favoured position. This concerns releasing the power of what is still secret inside information, and using it to improve the situation of every individual. We must hope that these changes can be achieved in negotiation.

However, we may, indeed, have to deploy surprising and very powerful incentives. A centralising statist might indeed want to change the legal rules of practice. For example, a statist might be tempted to ask what if it was not possible for a clinician – trained, after all, in public institutions with public money – to have any permit for any private clinical practice unless their fullest outcome data was promptly published by their NHS trust, or by an independent outcomes body? This would, of course, be an example of further state intrusion. Yet if voluntary professional publication continues to lag it may be a temptation to change the rules. Of course, such an initiative might have both expected and unexpected consequences. Some doctors would emigrate. Some become journalists. Some applicants might not enter the profession to begin with. But it may indeed become necessary to change the rules.

A decentralising dynamist would rather enable the market to achieve change, to deploy effective financial and social incentives to shift the situation through many degrees of the compass. Of course, there are many with economic interests to protect. But the delicacy and complexity of negotiations are not arguments in favour of fortifications. Nor for allowing the cloak of respectability to shroud new potentials.

Of course, the power and status of clinicians derives from the fact that they do something which no one else can do. But the issue here, too, shows that the power of 'experts' depends in part on the fact that they control, and often hoard, information. Some of this information, via the Internet, is now falling into other hands. This is gradually enabling comparisons to be made by customers. In some other areas of knowledge – notably term life assurance – comparison websites have simplified purchasing and much reduced prices. Here, Levitt and Dubner quote Supreme Court Justices Louis D Brandeis: 'Sunlight is said to be the basis of disinfectants.'[18]

Incomes and outcomes

There is then the question of pay as an incentive to the individual and as a measure of success. Will clinician's incomes be influenced by what consumers say? If the model of the individual taking willing revenues to a competing purchaser were adopted there would be this prospect, since purchasing decisions would impact on incomes. For the well-informed local purchaser could specify that they wish to buy a procedure from Dr Green but not from Dr Brown. And that the patient's values, preferences and views on appropriate outcomes are as follows. . . . Very direct incentives would include return business, retraining of the less satisfactory 'expert', or removal of the clinician or of the exit of the paying customer. Or both. A market structure of financially empowered individual choice (with the poor receiving tax transfers so that they are on the same footing as the middle class) will in fact offer a genuine rapprochement with clinicians. Indeed, of the three ways to manage clinicians the market is the most favourable means. The other two ways: central government targets, highly prescriptive procedures and artificial cost-containment or self-management, are each less attractive.

The challenge, too, is to find solutions which can lift professional morale by encouraging more autonomous, adaptive behaviour locally. Here, I suggest that free markets populated by mutual purchasing bodies and a pluralism of providers will have some unexpected effects. One is that they will be conciliatory to professional interests, in so far as this is legitimate in a free society. For the changes will promote the rewards and status of those professionals who continue to attract willing custom. The purchasing bodies will remunerate professional competence. Pluralism can be the context for a recovery of status and reputation. New investment in technologies and a more balanced team will enhance services. Settings, too, will change as services evolve. And so professional work itself will be a key locale of adaptive, creative development where the good is rewarded and the less good discouraged.

The alternative remains politicised controls, and centralised and simplified targets – simplification itself being necessary to political control. It remains a life of hierarchical decision making, and of market mimicry without individual empowerment. But citizen's juries, PALS, LINKS and other participatory devices unconnected to price or the control of money are unconvincing. They also stand in the way of professional development.

So we do need to align the driving values with a new alignment of incentives. Incentives should impact not only on the income of the organisation – the purchaser or the provider – but also on individual incomes. Medical staff should not be exempt. Indeed, their leadership is one of the predominant factors. Incentives must reach them directly. It is important to focus on this in future pay reform. Via incomes there can be a very direct customer input to encourage different responses from those who give service. This change will be very difficult to achieve given clinical resistance. But it can make a reality of 'co-production'.

Incentives can influence the money clinicians make, the work they do, their 'peer group' ranking, the wider social status, power and glory that they achieve – all the ways in which they can take advantage of their success. Payment by results needs to impact not only on the incomes of the institution, but also on the rewards of the specific individual clinician and the relevant clinical teams. Institutions like hospital trusts should take every cost-justified measure to improve productivity and quality. But the issue is not productivity, or volume, alone. It also concerns what we define as quality, and who decides what that is. In a competitive situation – including one with competing purchasers – it would be vital to count everything which different individuals, customers and clinicians, valued. And then for managements to take individual action concerning the personal productivity and the quality of *individual* clinicians and nurses and their incomes. Outcomes should be significantly defined and reported by the users of services. Incomes should be directly influenced by the experiences of *specific* patients. But how to do it?

We need to be clear what story we want the data to tell, and what we want incentives to promote. That is, what it is that we are aiming to achieve in the first place. This concerns the question of what is being measured, and how this may still be different from what we would really like to measure. When we clarify what we really want to measure then incomes should be much more closely tied to accomplishments. This is the distinction, if you like, between measuring GNP as volume and measuring the subjective value of what is traded. The measure of what is desirable to the cost-aware individual is separate from the measure of volume. This is a moral distinction. If the incomes of individual clinicians and their specific outcomes are to be much more closely linked this is to redefine what we mean by efficiency. Economic efficiency is one important consideration. But the link between inputs and outputs needs to be reconsidered in terms of the values of the recipient, the outcomes which individual clinicians achieve and those which the recipients prefer. Today the rewards for clinical outcomes are not coupled to performance, either in terms of volume (which is but one important test of productivity) and specific outcomes. Incomes are not designed to elicit appropriate behaviour or best outcomes, including those defined by patients and by patient experiences. They should be so if we are to identify and empower the features that individuals care about. And to encourage appropriate action to be taken to enhance their relative importance. The new science of genetics and the rapid evolution of pharma-technologies which will enable the treatment of the specific patient in new ways will re-emphasise these issues.

The more direct links between incentives and outcomes can help us achieve two necessities: to uncover the detail of individual clinical and customer realities, and to reveal and empower essential personal values. Economics offers a guide:

> Individual rationality, coupled with competition *and* prices, leads to efficient outcomes: that is, outcomes in which there remain no unexploited opportunities to improve everybody's welfare. . . . No matter which of the many efficient allocations you want

to achieve, you can always achieve it by first redistributing income in an appropriate way, and then letting competitive markets function freely. The critical feature in the formulations and proofs of these theorems is the existence of market prices. Without prices, there is no reason to expect efficient outcomes.

The missing element is the missing market. One which would directly link individual incomes and performance. And where in a properly informed market of enforceable contracts the customer is individually empowered financially. We reveal our priorities when we accept the missing market as 'a fact of life', or when we instead ask for a different perspective to prevail.[19]

Notes

1 Conservative Party, White Paper, NHS Autonomy and Accountability: proposals for legislation, 20 June 2007.
2 The Liberty Fund of Indianapolis, Indiana has in progress a 20-volume set of James M Buchanan's Collected Works. See James M Buchanan and Gordon Tullock, The Calculus of Consent (Ann Arbor, Michigan, University of Michigan Press, 1962); JM Buchanan and RD Tollison (eds.), Theory of Public Choice (Ann Arbor, Michigan, University of Michigan Press, 1972); JM Buchanan, The Limits of Liberty: between anarchy and leviathan (Chicago, Chicago University Press, 1975; JM Buchanan et al., The Economics of Politics (London, IEA, 1978), JM Buchanan et al. (eds.), Towards a Theory of Rent-Seeking Society (Austin, Texas, Texas A&M Press, 1980); JM Buchanan, Why I, Too, Am Not a Conservative (Cheltenham, Elgar, 2005); Gordon Tullock, The Vote Motive (London, Institute of Economic Affairs, 1976) and his Private Wants, Public Means (New York, Basic Books, 1970); WA Niskanen, Bureaucracy and the Representative (Chicago, Aldine-Atherton, 1971). See also Arthur Seldon, Capitalism (Oxford, Basil Blackwell, 1990); Peter Self, Government by the Market? The politics of public choice (London, Macmillan, 1993), and Brian Griffiths, Robert A Siroco, Norman Barry and Frank Field, Capitalism, Morality and Markets (London, Institute of Economic Affairs, 2000); Milton Friedman, Capitalism and Freedom (Chicago, Chicago University Press, 1962; revised edition, 1982); Milton and Rose Friedman, Free To Choose: a personal statement (New York, Harcourt Brace, 1980); their Tyranny of the Status Quo (San Diego, Calif., Harcourt Brace, 1983; London, Martin Secker & Warburg, 1984; Harmondsworth, Penguin Books revised edition, 1985.
3 John Meadowcroft, 'In the NHS, more can mean less', Economic Affairs, 26(3), September 2006, p. 81.
4 David Cameron, speech 'The NHS at 60', after visit to Trafford General Hospital, Manchester, 2 January 2008. Rosa Prince, 'Patients "will be able to choose their consultant"', Daily Telegraph, 3 January 2008, p. 10. The classic corrective to Mr Cameron's view on giving power to doctors is RG Evans, 'Supplier-induced demand: some empirical evidence and implications', in M Perlman (ed.), The Economics of Health and Medical Care (New York, John Wiley and Sons, 1974). The leading Cameron-supporter Nick Herbert MP has urged 'clear lines of accountability and the alignment of incentives'. But does this mean more than Mr Cameron's policy of trusting the professionals? Nick Herbert, speech to Reform, 'Conservatives are the party of ideas, progress and reform', 12 May 2008; Peter Riddell, 'Economy is key to revival of fortunes', The Times, 15 May 2008, p. 7.
5 Victoria Vaughan, 'David vs. Goliaths of bossy government', Health Service Journal, 28 June 2007, p. 18. See also David Cameron, 'The NHS at 60', speech to annual conference of NHS Confederation, Manchester, 2 January 2008.
6 Mulgan, Politics in an Antipolitical Age, op. cit., p. 67.
7 Toby Helm, 'Pay firms to find work for jobless, say Tories', Daily Telegraph, 5 January 2008, p. 1. I am aware that he has also offered an alternative, but 'power to the docs' seems to be his more settled idea. He told his party conference on 3 October 2007 that top-down targets must be scrapped, and professionals trusted, while emphasising outcomes. 'What we have got to do is make the NHS and doctors answerable to the patients and not the politicians.' But how? See Francis Elliott, '"Unscripted" Cameron delivers a textbook speech to the faithful', The Times, 4 October 2007, pp. 6–9.
8 David Willetts, Modern Conservatism (London, Penguin Books, 1992).
9 Over 90% of UK teenagers belong to a social networking website. A third of those keep at least four separate profiles running at once. Ninety-seven per cent of those currently at UK universities are regular Internet users. Bebo had 11 million users, MySpace 10 million and Facebook 4 million users in Britain alone in January 2008. Sophie Borland, 'One in four teens at risk over details on Facebook', Daily Telegraph, 7 January 2008, p. 2. Bonnie Malkin, 'Online baby boom reaches Facebook', Daily Telegraph, 26 December 2007, p. 7; Libby Brooks, 'Beyond the digital divide lies a new world of intimacy', The Guardian, 21 February 2008, p. 33. Dr Tanya Bryon, child psychologist and 'House of Tiny Tearaways' presenter was in late spring 2008 to report to the government on her commissioned review of the impact of new technology on childhood. The Internet, too, has proved to be a means of vast fund-raising in politics during the 2007–08 Presidential campaign in the USA. But this communication cannot be a one-way process. See also Robert Colville, 'The web will force politicians to be open', Daily Telegraph, 18 February 2008, p. 23, and his Politics, Policy and the Internet (London, Centre for Policy Studies, 2008).

10 Buck-Morss, op. cit., p. 277. See also the apposite discussion at pp. 238–56.

11 Mulgan, *Good and Bad Power*, op. cit., pp. 264–5.

12 The Quality and Outcome Framework (QOF), in which general practices participate, is a disease register which identifies patients who may be at risk. An audit of diagnosis is necessary to reassure on how this is working, especially for those with long-term conditions.

13 Giddens, *Mr Brown*, op. cit., pp. 89–90.

14 David Cameron, Speech to the King's Fund, London, 9 November 2006.

15 Giddens, op. cit., pp. 39, 88. Giddens also makes the point that 'unions working in the public sector may claim that, by definition, they are representing "the public", whereas in fact they might be acting against what is in the public's best interests – for instance, defending archaic work practices'. Giddens, ibid, p. 71. Ferdinand Mount shows, too, that Conservative as well as Labour governments have not had faith in 'ordinary' people being able to make choices, and still less faith in their institutions. The Balfour Education Act of 1902 placed both state and voluntary schools under political control. Conservative dominated governments of the 1920s and 1930s raided the National Insurance fund. The Butler Education Act of 1944 finally abolished fee-paying in schools and extended compulsory state education to age 15. Conservative administrations did much to expand the one-class council estates. All this helped to hollow out working-class life. Mount, op. cit., pp. 224–5.

16 Giddens, ibid., pp. 86–7. Examples of 'gaming' are legion. We know, too that there are many ways in which staff can resist policy initiatives, and dilute their application. In 1998 I suggested to Professor Paul Corrigan, then and now a key Whitehall adviser, that a small group be set up to consider each new reform from the point of view of 'gaming', to second-guess how managers would deal with new reforms. One example is 'patient-stacking': seriously ill patients left for hours in ambulances, or on trolleys, instead of being admitted immediately to A&E departments, to meet a government target on treatment times. See, e.g., Lucky Cockroft, 'A&E patients kept in ambulances to meet time targets', *Daily Telegraph*, 18 February 2008, p. 8. An interesting study of how institutional forces resisted health policy initiatives in the USA is Wendy Ranade, 'US health care reform: the strategy that failed', *Public Money and Management*, 15(3), July–September 1995, pp. 9–16.

17 Patricia E Natale, 'Harvesting global best practices: EMR: transforming patient care', address to Leadership Forum, Great Fosters, Egham, Surrey, 20 May 2007. This event was convened by the Cerner Corporation, a leading supplier of information technology with more than 6000 clients in 25 countries. British clients include Barts and the London NHS Trust, Barnet and Chase Farm Hospital NHS Trust, St Mary's NHS Trust and many others. I am grateful to Pat for our conversations.

18 Levitt and Dubner, op. cit., p. 60.

19 Landsburg, op. cit., pp. 76–7.

14

The messages of the aesthetic environment

'We shape our buildings; thereafter they shape us.'

– SIR WINSTON CHURCHILL

'Architecture, of all the arts, is the one which acts the most slowly, but the most surely, on the soul.'

– ERNEST DIMNET

'One might regard architecture as history arrested in stone, the movement of time congealed . . . at every point a building expresses the needs, the character of an age.'

– AL ROWSE

Every detail speaks. It says, 'You matter, but you do not.' It notes, 'You have clout, but you do not.' It tells 'You wait here, but you, please, come through.' It addresses 'sir', 'madam', or 'you'. The signs, doors, buildings and the 'Sellotape' culture of peeling and often incoherent notices say 'This is a public service.' It is not that the NHS has no aesthetic or cultural identity. Far from it. It has what Brenda Case Scheer in another context called 'the culture of aesthetic poverty'.[1] Indeed, its very identity reflects the powerlessness of patients.

Art and politics are *both* cultural productions.[2] The environment is one of the key areas which influence what the process of care feels like, sounds like, tastes like, what it is to the touch, to the seeing and the smelling. Signs and gestures, hints and slips, often unconsciously give the game away. Aesthetics is a form of cognition, as well as a cultural precondition. We talk of 'being in touch'. This emphasises those psychological categories which matter to patients: sympathy, compassion, respect, sensitivity, understanding the other's point of view, being 'in touch'. Form *is* content. It is in part about who and what we make feel 'real', alive, sensually responsive, the focus of the work of the services.

When we see so many grim but functional NHS facilities – and this, despite the recent building boom which has certainly made a difference – we can imagine the immense changes that competition would still generate. In the NHS the emphasis has been on low-cost function. Many NHS environments remain the accumulated detritus of dogma. So, too, are the attitudes that survive unchallenged within them. They are as manipulative as any so-called market faults, and more resistant to correction. The maintenance budget, too, is the easiest to cut. And when we ask, 'How many beans make five?' those who have to keep things repaired are not much more than half a bean in terms of status, alas.[3] There is no urgency placed by chief executives on this work. For very few patients can go somewhere else, and they have no control over tax-paid money.

Yet an emphasis on aesthetic values and on *the patient's experience* does not lower standards – even if they are hard to measure in the absence of the customer going somewhere else with their money. Indeed, such an emphasis raises standards. Indeed, it does so by changing them. It complements and supports other values. Such as patient safety and patient satisfaction. It is in part about who and what we make feel 'real', alive, and sensually responsive. And it adds a special dimension to them. Improving physical standards may be a terrible nuisance to management, but if service-users are individually empowered financially the changes can reflect what people are prepared to pay for and what can be achieved. With changed financial structures we can have *both* new cancer drugs and an attractive and welcoming environment in which to receive the treatment.

Professor Jon A Chilingerian (of Brandeis University and a former senior care manager) has reported that,

> Clinicians have learned that through the service process patients and their families experienced hundreds of *clinical moments of truth*. Research on the *satisfied patient* suggested that patients' overall evaluation of quality depends on the results of the processes, as an *experience*, at every point of contact. Quality measurement from this perspective requires mapping and surveying the patient's entire experience with the delivery system.

The dynamic President and Chief Executive of Swedish Airlines, Jan Carlzon, turned around a failing airline by focusing on this concept.[4]

When people like me in the 1990s sought to introduce art into hospitals, aromatherapy and soft music into pre-operation rooms, spent money on a welcoming mural in a refurbished outpatients department, invested in today's newspapers for waiting patients rather than give them five-year-old copies of *Punch*, renewed a rotting and rusting 50-yard long railing in front of the main entrance, I was criticised. This was 'waste'. It was not 'cognitive'. It was not 'medical'. It was not 'professional'. It was not 'necessary'. Never mind my non-absolutist suggestion that it was about helping individual patients affirm a sense of self and of being valued. No. Never mind my idea that every detail speaks. Especially on arrival. No. It did not represent any priority in terms of worthwhile difference of value or perspective. And in any case we were under no pressure to upgrade, were we? To socially engineer was a legitimate source of material value. To maximise flows in and out of the doors was, too. But these aesthetic 'details' were not worth attention, were they? For we were a knowledgeable elite, who knew best, didn't we? It was volume and cuts in waiting lists which were the sources of 'legitimate' (and political) value. Not even outcomes were the measure. This was, indeed, why we knew little or nothing of these. So why bother about such marginal inputs? *We* wouldn't live in buildings like this ourselves, of course. But this was a 'public service'. In an artificially rationed service I could understand how priorities were formed, and how the environment was made marginal. But this was not and is not inevitable. However, insistence and 'top-slicing' of budgets enabled these improvements to happen.

The objections, however, were puritan in tone, with an echo of the Marxist idea, too, that somehow mass markets and their personalisation are corrupting. This came strangely from doctors with large private practices. However, I was told by some that given limited budgets we had no business considering such human and aesthetic self-expression, or creativity, or design, or subjectivity, or self-affirmation among patients who were otherwise relieved and grateful to get a clinical service. And in any case they had no choices. My perspectives were superficial or presumptuous at best, self-deceptive and unnecessary at worst.[5]

We had to spend money on *real* things. True, we must spend on clinical work and on treatments. And we did, by the millions – although, as the Audit Commission showed, the NHS has persistently wasted billions in delivering its illogically managed and uncoordinated 'core' services. We do want services that work. We do care about cost. But we want generic standards to rise as well. We want very different minimum standards. We expect the evolution of the environment – what Virginia Postrel calls the revolution in 'look and feel'. For 'Form follows, and leads, emotion.' The space in which people encounter things is important in affecting them. The collective environment makes a difference to the individual. We should welcome meticulous attention to environments. So why must facilities be ugly and shabby, and inconvenient and unwelcoming, even horrifying, and filthy, too? The environment is a very real thing to a patient. It conveys messages even before anyone is articulate. The message is too often read as an omen or a warning sign. That shabby is as shabby does.

The challenge is to do everything possible to empower the self-responsible individual, and to trust in a society in which as we have more choices we have more self-responsibility for our actions and consequences. That is, in a society in which we are all deserving of equal respect and with an equal capacity for self-government. These issues are focused both by aesthetics and by better health outcomes. As Postrel writes,

> I have this image of my true self, not as a disembodied set of thoughts but as a visual, tactile creature, whose authentic identity is reflected in the sensory aspects of my person, places, and things. People can look at me and see something true about who I really am. I can see myself reflected in my surroundings. Surface and substance will match. This is the aim of aesthetic meaning – to capture and convey identity, to turn our ineffable sense of self into something tangible and authentic.[6]

The UK's leading art charity, The Art Fund, has as part of its mission statement that 'Art has the power to transform people's lives'. Of course, life-saving drugs and treatment are a fundamental essential. It is no help to be buried in a designer coffin. However, it is our environment and our relationships that then make that life saved worth living.[7]

Postrel again: 'Now, however, the quality-demanding elite is no longer so elite. It includes most of us.'[8] This is the success of liberal capitalist markets. But we cannot yet make these demands work for us in 'public services'. Alas, without individual financial empowerment the culture will still say *we*, the doctors, matter. *You*, the patient, do not matter as much. And the place where the work is done hardly matters at all. Regretfully, works management, maintenance staff, designers and architects have no status, save to put the cables to the operating theatres in the right place, and to keep them working. Who is in charge then? When I was Chairman of one of the largest NHS hospital trusts neither the Board nor the Executive team held the contracts for the consultants, whose every action initiated the largest part of our costs. These contracts were held by 'the Region'. One persistent result has been that a culture where you do not count as an individual – whether as manager, or as patient – is very daunting. Especially when as a patient what is happening is happening to *your* body. *You* bear the costs in risk, pain and time. It is *your* life to be lived. This is the scarcest resource in the world. *You* live or die with the results. The docs may do a great job. But you have to be there when they do it. You may well greatly benefit from the treatment, of course. But you are not just a statistic.

Our bodies *are* us. How we choose, too, says a lot about us. How we construct choice in society – and how we privilege it or deny it – does so, too. An NHS culture which suggests that the individual is of no consequence is scarily daunting. A rotting, neglected and 'irrelevant' environment is often frightening. We should instead pick up the gauntlet of John Ruskin's challenge of learning *to see*. An organisation which understands the importance of aesthetics in its places of work will appreciate the sensitivities of patients. It will see more. But an organisation that did so would already be competing for patients, for their willing revenues and their support and for the personal endorsement of their services. It would be an organisation which understands that sensory appeals are cultural, personal and personalised. That they create reactions without words. That they are intensifying. They are everywhere.

In the outside world cultural homogeneity began to break down in the 1960s. This shift has intensified in a multi-ethnic society. No longer could Henry Ford's successors tell us that we can have what we like as long as it's black. But not in public services. These increasingly look, feel and *are* left behind by the wider dynamist economy. The healthcare policies of all three leading political parties, however, remain too much gripped by the notion of 'one last push'. Of a change of government, to manage things 'properly'. Of even more money and some tighter management to correct what are actually wholly systemic and intrinsically endemic failures. This will not bake the biscuit.

Indeed, experience within the NHS is still like continuously crawling inside a Mobius strip. We are still in a world of grin and bear it. Of 'Wait there. What you grumbling about? Lucky to get it! Stop complaining and wait your turn!' Who among us has not heard that NHS mantra, waiting in A&E, or in outpatients, even with an appointment? When compared with the high-flown ambitions and the claims of 'the best health service in the world', the reality is often very grim indeed. Yet compare the dramatic changes in every aspect of our lives in the past 25 years with the fundamentally unchanging realities of state-provided, tax-funded services – protected still from any but marginal competition. Who has been lefty outy, and why?

Money talks, and preference walks

We know that money talks and preference walks.[9] If we want to get action on all these issues the most critical change required is to make purchasing itself work properly. An urgent change required is to introduce competing purchasing organisations. PCTs are presently local monopolies. Many encompass very large territories. There is no effective choice. They are not membership organisations. They are not controlled by consumers. They are part of the problem. They are not the solution.

My proposed patient guaranteed care organisations would provide the necessary re-balancing of power, both between the individual and competing purchasers and between purchasers and competing providers. This would influence production decisions, do much to determine patterns of demand, and by direct incentives encourage different lines of conduct and attitudes from providers. These competing purchasers would be obliged to attract willing members. They would make varied offers, in niche markets as well as in large markets. Singapore is one model. Another could be the German *krankenkassen* insurance funds, which have been encouraged to become independent profit-based organisations which compete for customers (albeit, with too limited movement).[10]

As the moral philosopher Adam Smith showed, by expanding markets to include more buyers and sellers trade makes greater specialisation as well as services to large markets possible. The chief benefits, typically, go to customers, not producers. The present structure of PCTs does not, alas, depend on competition between purchasers, nor are individual tax-based funds mobile. The hinge on which PCTs function is local monopoly. They are effectively government-created cartels. If the market were opened by individuals having control over their own funds which they could take to competing purchasers, services would improve and costs fall. Costs and returns would come into balance and customers would be better off.

Competition is about serving many different people in different ways which *they* define. This is what we mean when we consider competitive advantage. This introduces new economic and cultural moments, which lead to others, which lead to others. It is, too, about serving the coexistence of many different styles. It enables people to build their own identities. It delivers efficiency, rationality and a variety of truths. The living environment responds to these facts – and even the most ordinary facilities are tuned to a welcoming environment. Aesthetics, landscaping, lighting, 'look and feel' has a value. All this has been part of the evolution of a vast middle class, and of the experience of the empowered individual in the wider modernised economy. The market offers a fluid selection of ways which people will either endorse or refuse. Many choices coexist, with equal status. They are not part of a 'programme'. But the NHS still offers 'one best way', defined by 'experts'.

This artificial and anti-competitive situation currently protected by government is against the public interest. The shabby aesthetic environment speaks volumes, in a service mostly concerned *with* volume. It is both its mirror and its shadow.

Notes

1 Barbara Case Scheer, 'Sympathy with the Devil: design review and the culture of aesthetic poverty', Loeb Fellowship Forum, Spring/Autumn 1996, cited in Postrel, *Substance*, op. cit., p. 161.

2 References could be legion. Virginia Postrel's two works are essential. The work by Susan Buck-Morss, op. cit., is an important discussion of these issues, too, although it takes an entirely opposite political view.

3 I hope that my friends in 'estates' will agree with me. Many are very committed and reflective people. They should not treated as small beans. In 1993 I recommended to the then Secretary of State for Health, Mrs [now Baroness] Virginia Bottomley, that the estates and maintenance function should be represented at Director level on all NHS boards. This has not been achieved yet.

4 Jon A Chilingerian, 'Who has star quality?', in Herzlinger, *Consumer-Driven Health Care*, op. cit., pp. 443–53. His italics. See also Jan Carlzon, *Moments of Truth* (New York, Ballinger, 1987; reprinted, New York, HarperCollins, 1989).

5 See my *The Invisible Hospital and The Secret Garden*, op. cit. One supporter, however, was Tom Sackville MP, then a junior health minister, on whose Ministerial Group on Design and Health Care I served, 1993–98.

6 Postrel, *Substance*, op. cit., p. 108.

7 It's an important membership organisation with no government funding. To join see www.artfund.org.

8 Postrel, op. cit., p. 162.

9 See my article, 'Money talks, preference walks: who should assume responsibility for decisions about choice, culture, power and better healthcare?', *The Cerner Quarterly*, 4(2), 2008, pp. 52–9.

10 For krankenkassen ('sick funds'), see www.krankenkasseninfo.de.

15

Between the data and the deep blue sea

'For we wrestle not against flesh and blood, but against principalities, against powers.'

– EPHESIANS, V1, 12

'There is no truth, Saving in thine own heart.'

– WB YEATS

Information in the NHS too often occupies a secret space. It is too little revealed in the interests of the patient. It is not the immense flywheel that it could be in driving the democratic institutions of the civil state. It is not generally intended to empower.

There is too little useful published feedback on outcomes and the patient's experience. We know little of the effectiveness of individual clinical teams. But if we want patients to collaborate more effectively, then consumer understanding of what is happening or might happen and why is a necessity. We need to know about specific clinical outcomes, morbidity, survival rates and patient experiences. If we can also link information to incentives – for the individual patient and the clinician – we can significantly impact on care and results. Notably, in the enormous challenge of chronic care.

These ideas challenge the idea that somehow sickness is outside the control of the individual. That methods of treatment are limited and well defined. That treatment decisions must be filtered by 'experts'. Indeed, new technologies and the explosion of information concerning diagnosis, treatments and results on the net have demolished these assumptions. As John C Goodman (President of the National Center for Policy Analysis in Dallas) has noted, 'The information reality is that patients are becoming as informed as their doctors – not about how to practice medicine but about how the practice of medicine can benefit *them*.'[1]

The first point is that we want real information, and not just 'data' which only 'experts' can understand. Information should be published to facilitate choice, and not merely be collected for internal management purposes. For, as we have seen, choice *means* comparisons. It means risks. It means trade-offs. It means our personal values guiding our decisions. It means accepting that people may make decisions which we may not make for ourselves. It means good information, instead of its denial so as to manage demand. Information and knowledge are the essential levers if choice is to work for the individual. It is a condition of effective choice that there is a variety of providers, too, from which to select a preference. There needs to be extra capacity for choices to be real. Who then is to decide what is an appropriate or 'informed' choice?

Will we be allowed to make a choice which 'experts' might not make for themselves, but which is legal and possible? What will count as an 'unhealthy' expectation? Who decides who decides?

In the wider world we speak of 'comparing favourably with', and of estimating similarities. We judge positive and negative qualities. We compare and contrast, and express our specific preferences and values by the decisions we make. We do so in self-responsibility. Yet in health and social services we are too often in the dark. Inappropriate variation in clinical practice, unexpected and unexplained variation, remains a dark corner. Information is about benefits, risk and discovery. Yet there is so little information, for example, about the performance of individual doctors, clinical teams, or social services. We hear of the volume of work done. We do not hear of what works and what doesn't. We find it hard to judge the efficiency and effectiveness of services, or their safety. We do not normally have this information in advance of agreeing on a course of treatment, with a particular provider, with a particular medical team.

There is no public score-board and no tally of the things that matter most, which are outcomes and the patient's experiences. NHS data is politically constructed, and in those forms it is generally meaningless to patients. There needs to be transparency for open markets. We need a revolution of information, which modern IT is now equipped to deliver. We need information on the quality of diagnosis and treatments, outcomes and impacts. We need information on physicians, GPs, costs – remembering, too, that in open markets the lowest-cost provider is likely to be the most efficient and the best quality. Without full data professionals, too, find it hard to make comparisons and to improve. The vertical integration of the NHS – with government or its agents as single-payer, insurer, purchaser and provider – has disabled genuine information and its use. This is a necessary consequence of government setting funding levels and prices, controlling coverage and benefits, and rationing the processes for delivering care.

We cannot choose a doctor or a hospital treatment based on public, audited, open information on the quality of care we are likely to receive. We cannot evaluate a 'care-plan'. There is no link for practitioners between their incomes and their audited practice. 'Stars' awarded to NHS institutions by government do not tell us anything on how well intended results were attained for individual patients and their improved health. The information just beginning to be published by PCTs about GP performance needs to become more informative, too. We need to know about the patients' experiences. And about variations in referral rates. And about diagnostic patterns. Here, late diagnosis is important. It is sometimes due to reluctance by a patient to see a doctor at all. But hospital doctors know which GPs seem not be performing well in getting diagnosis right, and referring promptly. They see people referred by some GPs much too late. We need to find ways to formalise this knowledge. We know something about volume. But we do not know very much about primary care practice. Some of these GP practices are now very large. The people in them vary, in their skills and approach. We need specific information related to individual practitioners, and not a generalised league table. We should, too, not just collect and publish the information which is easy to get. We need the knowledge which is harder to find, and to measure and explain. Then, once this is published, people must have a choice of primary care practice and of a specific GP. This would be effected by the PGCA. On all this we need specific information, in clear English – and in clear, ethnic languages, too – in terms which patients will find useful and relevant. We should link scientific data and clinical comment with patients' expectations and experiences on what they most value. We need information on quality and also – but not only – on costs. What patients say about quality is central to the objectives.

The deficits of present information are significant – both for service-users seeking to make informed choices, and also for purchasers and for medical practitioners themselves. User groups strive to counteract what has been deliberately managed ignorance. But we need a national Disclosure and Information Commission to drive these changes forward in a competitive market. For patients and for managers, there remain systemic and fundamental gaps in publzic knowledge. Of both medical data, outcomes, experiences, and, also, of the basic financial knowledge of day-by-day operation. These include accounting at the service-line level. These are all deficits that no modern competitive business could possibly sustain. None could survive if there was no clear operational understanding of quality or of the management of revenues and of costs. Nor is information provided by a third of PCTs to general practitioners themselves good enough. The Audit Commission in 2007 found that only about a third of practices rated the quality, format and frequency of information as being good. The Commission for Health Improvement (now the Healthcare Commission) had previously found that some 75% of patients in some PCTs felt that they had not received adequate information about provision locally – including about GP practices. Information was, too, unevenly spread among ethnic groups.[2]

On financial management, Professor Bosanquet has said, 'At present the service is in the anomalous and indefensible position of spending £100 billion without knowing in any detail how it is being spent.' Thus, 'There is an air of unreality about the whole discussion of NHS finances.' Similarly, the information deficits in social care do much to prevent people accessing appropriate and timely services, as Stephen Burke, Chief Executive of Counsel and Care recently emphasised.[3] Generally, the lack of reality is underpinned by financial ignorance – something which could not exist in a market. The service does not know the impact of enormous new sums of money on any specific policy objectives.

In trying to find and to use information in order to make personal choices both consumers and medical practitioners are thus too often, indeed, caught between the devil and the deep blue sea. We may have two (or more) courses of action, but each may be dangerous. There may indeed be a safe harbour, but we have no independent maps when public data is so poor. Then indeed the devil may take the hindmost. Or, as Dr Johnson, wrote, 'To be tax'd, and beaten, is the devil.'

Ignorance no accident

Consumer ignorance in 'public services' is no accident. It is no surprise that exercising choice based on the limited information about the comparable performance of public service providers is far from straightforward. Indeed, it has been a prerequisite of the NHS and an integral result of its entirely artificial processes of rationing, deficit and denial, of deterring informed demand since the sources of funding have been so limited – and so narrowly based. The larger and more concentrated the state, the less there will be informed customers. It is no surprise that public information is so poor. It has been a *requirement* of a rationed system. It no shock, either, that special interests holding power over us suggest that measurement is too complex for 'ordinary' people to understand. Meanwhile, we have more information about the quality and price of breakfast foods than we do about doctors and hospitals. It may be the case that some elements of performance (such as what counts as an appropriate outcome?) may be difficult to define, measure and compare. And that professional, political and lay ideas of successful outcomes may differ. Performance measures, too, where they exist, may not enable users to consider alternatives easily. They may be very technical. But this is where advice and counselling comes in. Of course it is true that people vary in their tolerance and acceptance of risk. And the information available may be of no help to the individual seeking to consider the risk to which he or she is open, given their own circumstances. But we have already seen what we want the data to tell, and the incentives necessary to ensure that measurement and publication actually happens. Research, too, shows that better patient information (and emotional support) can lead to shorter stays, less medication, fewer adverse side-effects, better 'compliance', and higher levels of satisfaction.[4]

We should contrast the denial of information about 'public services' with the proliferation of information in the wider economy. We should consider its purposes, too. And its results. The difficulties that the poor and the weak experience in accessing NHS and social services is one of the most marked characteristics of 'public services' which were intended to help them most. In open markets, by contrast, there are direct incentives to serve everyone as well as possible. In addition, in open markets, managers cannot evade the real rules of economic life. Yet in the NHS, many managements spending millions of public pounds have no incentive to provide the data that users want, or to take any interest in doing so. They also still lack such simple systems for monitoring results as profit and loss accounts. They do not have monthly and quarterly monitoring of costs and revenues, nor estimates of the value added by additional employees. There is not sufficient knowledge of margins and of other such basic management factors – as was recently pointed out by Reform.[5] NHS hospitals, for example, do not know how well services have impacted on their patients, for these are not tracked over time – not even on a sample basis.

By contrast, it is a truism – but still true – that in open markets producers survive by gathering and spreading information. They seek to inform consumers. They depend on reputation. They manage knowledge of what they are providing, and what customers think of it. 'Branding' is one important guide to what consumers can expect. This is why there is such investment in its defence, and promotion. Its success reflects decisions that other unknown consumers have made, cumulatively and over time. Independent third-party appraisals are an important element. So, too, is word of mouth. Each guides the decisions of others. Markets have discovered and evolved genuine guidance for consumers to make sovereign decisions of their own. Firms which flourish are those that produce goods and services which people want, like, tell others about and which they are prepared to pay for. Those who do not do so vanish. Markets, too, empower the silent and not merely the politically active. 'Voice' is most effectively achieved by 'choice', whereas in the NHS we are offered these by many as alternatives. Of course, neither choice nor voice can remove all uncertainties. These exist in every case, in the minds of every doctor and patient, and there are no certainties about treatments or outcomes. We have to make individual decisions for ourselves. But this does not mean we should be without the guidance of public data.

Reputation a vital guide

The success of informed markets in meeting the wishes of consumers is a reality in all our lives. This historical truth is not invalidated by the idea that in any market there will necessarily be some asymmetries of knowledge. People compensate for this in many ways – by study, by paying for advice, by consulting advocacy services, by reading *Which?*, by listening to word-of-mouth and reputation or by going online. Informed markets have changed all of our lives, and go on doing so. They have this capacity in healthcare, too, if we would only let them do so. This is the case even though statists still wish to suggest that somehow modern consumption is a conspiracy against the 'real interests' of the 'falsely conscious' consumer. That somehow all advertising is deceptive, all promotion a swindle, all satisfactions a con. It is striking, however, that the removal of centralised tyrannies in societies based on these preconceptions always results in individuals wishing to become customers.

As Virginia Postrel shows,

> As soon as the Taliban fell men lined up at barbershops to have their beards shaved off. Women painted their nails with once-forbidden polish. Formerly clandestine beauty salons opened in prominent locations. Men traded postcards of beautiful Indian movie stars, and thronged to buy imported TVs, VCRs, and videotapes. Even burka merchants diversified their wares, adding colors like brown, peach, and green to the blue and off-white dictated by the Taliban's whip-wielding virtue police. Freed to travel to city markets, village women demanded better fabric, finer embroidery, and more variety in their traditional garments. ... Liberation is supposed to be about grave matters: elections, education, a free press. But Afghans acted as though superficial things were just as important. As a political commentator noted: 'The right to shave may be found in no international treaty or covenant, but it has, in Afghanistan, become one of the first freedoms to which claim is being laid.'[6]

These examples are not trivial. As Postrel shows, they challenged many widely held assumptions about aesthetic value. They also open up fundamental questions about information, preference and self-realisation. By contrast, in the NHS the lack of information in forms which the layperson can understand and consider is deliberate. It misunderstands or misplaces the wishes of the consumer. It clearly hinders the test of predictability. That is, of the user being able to find out about the likely effects of a service in advance. As I will show in my chapter '*My* body, but *your* decision? 'Concordat', and shared decision making', on 'concordance' between doctors and patients, there is in shared decision making and in the use of decision aids still a structure of highly restrictive practices among healthcare professionals. Especially so in the limited sharing of information and knowledge, including that necessary respect for the special knowledge which only patients bring to the situation.

Discovery, only by chance

Too often, discovering any information that the individual may believe to be necessary information has been a matter of chance. For example, consultations with people caring for an elderly or a disabled relative in Birmingham identified lack of information about what help might be available to them. This has been pointed out as one of the most significant problems.[7] This matters even if we accept the distinction between 'search goods' (which can be tested before purchase, like cars) and 'experience goods' (such as holidays, or medical treatments, on which a judgement about satisfaction is necessarily retrospective). For we do want to know what happened to other patients 'like me'. As we have seen, we know from the work of RG Evans, ML Barer, R Marmot and others that participation in active decision making improves outcomes.[8]

Yet as Dr Marian Barnes and David Prior rightly say,

> Access to any service depends on knowing that it exists, that it is relevant, and that one is entitled to use it. Choice between services depends on having such information about different options, and on having additional information about significant differences

between services in terms of their essential characteristics, and/or effectiveness of their performance.

As to available options, these are enlarged by competition, and by more effective purchasing. Similarly, alternatives which people feel will meet their case are also stimulated. As to experience in choosing, this is in part about learning to choose, in part about the evolution of assistance and advocacy. Barnes and Prior recognise this in 'the world confronted by impermanence, ambivalence and diversity'. As they say, 'Individuals are faced with the need to choose all the time: it is a condition of being in the contemporary world'. Giddens says that 'we have no choice but to choose'.[9]

Publication drives quality

A special issue of *Economic Affairs* concerned with pharmaceuticals and government policy recently demonstrated that restrictions in information and services contradict the rhetoric of the NHS about access and equality and indeed remain a strong feature of it.[10] In addition, as I outlined earlier, when government confers benefits on a special interest, the recipients are a relatively small group in society. They are better informed. But the costs of such benefits are spread widely, thinly, and over the population as a whole. One result is that a few have a powerful incentive to lobby intensively, but the many usually do not bother to inform themselves about it, or to take any actions. This is one of the reasons for consumer ignorance in public services, for which the consumer is usually falsely blamed. As so often, when evidence replaces faith and assertion we learn to choose. One argument often made in the past has been that publishing clinical data will lead to patient selection, with doctors tackling only simpler challenges. Recent data suggests that this is not the case. And that publication drives quality and does not lead to patient selection.[11]

Dr Nigel Beasley, a Consultant ENT Surgeon and the National Clinical Lead for Hospital Doctors in the NHS, has powerfully put the case that the use of new electronic information systems is making a radical difference.[12]

This book urges that we need to connect direct incentives to these technologies. These offer data for action. Data which is alive, living, real, useable and current. It is essential that we use this data appropriately, and that we work with patient-defined values. For, as Dr Beasley has noted, the NHS's own Health Modernisation Agency (now closed) said three years ago that in terms of modernisation the NHS was not succeeding, either horizontally or vertically. There was poor integration. The service was good at introducing pilots but poor at spreading their adoption. National leaders were more optimistic about change than frontline staff. There was limited strategic cooperation. Projects were under-conceptualised, and often lacking in reflection and analysis.[13] However, improvements in IT are making a large contribution in improvement and change. For example, the 'Publication of cardiac surgery mortality data in the UK has been associated with decreased risk adjusted mortality . . . .'[14]

But, as ever, the challenge is not just about technical competence. It is cultural. Clinical leadership, for or against change, was and is critical. Clinicians, alongside others, need to consider how to improve their performance. This can be centrally led, with specific goals for formal structures. Or the service can look to the 'social movement' approach, to release energy from the bottom up. It is important that clinicians are leaders. Incentives are an important part of the picture.

It was and is essential to motivate people to be more aware of their practice, and to self-examine and self-assess as well as to be audited in a marketplace. But we need more. We need people not only to change, but to welcome change and to lead it and be its champion. This is, in part, to answer the question 'What's in it for me?' It is, too, to try to achieve change 'with people' rather than 'to people'. An important aspect here is that people should be helped to see that *their* motivations and *their* outcomes will be more readily achieved by changes, as Pat Natale stressed.

Since new IT has a pivotal role and very particular potential, involving clinicians in the design of the IT framework for analysing practice and encouraging change locally is critical to local ownership. The best local prompter (or the most intractable obstructer) is likely to be a respected local clinician working in partnership with managers (and the Trust Chairman!). In my model of individual financial empowerment he/she will be encouraged to act positively both by changing economic realities as well as by clinical perceptions of better practices. This is not only about boundaries, but also about convergence. Here good feedback is crucial. The necessary information has to be as close to real-time as possible. Clear definitions of evidence that matters and a system of immediate challenge and comparative frontline audits – for example, of drug usage, and of clinical pathways – on a regular and frequent basis are persuasive elements in terms of lived experiences. For example, if a clinician or a nurse is evidently not following an agreed protocol. Meaningful and valid feedback, which is seen as relevant to those doing the jobs and which chimes with their individual values, is clearly motivating. This means having the latest information, and in real time – using it for better management.

Persistent reinforcement of change is also necessary – using direct incentives and public information for accountability. Otherwise, we roll stones uphill and they roll back again, since old habits die hard, if at all.[15]

New IT shows that people can be moved in several different ways. Technically, yes, but also and crucially in terms of their emotions and values. And by economic and social incentives. The data must be perceived by clinicians as valid if it is to motivate them to change practice. In addition, it takes time to persuade people that data is credible. Here, its source and timeliness are vital to its perceived validity. Benchmarking, too, improves the meaningfulness of data and its feedback. When the data is in hand, leading physicians can enhance this effectiveness both in feedback and in shifting practices. Persistence matters, too. For feedback must insist and persist if we are to sustain improved performance. IT systems achieve this rapid feedback in ways which paper-based systems did not. They also offer the prospect of transferring leadership across the organisation. The key clinical values and drivers must be better, safe care and a culture of constant improvement owned by the staff. Here, permission to change is essential for the encouragement of local variation, the focus on a better patient experience and better outcomes.[16] It is, however, vital to decide *with* patients what is to be measured, and why.

Official websites and a Quality Chartbook

However, alas, open access to reliable data is still evaded or suppressed. There is little or no guidance on quality. Indeed, there is little investment in its measurement.[17] There is, as I have said, no coherent guide to the individual performance of doctors, or of their clinical teams and their outcome records, although some surgeons like the heart specialist Ben Bridgewater in Manchester advocate publication.[18] Patient literature meanwhile is inadequate. Official websites – such as NHS Choices – are not designed to fully inform users. It is surely inconceivable that if service-users did control funds, and if they joined together in cooperative mutual purchasing organisations, then no such information deficits could exist for long. It is the neglect of free choice which has allowed official providers to evade the key responsibility of knowing who does what well, who is best, who needs help, retraining or discipline, and of having to inform us. Yet, in my experience, every doctor knows to whom they would not send their daughter. As I pointed out earlier, this informal information is usually locally based and well-founded. But it is not public information. Middle-class people can sometimes get access to such local knowledge, which is again one of the class biases of the system.

Recently, a standard academic assessment of the quality of care in England highlighted how poor much data still remains. A number of other authorities have said the same thing, including the government's own Health Commission, and the Picker Institute of Europe, as well as Sir Derek Wanless, the former adviser to Mr Gordon Brown. A chorus of others have drawn attention to poor data, too, such as Dr Andrew Vallance-Owen, Medical Director and a leading figure in healthcare debates from the insurer BUPA. So, too, the respected information consultant Dr Anna Donald, and Vanessa Bourne (a former Chairman of The Patient's Association), and Ruth Thorlby (of the King's Fund).

A standard periodic academic assessment of the quality of care offered in England is *A Quality Chartbook: patient and public experience in the NHS*, by Professor Sheila Leatherman and Kim Sutherland.[19] The most recent report showed much neglect of involving patients in decisions about their care, and about self-care. In UK primary care only 29% reported that their doctor had told them about treatment choices, and asked their opinion. Drawing on the Health Care commission's large-scale surveys in England they showed that only half of inpatients and 40% of people with mental health problems were fully involved in decisions about their care.

The government publication *Our Choices in Mental Health: a framework for improving choice for people who use mental health services* was explicit about necessary choices and their support.[20] However, Leatherman and Sutherland reported that fewer than half of inpatients surveyed indicated that danger signals and medication side-effects were explained to them before discharge. In diabetes care both well coordinated and improved self-care is a key intervention to help improve good glycaemia control. Yet only 10% indicated that they had participated in education and training programmes. Of those who had not participated, the vast majority had not been offered the opportunity to do so. The fragmentation of diabetes care is already well known to be a cause of serious consequences including death and disability, as well as higher costs.

Second, the Picker Institute, which runs the Advice Centre for the NHS Patient Survey programme for the government (strapline: 'Making patients' views count'), recently dismissed as 'hollow' the rhetoric of the NHS about becoming 'patient-centred' (itself a very vague term). Its report, *Is the NHS Becoming More Patient-Centred?*, noted that the number of patients who said they were closely involved in decisions on their care has fluctuated by only 1% from 2002–06. There was, too, 'a worrying deterioration' in the availability of hospital staff, despite the unprecedented new investment. Some 22% of patients in 2006 were unable to find a member of staff with whom to discuss their concerns. This was an increase of 5% from 2002.[21] Hardly possible in an open market?

Dr Anna Donald, co-founder of health information provider Bazian, recently wrote: 'Patient websites are seldom designed to meet the average levels of functional literacy.' The DoH's own flagship NHS Choices website – in which £15 million was invested and which since July 2007 has given patients some limited clinical and service information to help with decisions on where to have treatment and with which GP to register – was itself criticised for massive inaccuracies.[22]

Dr Angela Coulter, European Head of the Picker Institute, believes that the huge demand for information is 'largely unmet and what there is does not gear itself to the demands of the patient'. Information on two official websites, NHS Choices and NHS Direct, tends, too, to be 'didactic, rather old-fashioned and paternalistic', instead of recognising patient's roles in making decisions about their healthcare. Vanessa Bourne, head of special projects at The Patients Association (and a former Chairman as well as an influential figure in the National Association of Health Authorities and Trusts, predecessor of the NHS Confederation) thought that the NHS Choices website 'does not answer the questions that patients want to ask – it answers questions that the service thinks patients ought to want to ask.'[23]

Again, we hit the submerged rocks of the culture. Yet we know that good information and educational resources can be highly beneficial both in terms of supporting autonomy and in terms of clinical and social outcomes.[24] There is, of course, some very good general news; for example, in positive improvements in cardio-thoracic surgery and care. But the 'ordinary' patient has difficulty in knowing which doctor does best. Some GPs advise. But the reports already quoted here are not encouraging on that count.[25] Sir Derek Wanless, in a retrospective review of his two earlier reports for the government, decried the continuing failure to collect data and to measure quality. Nigel Edwards, of the NHS Confederation, emphasised this.[26]

One key area is basic safety. This is a major issue and of great concern. The Chief Executive of the Health Commission, Anne Walker, called for all health and social care providers to publish comparable data and information on safety and quality. The Medical Director of BUPA, Dr Andrew Vallance-Owen, called for more. In January 2007 the Healthcare Commission was critical, too, of the quality of clinical data available from the Independent Sector Treatment Sectors with which the NHS contracted.[27] Both the NHS and the private sector should provide data measuring clinical outcomes and success rates, to allow patients to make informed 'real choices'. To do so, agreed definitions for performance indicators were necessary. The government commissioned a feasibility study on this in 2005, *but it has not been published.*[28] The NHS's own information partner, the Dr Foster Intelligence organisation, in a report accompanying its 2007 hospital guide *How Healthy is Your Hospital?*, said that 'The NHS currently lacks measures of patient safety that allow national and local comparisons.'[29] Yet the National Patient Safety Agency *Safety First* report acknowledged that the National Reporting and Learning System is receiving 60,000 incident reports a month, even though there had been other improvements.[30]

As we see, NHS data has never been gathered and published in order to facilitate choice. Indeed, until Mr Blair and Mr Milburn pushed the 'choice agenda' forward – and against great resistance from special interests – choice and thus enhanced and knowing demand was discouraged. It could only make life more difficult for managers. Instead, data on volume (but not on quality) was only collected as a historical, reflective exercise, rather than as 'real-time' information to be actively used as a key management tool to drive progress and performance. In an open, competitive system, live and current data would be a necessary key lifeline.

What of primary care and our knowledge of its work? We know much less than we would like. Health Secretary Alan Johnson has made the improvement of primary care and access a priority.[31] However, Ruth Thorlby, King's Fund Health Policy Fellow, has pointed out that there is very little data on important aspects of primary care, considering all the millions of GP appointments.[32] Evaluating the London pilot choice project on elective care, The King's Fund, the City University and the RAND Foundation found that patients wanted to choose hospitals on the basis of quality care, but there was too little data. Patients wanted results at the level of the individual clinician or clinical firm.[33] The National Patient Safety Agency also criticised information as the basis of choice presently offered to patients – on MRSA rates, hospital food and how hospitals manage risk – as 'meaningless' to the general public.[34] The rigorous development of the government's pivotal policy of 'payment by results' project has also been restricted by what one commentator called 'the paucity of information systems'.[35] The multi-billion pound centralising NHS IT strategy is still some years from full operation. And it is not intended to measure quality. Nor will service-users control the data. The Institute for Public Policy Research spoke out in March 2007 concerning secrecy about unsafe hospitals and poor quality.[36] Yet the problem of variation in quality and of erratic medical practice and clinical error, too, is profound. Indeed, it is one of the biggest priorities facing care services.

Finding information

The figures we do have indicate the difficulties the NHS has in spreading best practice, even when we have the publication of revealing figures. There is, however, some effort now being made to try to discover patient satisfaction and the impact of NHS interventions in terms of quality, or well-being. This must surely depend on capturing what patients say about their experiences, and about results over time. In 2005 the Office of National Statistics set up a new Centre for the Management of Government Activity to measure output, periodicity and quality. But it found immediately that there is little data available and existing information is not useable concerning quality. It only measures activity and does not take into account quality changes and improvement.[37] There are, however, overseas examples which are part of the necessary guidance for change in the UK. From 2007 all hospitals in the USA were reporting on a consistent set of measures for patient satisfaction and some common care outcomes.[38] The British healthcare insurer and provider BUPA has long used patient-reported surveys to measure quality, and has the largest database in Europe, of 100,000 patient records. The Centre for Health Economics, York, NICE and the DoH are now using this data to model output in terms of quality change and patient satisfaction.[39] Thus far, however, the information guides no British patients in terms of current and future decisions they may make. For example, unlike many outcome information initiatives in the USA, there are no public website tools using this information to guide consumers.

In the dark as we are concerning performance, it is a surprise perhaps that the US research organisation the Commonwealth Fund has ranked the NHS the best in the English-speaking world in terms of value for money (but *not* in actual service provision).[40] However, the healthcare press and daily media regularly cites such deficits as poor cancer care; one in five patients leaving hospital malnourished; lengthy hospital waiting times; inadequate public health outcomes; MRSA and hospital-acquired infections/avoidable deaths.[41] In such a picture the importance of much better information to help patients take the best available pathways is of great concern.

Here, a wise comment by Geoff Mulgan concerning policies and programmes seems to me to be apposite and fundamental:

> If we cannot be certain that a system is trustworthy, that our principles are universally applicable, or that our chosen means will deliver the desired ends, then it follows that we should always favour the coexistence of more than one system over just one, however perfect and appealing it may seem. The coexistence of more than one system reduces

the scope for damage when things go wrong; it makes a society better able to adjust to unforeseen circumstances; it creates competition between systems, a competition that should be philosophical as much as economic, forcing each to live up to its ideals, or to adapt; and it gives the individual or group a degree of philosophical choice about the right ways to live and work. . . . Such a pluralism brings with it a distinctive idea of what the state is for. Rather than applying uniform rational principles, its task becomes one of overseeing the balance between systems, redistributing resources and creating the conditions for a variety of groups and institutions to organise themselves. Rather than engaging in social engineering (the old mechanistic metaphor), the state's legitimate task becomes one of creating the space for social experiment.[42]

The intention here is thus not to set out a holistic blueprint. It is instead to endorse the encouragement of balancing forces, of countervailing powers, of choices to prompt a transformation by shifting structures, by adaptive balances, by avoiding any notion of finality. Or, in EF Schumacher's terms, of encouraging the social necessity of a much better mix of 'stability and change, tradition and innovation, public interest and private interest, planning and laissez faire, order and freedom, growth and decay'.[43]

Liberal economics

If we want good information, if we want better outcomes, if we want individual and self-responsible choice, we need to take much more seriously the insights of liberal economics. For here there is no sheltering from the informed public. The economist Professor Colin Robinson, introducing volume 4 of *The Collected Works of Arthur Seldon*, summarised Seldon's illuminating approach to these problems:

Seldon's main and recurring argument is that non-market provision, financed by taxpayers, leads to a fatal disconnection between suppliers and consumers. Suppliers do not depend directly on consumers for payment and therefore have no reason to discover what consumers want, to provide for existing demands, or to innovate to meet the demands of the future. Furthermore, because suppliers do not face any competition, efficiency standards set by rivals do not exist. Consumers see a price at zero at the point of service delivery, and so their demands inevitably expand far beyond what they would have been had they been charged the full cost of the service. In the absence of any price mechanism, the mismatch between supply and demand is not automatically corrected, and thus the state must resort to rationing by a bureaucracy insulated from the market, which, over time, develops a high-handed attitude toward those it is supposed to serve, regarding them as supplicants rather than as valuable customers.[44]

Seldon also considered alternative funding mechanisms to taxation: he advocated a reduction of taxation, and with tax transfers to the poor to enable all to pay charges or insurance contributions at market levels. He also considered tax rebates, subsidies, cash grants to consumers, and vouchers. His analysis can be found in the studies collected as volume 4 of his Collected Works, *Introducing Market Forces into 'Public' Services*.[45] The individual sum spent for each citizen on the NHS now amounts to some £2000 per annum, which would rapidly establish a very handsome HSA. We could also pass funds (or tax transfers, for the poor) back to individuals, and purchasers could then compete for these funds.[46]

Here, Dr Anna Donald recently wrote:

A reform that would make the NHS easier to run is to divide the whole thing into one insurer-gatekeeper and many provider units. In most countries, this division of labour is normal: a national insurance body makes decisions about what mostly will be covered, while local providers deliver care with reasonable degrees of flexibility. The NHS is unusual in that insurer and provider functions are still carried out at all levels, so frontline workers sometimes make on-the-spot coverage decisions. This is like your mechanic having to mend your car and deciding whether your insurance should pay for it. Such an old-fashioned arrangement, a legacy from the NHS's pre-war origins, is inefficient and inequitable, resulting in postcode lotteries. Sorting it out would make the whole system easier to manage.[47]

Meanwhile, it is one of the most critical consequences of a non-priced, rationed, 'expert' and centralised system of controls that the public information on quality and clinical performance and the outcomes of treatments which an open system would publish as an operational necessity is not available. There has been no incentive to gather it. This has had a long-term impact on quality, and on millions of lives. It is one of the great demerits standing in the way of real choice. This huge deficit of data does not, however, hinder NHS representatives from making grand claims. Dame Gill Morgan, Chief Executive of the NHS Confederation, speaks of the NHS as now 'providing fantastic clinical services'.[48] But how do we know? How does the individual and potential user of services know? What are the measures? This is merely rhetoric unrelated to the hard-rock of reality. Who does what well? Who says so? We do not know? Whistling in the dark will not improve the position.

Class, again

Class matters here. It is evident that one of the reasons why the middle classes have done best from the NHS is that they are much better at getting information, both via patient groups, websites, and by formal and informal contacts. Even so, the former Conservative Secretary of State for Health, Stephen Dorrell, was reported to have forbade the use of the word 'choice' (and 'internal market') when conducting his party's latest review of health policy, although he spoke of informed local decision making and criticised years of micro-management by politicians as 'proxy consumers'.[49] The clear implication is that even if his party was in favour of choice, it would be *sotto voce* in order not to frighten voters. And 'choice' would actually mean more power to local government or to elected bodies. However, the role of politics should be to guarantee the discipline of protecting competition, to encourage better provision of services by independent purchasing and otherwise to depoliticise healthcare. This would be achieved by free markets and by good information. Other proposals, such as to run the NHS with an 'independent' board (on the lines of the BBC Governors) will not do this. The only way to take the NHS and social services out of politics is to take them out of the state and into genuine markets.

The most important information is the reporting of outcomes by individuals. Here, patient groups gather experiences, and these are important in guiding some choices. For it is only consumers who can say what worked for them. They are the only ones who experience the services. Their experiences are the most important and definable product of services. It is this knowledge which should inform all processes, to improve outcomes. It is the uncovering of surprising, unexplained and unnoticed variation, too – explaining it when justified, correcting it when not – that is essential, as Dr William Pickering has emphasised.[50]

No doubt services are complex. No doubt measurement is not the answer to everything. No doubt there are methodological problems in measuring outcomes. But without good outcomes, without the knowledge that patients uniquely hold, what do we get for the billions spent? For example, evidence indicates that there is a greater than 10% difference in survival rates for breast cancer between apparently comparable hospitals. Why? What do patients say happened to them? In addition, very many suffer from long-term conditions. How well are they treated? What do they say? In talk of 'patient value', this is what matters.[51]

We need individually financially empowered real choice and incentives to align professionals, patients and opportunities. And we need good published and audited information to optimise comparisons, choice and quality. This needs to be physician-specific and patient-specific. This is in some respects difficult, but it is not impossible. Indeed, in America there are very instructive models which we could follow. The Foundation for Accountability (FACCT) began in 1995 to design programmes to measure the results of care, medical practice and the consumer's experience. The project has been developed, tested and validated for a number of conditions, including breast cancer, diabetes, major depression, asthma, HIV/AIDS, child care and care at the end of life. Nursing homes ratings have been published since 2002. The National Quality Forum is a statutory organisation to develop reporting standards. Most states have published good data, as have several private purchasing consortia. The National Committee for Quality Assurance (NCQA) – an independent agency – publishes a set of some 60 'effectiveness of care' indicators. Online doctor directories include patient ratings, too. Some, such as the Massachusetts Health Quality Partners, are developing methods for evaluating individual physician performance. Care Counsel provides expert advice on nurses to consumers. Consumer's Medical Resource enables consumers to get expert second opinions on their physician's treatment recommendations.[52] We can have it, too, if we really really want it.

Consultation no substitute

Until there is individual, financially empowered choice the NHS seems unlikely to make the necessary investment in publishing good information. Instead, it engages in constant 'consultations' about planning – but wastefully, unresponsively and with little public confidence in the results. One thoughtful senior NHS manager, Sophia Christie (Chief Executive of Birmingham East and North Primary Care Trust) recently wrote:

> Our most likely reason to engage with local people is when we have to do a consultation. Most are initiated as statutory requirements once a decision has been reached. We seek to minimise the scope of consultation and the constant claim is that nothing much is changing and local people will notice no difference, which generally begs the question 'Why bother?'[53]

Formal public meetings only engage the sort of people who like attending formal public meetings. Those trying locally to influence policy were usually unrepresentative. There are those who have the personal and social capital to engage with local health policy and services, to meet for several hours a month in formal settings and to be able to tackle, analyse and articulate challenges to the highly paid, highly educated professionals who run local services. This is a group largely unrepresentative of the majority of the most vulnerable service-users.[54]

And even despite all this effort the NHS does still not invest seriously, systematically, and professionally in consumer research about satisfactions, outcomes and what worked for the individual. If consumers (patients/service-users) controlled individual savings funds this would happen like lightning itself. And it is the improvement of quality and access which is the most fundamental challenge. Here, in its sixtieth year, the NHS still has not taken the single major step towards the proper and unrelenting pivot on patient-defined value and choice by measuring and publishing information in a democracy on risk-adjusted care outcomes. Every organisation should be trying to improve all the time. Why are such deficits still in place in terms of information after 60 years? The NHS does not have the information because it has not been required to do so by competitive pressures. And it does not believe that we *should* have the information because of its ideology. Yet if the knowledge was gathered and issued it would necessarily have the profoundest effects on purchasers and providers, and on what individual customers would accept. Even imperfect measures would be a strong start, with 'good enough' outcomes metrics (to use the jargon) prompting much better metrics.

The public sector borrowing requirement has risen to the level of £43 million for the year 2008–09. This is exerting inflationary pressures on interest rates and on the wider economy, which produces the wealth to pay for state services. Yet, still, as Harry Telser and Peter Zweifel recently noted, 'In the present allocation of resources in healthcare, preferences of consumers as the ultimate financiers of healthcare services are judged to be of little relevance.'[55] This, despite the innovation of personal budgets in social care. The problem was again recognised by the Communities Secretary Hazel Blears MP, who on 5 March 2008 promised a white paper on making local organisations – including the NHS – more accountable. Ms Blears proposed a statutory right to information, but she did not acknowledge that the market would otherwise generate as part of normal life that which bureaucracies conceal.[56] Ms Blears' proposals are not the correct radical solution. Information and the control over money is the only known means by which consumers can control producers. This is why both are held back. If each were available to the consumer the provider would have to satisfy them in order to prosper. Meanwhile, the NHS struggles, in benign paternalism, to provide choice. But until the beginnings of personal budgets those working in the NHS and in social care have fought entirely shy of the only means by which this can be achieved. This is a direct use of economic instruments, but it remains very limited. Similarly, there is more information available than formerly on the Internet, on care and care programmes, and on the accreditation of professionals. But the information is insufficient or ill-cast to help patients choose between treatments and between professionals. As the Picker Institute survey showed, people dislike the limits and they want more choice – particularly the poor.

We need the fullest information to realise the market, together with individual financial empowerment. No detail is too small. No Tarot cards are needed to guide the way. In a world literally spoilt for choice in every other area (save for deficits in state education, which parallel those of the NHS and social care) the egalitarian necessity of focusing on the consumer's experience is not merely theatrical or political. It is fundamental to quality and to improvement. It can be extremely fruitful in therapeutic terms and in terms of endorsing a free society. It will unavailingly become so if the patient controls the money. The alternative is a sterile stability, no quieter a life, and a continuing decline in prospects and standards.

In English-speaking countries in particular there has been a wish and a new moral consensus – if not yet a sufficient instrumental commitment – during three decades of root-and-branch reform to try to put the customer or citizen in charge to reshape public services. But we in England still have no clear, unequivocal and universalised code by which to structure choice in public services. We do not yet have the necessary clarity of language. We have not yet made the necessary commitment to ensure that choice, financial empowerment and the necessary information are *individually* real for everyone, hence much of the interest and importance of the debate. We live in an information society. But where is the information? Markets depend on comparisons. They ensure that we have the information. State-run services and 'quasi-markets' do not.

Notes

1 John C Goodman, 'Designing health insurance for the information age', in Herzlinger, *Consumer-driven Health Care*, op. cit., Chapter 11, pp. 224–41; see also JC Goodman and GL Musgrave, *Patient Power: solving America's health care crisis* (Washington, D.C., Cato Institute, 1992).

2 Audit Commission, *Putting Commissioning Into Practice: implementing practice based commissioning through good financial management* (London, Audit Commission, 2007); Commission for Health Improvement, *What CHI has found in: primary care trusts* (London, CHI, 2004).

3 Stephen Burke and Cathie Williams, 'Coded message', *The Guardian*, Society section, 5 March 2008, p. 6.

4 SE Levitan, *Providing Emotional Support: Picker/Commonwealth Report* (Boston, Beth Israel Hospital, Winter 1992), 1. See also Chilingerian, op. cit., p. 448.

5 N Bosanquet, A Haldenby and H Rainbow, *NHS Reform*, op. cit., pp. 28, 51–2.

6 Postrel, *Substance*, op. cit., pp. ix–x. See also Peter Beaumont, 'Iran's young women find private path to freedom', *The Observer*, 16 March 2008, pp. 42–3.

7 Older people in Fife, too, who were involved in a project to explore their experiences of growing older and using services intended to enable them to stay living at home also highlighted lack of information and efforts to access it and services and an 'uphill struggle', or 'a fight'. 'Having exhausted their energies simply trying to find out what is available, people may feel little inclination to seek information about alternatives, or to question solutions which are offered.' M Barnes and G Wistow, 'Consulting with carers: what do they think?', *Social Services Research*, 1, 1992, pp. 9–30. I owe the reference to Marian Barnes and David Prior, 'Spoilt for Choice? How Consumerism can Disempower Public Service Users', *Public Money and Management*, July–September 1995, 15(3), pp. 53–8.

8 See RG Evans, ML Barer and R Marmot, *Why Are Some People Healthy and Others Not?* (New York, Aldine de Gruyter, 1994). Also, R Marmot *et al.*, 'Contribution of job control and other risk factors to social variations in coronary heart disease incidence', *The Lancet*, 350, 1997, pp. 235–9; Michael Marmot, *Status Syndrome* (London, Bloomsbury, 2004); Bruno S Frey and Alois Sutzer, 'Happiness, economy and institutions', *Economic Journal*, Royal Economic Society, 110, 127, October, 2000, pp. 9128–38. I owe the last two references to Geoff Mulgan, *Good and Bad Power: the ideals and betrayals of good government* (London, Allen Lane, 2006; Penguin Books edition, 2007), p. 71.

9 Anthony Giddens, *Modernity and Self-Identity* (Cambridge, Polity Press, 1991), p. 81. The classic statement is, of course, Isaiah Berlin, *Four Essays on Liberty* (London, Oxford University Press, 1969). Also Barnes and Prior, 'Spoilt for Choice?', op. cit.

10 *Economic Affairs*, 26(3), September 2006. Guest editor, Tony Hockley of the LSE.

11 Ben Bridgewater *et al.*, 'Has the publication of cardiac surgery outcome data been associated with changes in practice in Northwest England?', *Heart*, January 2007. See also Ben Bridgewater *et al.*, 'Surgeon specific mortality in adult cardiac surgery: comparison between crude risk and stratified data', *British Medical Journal*, 5 July 2003, 327, pp. 13–17; Ben Bridgewater *et al.*, 'Mortality data in adult cardiac surgery for named surgeons: retrospective examination of prospectively collected data on coronary artery surgery and aortic valve replacement', *British Medical Journal*, March 2005, 330, pp. 506–10.

12 Nigel Beasley, 'Managing in the UK Health Economy', address to the Leadership Forum convened by the Cerner Corporation at Great Fosters, Egham, Surrey, on 20 May 2008.

13 Paul Bate, Helen Bevan, and Robert G Bevan, '*Towards a Million Change Agents*'. A Review of the Social Movements Literature: implications for large-scale change in the NHS (London, NHS Modernisation Agency, 2004).

14 Ben Bridgewater, Antony D Grayson, Nicholas Brooks, Geir Grotte, Brian M Fabri, John Au, Tim Hooper, Mark Jones and Bruce Keogh, 'Has the publication of cardiac survey outcome data been associated with changes in practice in north west England: an analysis of 25 730 patients undergoing CABG surgery under 30 surgeons over eight years', *Heart*, 19 January 2007, 93, pp. 744–8. See also MR Ward and B Bridgewater, 'Implications of publishing surgical results', *Heart*, 11 September 2007, 93, p. 1136; FL Grover, Joseph C Cleveland Jr., and Laurie W Shroyer, 'Quality Improvements in Cardiac Surgery', *Archives of Surgery*, 137(1), 1 January 2002, pp. 28–36.

15 JM Eisenberg, *Doctors' Decisions and the Cost of Medical Care* (Ann Abor, Mich., Health Administration Press, 1986), pp. 116–17; also, Millenson, op. cit., p. 553.

16 See also EH Bradley, ES Holmboe, JA Mattera, MJ Radford, and HM Krumholz, 'Data feedback efforts in quality improvement: lessons learned from US hospitals, *Qual Safe Health Care*, 2004, 13; pp. 26–31; T Greenhalgh,

K Stramer, T Bratan, E Byrne, J Russell, Y Mohammad, G Wood, and S Hinder, *Summary Care Record, Early Adopter Programme: an independent evaluation by University College, London* (London, University College, 2008); Chris Ham, *Integrating NHS Care: lessons from the front-line* (London, Nuffield Trust, 2008). I owe these references to Nigel Beasley.

17 A recent study showed that the public would like to know more about the quality and range of NHS work but current sources of information do not enable them to make assessments. Instead, information is provider-led. Martin Marshall, Jenny Noble, Helen Davies, Heather Waterman and Kieran Walshe, 'Development of an information source for patients and the public about general practice services: an action research study', *Health Expectations*, 9(3), September 2006, pp. 265–74.

18 Ben Bridgewater, 'Why doctors' outcomes should be published in the press', *British Medical Journal*, 19 November 2005, 331.

19 Sheila Leatherman and Kim Sutherland, *A Quality Chartbook: patient and public experience in the NHS* (London, The Health Foundation, 2007).

20 Department of Health, *Our Choices in Mental Health: a framework for improving choice for people who use mental health services* (London, Department of Health, 6 November 2006).

21 Angela Coulter *et al.*, *Is the NHS Becoming More Patient-Centred?* (Oxford, Picker Institute, 2007). See also A. Coulter *et al.*, *Assessing the Quality of Information to Support People in Making Decisions about Their Health and Healthcare* (Oxford, Picker Institute, 2006).

22 'Massive inaccuracies mar GP patient choice website', *Health Service Journal*, 9 August 2007, p. 5.

23 Alison Moore, 'When will NHS digital dreams become a reality for patients?', *Health Service Journal*, 16 August 2007, pp. 12–13.

24 Anna Donald, 'On consumer information', *Health Service Journal*, 31 May 2007, p. 15.

25 Paul Robinson, 'Outcomes improve in cardiology', *Health Service Journal*, 31 May 2007, p. 16.

26 Sir Derek Wanless, John Appleby, Anthony Harrison, and Darshan Patel, *Our Future Health Secured? A Review of NHS funding and performance* (London, King's Fund, September 2007); Nigel Edwards, 'The NHS wasted its big chance: will it learn from its mistakes?', *Health Service Journal*, 20 September 2007, pp. 14–15.

27 Helen Mooney, 'Data on ISTC's clinical quality is "extremely poor", finds probe', *Health Service Journal*, 18 January 2007, p. 5.

28 Helen Mooney, 'Call for comparable data across care services', *Health Service Journal*, 20 September 2007, p. 12.

29 Dr Foster Intelligence, *How Healthy is Your Hospital?* (London, Dr Foster Intelligence, 2007).

30 Victoria Vaughan, 'Johnson wants competition to prop up poor GP access', *Health Service Journal*, 26 July 2007, p. 5. The National Patient Safety Study Agency into avoidable patient deaths estimated the number as between 800 and 34,000 a year. This is an extraordinarily vague assessment, partly attributed to staff reluctance to admit to various forms of medical error. Dr Pickering's call for unannounced inspections and a regulator able to call for any clinical notes at any time is instead the right call. The Confidential Enquiry into Maternal and Child Health, in its seventh report in 2007, was 'struck by the number of healthcare professionals who failed to identify and manage common medical conditions or potential emergencies outside their immediate area of experience' – for example, failing to spot fatal conditions such as blood poisoning. A research team led by Professor Trevor Sheldon has suggested that more than 90,000 patients die and almost 1 million are harmed each year in England because of hospital blunders. These include errors during surgery, falls, infections and complications. He examined hospital notes from one hospital over six months and said the results were representative of what was happening across the country. However, the truth is that until Dr William Pickering's proposals are implemented no one can know the full extent of these difficulties, or who is responsible for them. See Pickering, op. cit.

31 Victoria Vaughan, 'Johnson wants competition to prop up poor GP services', *Health Service Journal*, 26 July 2007, p. 5.

32 Rebecca Evans, 'Why minorities still stand out from the primary care crowd', *Health Service Journal*, 2 August 2007, pp. 12–13.

33 Peter Burge *et al.*, *Understanding Patients' Choices at the Point of Referral* (London, King's Fund, City University, and RAND Foundation Europe, 31 May 2006); Angela Coulter *et al.*, *Patients' Experience of Choosing Where to Undergo Medical Treatment: evaluation of London Patient Choice Scheme* (Oxford, Picker Institute Europe, 2005). See Diane Dawson *et al.*, 'The effects of expanding patient choice of provider on waiting times: evidence from a policy experiment', *Health Economics*, February 2007, 16(2), pp. 113–28 uses econometric methodology to estimate the impact of the project on waiting times. Average waiting times shortened in the London region, and converged among London hospitals.

34 Daniel Martin, 'NPSA attacks 'meaningless glossy menus', *Health Service Journal*, 12 October 2006, p. 6. Even so, patients were going to other countries for treatment in Spring 2008 through fear of MRSA, and also avoiding NHS waiting lists. See www.treatment abroad.com.

35 Noel Plumridge, 'On payment by results', *Health Service Journal*, 10 May 2007, p. 15; Comments by health minister Mr Andy Burnham at publication of DoH consultation paper *Options for The Future of Payment by Results: 2008–09 to 2010–11* (London, DoH, 2007). Helen Mooney, 'Poor data threatens future of PbR system, warns minister', *Health Service Journal*, 22 March 2007, p. 5. National Audit Office, *NHS Connecting for Health* (London, National Audit Office, 15 May 2008) said that the system would not be ready until 2014 at the earliest.

Privately, experts say that in its present form it will never work at all. So far £3.6 billion of a projected total cost of £12.7 billion has been spent. See also first leader, 'A Question of Trust', *The Times*, 16 May 2008, p. 18.

36 Charlotte Santry, 'IPPR: honesty over unsafe hospitals is the best policy', *Health Service Journal*, 8 March 2007, p. 7.
37 Philip Lee, 'Public Service Productivity: Health, February 2006', Office of National Statistics article at www. statistics.gov.uk.
38 Rebecca Allmark, 'Money no excuse for hampering progress', *Health Service Journal*, 26 July 2007, p. 18, reporting on analysis by Dr Mark McLellan, former head of US Medicare and Medicaid Services and senior policy director for healthcare at the White House. See also www.policyprojects.com.
39 Mark Gould, 'In pursuit of happiness', *Health Service Journal*, 10 May 2007, pp. 22–3.
40 Karen Davis, Cathy Schoen, Stephen C. Schoenbaum *et al.*, *Mirror, Mirror on the Wall: an international update on the comparative performance of American healthcare* (New York, Commonwealth Fund, May 2007). 'UK healthcare ranked best value for money', *Health Service Journal*, 24 May 2007, p. 8.
41 The Health Commission recently found that the top five overall issues in patient complaints were safety; poor communication; ineffective procedures; poor complaints handling; and dignity and respect. See www. healthcarecommission.org.uk. The NHS has a standing committee on malnutrition. See Malnutrition Study Group, *The 'Must Report': Nutritional Screening for Adults – a multidisciplinary approach* (London, MAG, 11 November 2003).
42 Geoff Mulgan, *Politics in an Antipolitical Age* (Cambridge, Polity Press, 1994), pp. 77–8.
43 EF Schumacher, *A Guide for the Perplexed* (London, Abacus edition, 1977), p. 127. I owe the reference to Mulgan, op. cit., p. 81. See also Niall Dickson, 'Darzi review must avoid national blueprint to enable best local solutions', *King's Fund B-monthly Update*, 28 February 2008.
44 Colin Robinson, Introduction to *Introducing Market Forces into 'Public' Services*. Vol. 4, *The Collected Works of Arthur Seldon* (Indianapolis, Ind., Liberty Fund, 2005), p. ix.
45 Robinson (ed.), *Collected Works*, vol. 4, ibid.
46 *Reform Bulletin*, 22 February 2008, at www.reform.co.uk.
47 Anna Donald, 'On lessons from Australia', *Health Service Journal*, 5 July 2007, p. 17. See the full analysis in Arthur Seldon, *Charge* (London, Maurice Temple Smith, 1977), reprinted in volume 4, *Collected Works*, op. cit.
48 Dame Gill Morgan also said that she disliked using the word 'customer'. Mark Gould, 'Someone to squeeze', *Health Service Journal*, 21 June 2007, p. 30. For an insight into the survival of the prevailing 'planning' mentality, of surprisingly unreflective and narrowly focused thinking – with one or two exceptions – and apparent unawareness of the economics of public choice literature. See 'Wish they weren't here?', *Health Service Journal*, 25 January 2007, pp. 22–5, where leading NHS figures discussed reform possibilities including an independent NHS board. Even a Civitas author speaks of our 'world class doctors, consultants, nurses and even managers'. But how do we know? See James Gubb, *Why the NHS is the Sick Man of Europe* (London, Civitas, 2008). On public choice theory, see note 2, in my Introduction: sources for courses.
49 Notably, in 2001 in Kidderminster in the Wyre Valley constituency when the proposed closure of the A&E unit promoted a citizen rebellion which saw a doctor, Richard Taylor, overturn a majority of more than 17,000 to evict the sitting Labour MP. Many local and national consultations seek views and then ignore them. Over 22,000 people 'e-signed' a petition on the Downing Street website over the future of The Royal Surrey County Hospital in Guildford. And 31,000 supported the return of dedicated military hospitals. In Worthing, Chichester and Hayward's Heath in Sussex, at Chase Farm Hospital in Enfield, and in many places in the UK, local campaigners sought to retain facilities slated for closure. Alan Milburn has drawn attention to the contrast between involvement in public protest and in charitable endeavours, compared with falling voter turnout. See two speeches: 'Empowering citizens: the future politics', speech to the Global Foundation, Sydney, 2 May 2006; 'A 2020 Vision for Britain's governance', St Chad's College, University of Durham, 24 May 2007. See also Milburn, speeches on charities legislation, House of Commons, *Hansard*, 26 June 2006, cols. 40–52, and *Hansard*, 25 October 2006, Report stage. Public consultations on closing 2550 post offices were also a 'sham', according to Labour MP Kate Hoey. 'Public consultation on closing 2500 post offices is 'sham'', *Daily Telegraph*, 26 February 2008, p. 6.
50 Pickering, op. cit.
51 See my chapter 'Cancer and the 'efficiency myth', above.
52 David Lansley, 'Providing information to consumers', pp. 419–27; Lawrence N Gelby, 'Care Counsel: consumer-driven health care advocacy', pp. 499–500; David J Hines, 'Consumer's Medical Resource: helping consumers evaluate medical treatment options', pp. 510–15, in Herzlinger, *Consumer-Driven Health Care*, op. cit.
53 Sophia Christie, 'On telling our story', *Health Service Journal*, 12 October 2006, p. 20. Christie also pointed out that taxpayers generally want less spent but individual patients want more. On social capital see works cited by Arthur Seldon and David Green. Also Robert D Putnam, *Making Democracy Work: civic traditions in modern Italy* (Princeton, NJ, Princeton University Press, 1993).
54 Michael White, 'On politics', *Health Service Journal*, 13 September 2007, p. 10.
55 Harry Telser and Peter Zweifel, 'A new role for consumers' preferences in the provision of healthcare', *Economic Affairs*, 26(3), September 2006, pp. 4–9.
56 Hazel Blears, speech 'Putting communities in control', to regeneration conference, London, 5 March 2008; 'Unlocking the talents of our communities – an overview', www.communities.gov.uk. Also, Patrick Wintour, 'Blears wants police, NHS and councils more locally accountable', *The Guardian*, 5 March 2008, p. 5.

16

'Coercion, contagion, learning, coaching'

'The essence of optimism is that it takes no account of the present but it is a source of inspiration of vitality and hope when others have resigned it; it enables a man to hold his head high to claim the future ... and not to abandon it to his enemy.'
— DIETRICH BONHOEFFER

'I'm an optimist, but I'm an optimist who carries a raincoat.'
— SIR HAROLD WILSON

There are still good grounds for optimism about change. In short, we have tried everything else, and it hasn't worked. We seem likely now to really try the market solution.

I believe that we can move swiftly with health savings accounts. Personal budgets already demonstrate that we can build experience which itself demands more boldness. We can support change – and accept some failures in the process of experimentation. We can draw on this experience of what works, what still doesn't work, and of what still needs to be done. The issue is not to force change into a given direction, but to measure as we go, to get the boundaries right, and then to let markets themselves enlarge the frontiers. We need to advance the necessary adaptive, trial-and-error change of learning as we go. This chimes best, too, with an Oakeshottian tradition of conservative scepticism. Services should not be a 'system' (like socialism, or communism). They should be rooted in an approach of trial-and-error learning, and of accepting surprises. This view also accords with what Nobel prize-winning economist Professor Ronald Coase called 'the problem of social cost', which is concerned with assessing and facilitating necessary trade-offs and improved costs and benefits.[1]

We can easily see that a system of 'one size fits nobody' will no longer serve. We can also see that culture is one of the critical determinants of social cohesion and improved services. This is then an enquiry into both the results and the legitimacy of the NHS and social care organisation. And about the possible catalysts for change. It concerns class and class power as well as rights and responsibilities, even though class politics is no longer at the leading edge of public debate. Culture, however, asks us to consider motive and incentive. It highlights results, which have to be explained. Notably, the systemic and deeply embedded inequalities in British health and social care which have continued during all premierships since Attlee's. Why do these inequalities of access still exist, and how could they be corrected? We do, after all, seek to live under a system in which service is spread fairly across all citizens, with a universal set of claims which apply to and benefit each of us, and where we are each officially promised – but not legally guaranteed – individual and personal services.

Sir Douglas Hague outlined the four ways in which any system can be changed: by *coercion* (or the pressure of competition or recession, or government action); by *contagion* (or the transfer of culture from outside organisations by the recruitment of new people); by *coaching* (when management seeks help to change); or by the evolution of a *learning organisation* (when an organisation learns how to define and establish an appropriate new and open culture).[2] As Sir Douglas said, the most desirable way of changing a culture is when the people in the organisation set out to do so for themselves. The NHS and social care reforms have engaged management in all four approaches. Three of the four 'effectors' – contagion, coaching, and the learning organisation – are regarded as relatively innocent even if time-consuming activities by many public sector managers and by medical professionals. No one thinks it is easy to run a hospital, a general practice, or any other healthcare institution. No one thinks they are easy to change. Yet coercion, contagion, coaching and the idea of the learning organisation depend on irresistible prompts, I suggest, such as cash in the hands of the consumer. Politics alone has not managed to do it. 'Leadership' alone has not managed to do it. Much talk about 'the learning organisation' and of fashionable management gurus invited to address NHS conferences have not managed to do it. If we want economy and efficiency and effectiveness, if we want responsiveness and personalisation, too – that is, if the three e's are to 'elp – it is choice and the possibility of the rapid defection of financially empowered consumers which offers the biggest encouragement to change from a controlling 'kultur' to a 'culture' of consumer satisfactions. A culture which manages to change by itself will, too, be better equipped to change again as trial-and-error endeavours reveal new opportunities and challenges. We all have to learn how to learn, and to have the confidence to un-learn, too.

Choice offers *positive* new ways to engage with the users of services. With their explicit and their tacit knowledge. With their personalities, their wishes and the trade-offs they alone bring to the discussion. With the individual choices which they alone may wish to make. Choice might be seen as coercive. Yet it is actually the prompt which is at the heart of the learning organisation, since it concerns everyone involved – including the users of services – actively *learning together*. The NHS, social care and government have to move beyond systems of volume and financial management to a culture of more venturesome and imaginative concern with consumers and their wishes. Including taking risks inventively, in welcoming the unknown future. This is not the same as taking unconscionable risks with lives. Indeed, it asks for investment in new possibilities which can improve lives. For example, asking people what they *want* from services, and then delivering this.

In the private sector, there is no alternative but to respond to empowered choice, to changing environments, to new cultures. I suggest that the choice agenda is beneficial to everyone, including medical professionals – who otherwise reject external surveillance, the centralised measurement of performance chiefly by volume, over-bureaucratic rules, government targets, and 'intrusive' micro-management by local executives who they do not feel are properly educated.[3] For medics, indeed, choice and the more open market is the creative means to professional fulfilment. It is normal in their private practices. For those with a private practice it is a key source of their living standards and their professional satisfactions. It is the alternative to unimaginative, bureaucratic approaches which do not meet the nature and complexity of the innovations necessary. Choice is the prompt to doing so, as well as for professionals to develop new attitudes and to value interpersonal skills which matter so much in healthcare. In addition, it depends on pluralism.

It is vital that we find ways to continue to change the system when it is failing its clients. But it is very difficult to close public sector institutions. The local, democratic and cumulative power of consumer choice would, however, make such alterations legitimate. One dilemma here concerns democracy itself. What should the local policy be if local people demand to keep St Hilda's on the Hill open, even if it is not efficient or effective? If enough people value what they identify as benefits, if they join a mutual purchasing organisation which spends their savings fund at St Hilda's with their support, we have a proper test of value and preference. But without this system in place there is uncosted and politicised demand, and no proper evaluation of opportunity cost. Instead, there is an evasion of realities. It is evident that it is easy to orchestrate a media campaign to prevent change. This is an aspect of 'media democracy' at work. However, doctors and managers may argue that there are very good reasons in terms of improving services for change to happen. Change, however, is often identified by the general public as denial, reconfiguration as 'cuts', reorganisation as the unacceptable loss of convenient local access. The debate hardly turns on outcomes at all. If it did, legitimacy would more easily be seen in recommendations for change.

This is, indeed, an area of considerable dilemmas. Ultimately, it ought to be local purchasers (representing their members, financially empowered consumers) who decide the fate of St Hilda's, although electoral pressures will be considerable and politicians will do their best to persuade purchasers to protect the hospital. No doubt knighthoods and quango appointments will be quietly mentioned. But if consumers control the individual funds they will directly and cumulatively impact on such services. Some issues of strategic decision making, however, may have to remain national. Such as where do you put A&E? This then will have to be argued through and voted upon.

Notes

1 Ronald Coase, 'The problem of social cost', in *The Firm, the Market, and the Law* (Chicago, University of Chicago Press, 1988), pp. 95–156, reprinted from *The Journal of Law and Economics*, 3(1), October 1960, pp. 1–44.
2 Hague, *Dinosaurs*, op. cit., pp. 113–14.
3 Sir Gerry Robinson, the 'management guru', in his programmes based on Rotherham General Hospital, in South Yorkshire. *Can Gerry Robinson Fix the NHS?*, a fully funded Open University project, broadcast on BBC2 on three consecutive nights, 8–10 January 2006, and *Can Gerry Robinson Fix the NHS? One Year On*, broadcast on BBC2, 12 December 2008.

17

Are you being *personal,* or what?

'*What shall I do? I guess you will have to find your way like the rest of us. That's what it means to be free.*'

-- ISAAC ASIMOV

'*It's about choice, it's about control, it's about autonomy.*'

– FRANCES HASLER

In the short term at least, there are but two ways to keep social care 'free'.[1] We can either increase taxes on the young and employed, or drastically curtail the quality and availability of care for those receiving social care. In the medium and long term we need to set in place a stable, evolving, funded system. This turns on incentives once again. Meanwhile, we stand on a burning deck.

In funding this care we are in a situation of grave emergency. Where is the money to come from? How much will be needed? On what basis is it to be raised? What impact will raising it have on the crucial variable, which is economic growth for savings and investment, if we are to pay for the provision of social care?

I again focus on a preference for a savings model for all as the viable and stable solution for the future. We need to ask which incentives we can deploy to encourage people to look ahead to the time when their long-term elderly care must be funded by someone. Will that someone be the state, taxing and spending? Or the individual? Or the family? And what of those who make no effort to do so? Or those who do try, but cannot save enough? Or those who miscalculate their own longevity and the necessary costs of care? Some families might be prepared to look after their own funding, or use housing equity. Others may spend all they get, and live life as sufficient as the day thereto. Many will never earn enough to save or invest long term for care, however well intentioned they are. There needs to be a safety net, but with edges not so smooth and silky that they discourage personal effort and thus increase the burdens on us all. The emphasis should be on private funding linked to the financing of an HSA, with subsidy for the poor.

As I said in the Introduction to this book, the current enquiry by government has lifted the lid on a box of conundrums. This, indeed, is an area which is a veritable zoo of dilemmas. There are a lot of awkward animals. Perhaps it is a sufficient statement of intent to want to encourage a savings model for all, and to construct a back-up net for those who for whatever reason cannot manage this. Or, at the very least, to take the view that all individuals and families *should* be in a position where they are responsible for making plans appropriate to their circumstances and family situations. This could include the use of savings, augmented pensions, housing equity or the support of carers from within the family. It may be, though, that with the best of intentions not all problems are fixable by a government plan. We may have to rely on adaptive change, not all of it predictable.

There is a real problem here concerning savings and funding. I recognise the difficulty that some people would have in funding private provision, and give details below. The mathematics is daunting for those on low incomes. I recognise a role for the state. I think it will inevitably be necessary for tax-based funds to be available to those who have not provided for themselves, or who have not provided sufficiently. The disincentives to save are obvious, as are the individual challenges. However, when the time comes I would give tax-subsidised personal accounts for such people when in need of care. How to set the levels will always be problematic and controversial.

These questions once again pose the fundamentals of how government, voters and the economy interrelate in a very complex area of finance and provision. This again concerns the underlying choices of how we view ourselves, one another and the state. How interventionist are we to be, and what are the market-based solutions? What would be the basis of the best policy, and how close to it can we get?[2]

The innovation of health savings accounts would enable us to address the funding of elderly care, together with every other area of health and social care. We need to unveil positive and to suppress negative incentives. The governing principles should be that we are responsible for ourselves, and that we should take responsibility for our actions. That we should make the price of all services transparent, and cease to suffer from the disadvantages of suppressing price signals. We should actively enable as much competition and choice as possible. We should use positive incentives to encourage saving, and do all we can to avoid embedding negative incentives which deter self-provision. We need to move away from a system which relies on transfers between generations – as in pensions provision – to individual lifelong savings where at all possible. Any reforms, too, need to be cautious about embedding new rights which will be difficult to fund or to amend as the voting power of the elderly increases. A health savings account would integrate these principles into a sustainable policy, with incentives to save and to avoid the marginal consumption of our own resources.

The revelation of personal budgets in social care has put the rationing of social care for the elderly out front. It is now exerting upward pressures on financing. There are once again insistent redistributive bids, demands for rights irrespective of contributions, an insistence on undiscriminating cover for all. There is too little concern for how the productive economy is to fund these charges. Or what the psychological, social and economic impact is of continuing to insist on statist ideas when dynamist approaches are instead essential.

Politics and the elderly

These are moral, economic and political problems. I explore the complex economic challenges below. Politically, we know that the elderly vote in large numbers, and that they are likely to vote as a force for specific and costly policy objectives. In addition, as Professor Philip Booth has emphasised with regard to pensions, governments now especially target the elderly voter and design platforms to attract those whom they see as the median voter.[3] In a democracy, reform of elderly care is likely to continue to be very difficult because of the temptations of this politics. Difficulties over reforms of pensions policy in every democracy have demonstrated this. There is the risk that change will set up strongly entrenched interests, that new entitlements will accrue to many, and that future change will be very difficult in a system of political voter-bidding. At least in the short term, we need to try to set in place structures which will be impervious to voter behaviour and to political temptation. Professor Booth has drawn attention to the dangerous example of what some have proposed as a citizens' pension. This reflects the danger ahead in some formulations of possible elderly-care policy. For example, as proposed recently by the Liberal Democrat leader Nick Clegg, who called for a care guarantee of £2 billion for personal care payments for all elderly people requiring care 'based on need and not on ability to pay'. This call, however, does not deal with how to pay for this.[4] The ragged rocks ahead include elderly-care cover funded at any necessary level irrespective of contribution; any increase in funding received by all; any projected increases in state benefits openly manipulable by the ageing median voter; increases voted for by the recipients who then pass the cost to the working young; disincentives to save; the continued expectation that 'government must do something about it', and that 'it is not my business to do anything.'

This is an area of particularly difficult dilemmas. Incentives can have both positive and negative effects. Voluntary activity can leave ragged edges. State compulsion and provision can destroy morality and self-responsibility. The use of the means test is a necessary instrument, but here, too, there are many shades of grey. For example, Dr Oskari Juurikkala has argued that, in terms of public pensions provision, means-tested benefits are among the strongest causes of low savings rates and early retirement.[5] I try to offer a path across these policy swamps, with some stepping stones. Perhaps sometimes I am too specific, and at other times too general. However, I hope I have suggested a direction of travel. This is not an easy topic. It is particularly unyielding if we seek tidy solutions. But the proposal for more taxation to fund ever higher costs is almost certainly unsustainable, and unwise.

Empowerment through savings

The signposts to the future of ageing, and the economics of the economy itself, and of savings, pensions and elderly-care provision, are dauntingly clear in some respects. The Institute of Economic Affairs is conducting an 'Empowerment Through Savings' project, sponsored by the Templeton Foundation. This is examining the economic problems and dilemmas that are arising as a result of ageing. Professor Philip Booth (Editorial and Programme Director at the IEA, and Professor of Insurance and Risk Management at the Cass Business School in London) and Mr Nick Silver (lead consultant on the project and a consulting actuary) recently summarised some of the issues. *Economic Affairs* brought together a series of important articles addressing the dilemmas.[6] Here Booth and Silver emphasised, rightly in my view, that responses to ageing require flexible labour markets, high quality education, and a good institutional framework which will ensure that individuals can respond personally in the best possible way to the circumstances which they face. And that we have positive incentives for personal action. An activist, politicised interventionist policy which deters individuals from responding to price signals, which deters savings, and which increases structural costs would be unwise. Clearly, funding, savings, pensions and elderly care provision all have very long-term implications. An ageing labour force changes the returns to capital (including those to human capital). So, too, do changes in the extended family, the survival or decline of small family businesses and such economic issues as the stability of the value of money in terms of predicting future yields to pay for care.

The political problems of 'voice' – which is often offered by statist commentators as the alternative to individual financially empowered and responsible 'choice' – are challenging. As Booth and Silver say, 'public choice' is already making meaningful pension reform very difficult in democracies. It may do so, too, concerning the funding and provision of elderly care. 'Large blocks of voters with aligned interests are emerging who may support the expansion or resist the contraction of the state pension system. Booth quantifies this effect and the results do not make comfortable reading.'[7] The evolution of personal budgets, and the cohesive purchasing in my proposed PGCAs, may indeed make this problem the greater if politicians continue to buy off older interest groups.

Then there is the question of whether the economy can and will support and encourage savings which, if they decline, can lead to a fall in economic growth. If returns on capital fall, how do we fund elderly care? If birth rates fall, the problems worsen. If there is a move away from state provision, do we adopt a policy of compulsory private savings for elderly care (and for pensions)? If voluntary, which incentives work best? In terms of private capital accumulation, and the payment of care by equity release, what would happen if returns to housing wealth were taxed in the same way as returns to other forms of capital (as Dr Nicholas Misoulis has suggested)? What then of 'equity release' plans as a means to fund elderly care?[8] There are other issues, too, concerning international capital flows and the accelerating movement of people and of capital. What will be the impact of immigration, new medical technologies and genetics and changing birth patterns on earnings, savings, investment and calls on services?

These are all important questions which focus us on funding the 'choice agenda' and 'personalisation'. Personal budgets help us to enquire within about what individual choice means *in practice*. They take us beyond the language of consensual pragmatists, to start to transform health and social care purchasing and provision. They also open up crucial issues of funding. For example, for those who are self-funding elderly care already, but who do not have enough money to live decently. And for those struggling with local authority accreditation regulations and diversionary tactics to deter demand. There is also the issue of how to make individual purchasing decisions really effective in social and long-term elderly care. I suggest, again, through collaborative, mutual purchasing organisations – my PGCAs.

Culturally, a big issue also is how to carry staff with us in change. Encouragingly, Patrick Duffy has pointed out that social workers who have had to do assessments for the sake of doing assessments now realise the fulfilment of sitting down with people and helping them to live their own lives and make their own choices. Yet the risk remains that a complex, bureaucratic system will still emerge, instead of the simple, universal one which could evolve without 'experts' taking back control.

The 'choice agenda' reprised

All this re-emphasises the choice agenda, and in complex ways. As we have seen, the choice agenda dramatises the key questions. Who decides who decides? Who rules? Who will help choice happen? Who takes which actions if they do not like the results? For the individual there are essential questions to face about elderly care, looking in the mirror in the morning. Care which is personal, or patronised? Personalised service, or pre-packaged? Paying customer, or rationed recipient? Actual buyer with your own lifelong health savings account or other cash funds, augmented pension or house-equity release, or a benefit beneficiary? Thoughtful and aware investor in your own future care, or the eventual recipient of what a safety net can offer? Quality-controller as the service-user, or take what you're given? To value independent living and decision making, or to put up with individual begging or a shaky safety net from cash-strapped central or local government? The mere possibility of only very basic care or the certain promise of a fund you own for best care in your own home, in a residential or nursing home, in a hospital, or in another specialist facility, as you choose? Who is to define and decide the answers to these questions? On the basis of which principles? How are savings and services to be funded? By whom, and with which suitable incentives and guarantees? How can we be fair to all, in a socially coherent society of justice and self-responsibility, and without introducing disincentives to save?

My emphasis, which the reader will now expect, is that it is vital to empower the self-responsible individual to actually control the money, but also to consider how then this spending can be most effective. This changes the debate in several ways. On whose terms is choice to operate? Is choice to be allowed to have a dynamic of its own? Is there to be a new respect for individual decision making? Will we permit competition as a democratic structure? Will we express in policies an intellectual belief in the capacity of the individual to decide how they wish to live their own once-only life? Who will pay the bills?

The introduction of personal budgets has opened wide large windows into these questions. A new social situation is becoming clear. New initiatives are being proposed, some of which focus on the real choices before us. For example, the International Longevity Centre in London (which specialises in policy on longevity, ageing and population change) published in February 2008 *A National Care Fund for Long-Term Care* by James Lloyd (Head of Policy and Research). This proposed a social insurance fund, which would be limited to cohorts of 65 years or so. It would be means-tested, and would pay for care to a standard benchmark which the fund would cover for all enrolled members. There would be automatic enrolment, with the right to withdraw. There would be total flexibility on how contributions would be paid, including deferral of payment until after death, when the person's estate would be charged. This plan would rely on a fully fledged market in complementary private insurance, with long-term care insurance enabling the individual to select a preferred level of cover and benefits. This is an imaginative series of proposals. It makes a serious attempt to address the issues, which mere demands by pressure groups for billions more tax-paid funding do not.[9]

Dilemmas in funding – practical and moral

How interventionist are we to be? It seems that there should be a means test, to enable funding and provision to be targeted for the poor. More dilemmas. Do we slacken the present means test, in order to discourage 'gaming the system' by making sure you do not have sufficient chargeable assets when care has to be funded? Dr Juurikkala has suggested that, in pensions policy, the provision of means-tested benefits has been intended to reduce the size of state pension systems and target help on those who need it most, but that such systems have strong disincentives to work and to save. They raise marginal rates of taxes, and impact on work effort and savings. Dr Misoulis, when considering pensions, said the following, which is relevant to our discussion:

> A compulsory minimum level of saving could also be introduced, in order to discourage reliance on means-tested benefits, which in effect allow people to free ride on the savings of others, reduce the after-tax actual yields people receive, and discourage people from saving. For this compulsory minimum to have the desired effect, though, it must be perceived by the economic agents for what it is, *saving*: neither taxation, nor pay-as-you-go. To that means, it should be deposited in a fund of the individual's choice, and

the government's involvement should be strictly limited to ensuring that the minimum saving has been put aside. Of course, an alternative to this policy would be to reduce means-tested benefits. Politicians have to balance the desirability of this course of action with the desirability of compulsory saving, but the two issues of means-tested benefits and compulsory saving are intimately linked.[10]

Diluting the means-testing criteria would perhaps have benefits. But it would also reduce the extent to which the better off had an incentive to save and to provide for themselves.

We might adopt the following position on these vital dilemmas.

First, the state should provide money which delivers sufficient resources to the poor to ensure that they are kept in dignity. But it should do no more as there should not be disincentives for effort. Dignity or 'basic needs' are the key words. There should also be some deliberate uncertainty built into policy. Funding should be confirmed or held back on an asset-tested and income-tested basis. This is not actually very different from the current position. However, a long-term commitment to encouraging self-funding by savings (whether in cash, or investments such as the release of housing equity) would change the balance of costs.

Another dilemma is how best to protect the morality of voluntary care and family support. If you allow the personal account money to be paid to family carers you bring non-market family care into the market and commodify it. In addition, if you adopt the imaginative policy of offering tax credits for those voluntarily helping family members – and who do not wish to be paid – this would be a commodification of charitable moral care. As to the holder of personal budgets, a moral policy would be to allow the cared-for person to do what they like with the money they are given. But this, too, can conflict with other moral obligations. Thus, if they use family care then they keep the money for living costs or give it to the family member who is caring for them; for example, to a personal assistant. There are now many family members thus employed (but 'commodified'?). However, what if people do not then spend the personal budget to ensure care for themselves? We then enter the territory of inspection. Would the local social services have to be able to apply for a legal order to stop the payments and provide care directly? This increases costs, employs busy-body 'jobs-worths', and intrudes upon private life. But the personal budget is public money – albeit tax-funded. We have to be careful about defining 'appropriate' decisions about funding and care, and a public but contestable document or contract may be advisable. There are no easy solutions, save that of just increasing taxes and spending more money indiscriminately. But that is not an easy solution at all.

In addition to the global problems which Professor Booth and Mr Silver described, there are localised issues which are a subset of the larger dilemmas. First, passing the control of money by personal budgets to service-users has shown that major and positive results can be achieved in financially empowering choice. Second, the personal budgets project demonstrates how enfeebled the funding model for social and long-term elderly care actually is when provided by the state.

Third, it also shows that even those who have self-provided have often underestimated costs and the lengths of their lives. Fourth, even when individuals have control over savings and other funds we need to encourage the evolution of member-owned, mutual local organisations to help the individual to successfully purchase services. Fifth, we have to address the issue of the safety net for those who do not or could not provide for their care.[11]

The 2008 fundamental review of eligibility

In the absence of appropriate saving and funding mechanisms a recent report to the Commission for Social Care Inspection by Melanie Henwood and Bob Hudson, *Lost to the System? The Impact of Fair Access to Care,* clarified some of the many difficulties in elderly care faced by several different kinds of people. These include those who do not qualify under strict local authority criteria for elderly care. But they include also those already in control of savings which they have self-funded and whose assets exclude them from applying to local authorities even if they wished to do so.[12] Many with no funds of their own have more difficulties securing suitable services than may be supposed, despite the success stories in personal budget pilot schemes. Many vulnerable, isolated and elderly people are excluded by local authority eligibility criteria for social care. And those who are self-funding can still find themselves in difficulties in securing appropriate services.[13]

The fundamental review of social care eligibility criteria initiated in early 2008 by care minister Mr Ivan Lewis will be insufficient if it merely looks at shifts in eligibility wording, or moves definitions in the margins, or entertains demands for more tax-based funding. It must instead be founded on a total and a radical review of elderly care funding in the context of health and social care services as a whole. It should willingly embrace a national enquiry into the potential of a British health savings account, and of tax incentives to bring this reform into being.

Mr Alan Johnson has drawn attention to a £6 billion 'black hole' in funding care for the elderly.[14] Mr Gordon Brown has proposed a new compulsory tax-based social insurance scheme for non-medical care for the elderly, rather than a voluntary structure with tax incentives for savings. Mr Brown's proposal means that younger workers will fund the care of the elderly through an 'ageing tax'.[15] This plan – supported by the NHS Confederation – is now open to a six-month consultation, to be followed by a Green Paper.[16]

Hypothecating inheritance tax for care is one other possibility. In Germany and Holland payroll taxes are the norm. In Scotland, there is presently universal free care, but Audit Scotland has warned that this is unaffordable. Another approach is that suggested by Stephen Burke, director of Counsel & Care, who has said that all care could be free with a levy of 2.5% on every estate over £10,000 after death.

The enquiry into eligibility needs to go to root-and-branch reform. Otherwise, the risk is that it will merely lead to increased demands for 'the government to do something', and the taxpayer to pay the bills. We need to move rapidly towards a longer-term funding solution where everyone is funded and empowered by savings in cash, capital, housing and the like (or tax transfers for the poor) to ensure individual purchasing power for good elderly care. Personalisation should be for every person. Access should be possible for all. But this will not be achieved by a system based on raising taxes in a compulsory structure.[17] Nor on one where local government is the rationing agent. We need direct tax incentives to encourage voluntary saving, while leaving people free to make their own decisions about what savings mean and how they can be structured.

To an extent there is always likely to be a parallel system of savings-funded and tax-based state-funded care, since many will not save, not be able to save, or be too late to save. The necessary long-term reform is to encourage many more to save, and to bring significant additional funds into the system. In the interim, there will need to be state funding for those too late to join a new funding structure. A general commitment to increased savings would help finance that by the investment of these savings in the growing economy. I say more on this, below.

How eligibility doesn't work now

The responsible minister, Ivan Lewis, announced at the end of January 2008 an enquiry into these issues following the Third Annual Report to Parliament on *The State of Social Care in England 2006–07* by the Commission on Social Care Inspection [CSCI] on 28 January 2008. In March 2008 he announced that local authorities would be invited to bid for a share of £80 million to enable older people to stay together in their own homes.[18] The CSCI report drew attention to the current postcode lottery between local authorities, difficulties with means testing and serious problems with the management of eligibility thresholds and access. Personal budgets will only succeed if they are properly funded, if user support services can secure sufficient income, and if the initiatives retain legitimacy. Financial reform is very urgent.

The CSCI report showed that those who do qualify for council support in social care and who get it are realising a better quality of life, but that there remains a seriously deficient postcode lottery in social care. Nearly three-quarters of local authorities have refused help to anyone whose needs they define as not either 'substantial' or 'critical'. Thus, those classed as with 'moderate' needs – consider, this means those who cannot carry out routine tasks such as getting out of bed, bathing and doing the washing up – are excluded. You can starve quietly at home, with only 'moderate' needs. Another 275,000 pensioners with less intensive requirements, such as needing help to go to the shop, are excluded. Some 6000 elderly people with 'high support needs' – those who cannot bathe or eat without assistance – receive no services and no informal care. CSCI estimated that 450,000 people do rely on family and friends, even though they have been assessed as needing more help. For many with close families and younger friends, help may be at hand. But this is a society where many now have neither. This, despite the report that informal care takes up some 70–80% of the total cost of social care. In dementia care relatives at home provide 37% of the care, which saves the state some £5 billion a year.[19]

The difficulties reflect some huge shifts in family structures. In 1945 in Wolverhampton 51% of older people lived in households comprised of two or more generations, and in Bethnal Green 41% in 1954–55. In the early 1950s each older person had an average of 13 relatives living within a mile; 53% of older people had their nearest married child living either in the same dwelling or within five minutes' walk. Today, many old people live a lonely existence, even though a majority live within five miles of where they were born. It is perhaps a surprise that the informal sector has held up as well as it has. One reason may be that electronic communication involves many older people, in part prompted by developing the skills needed for genealogical research. It is important, for both moral and financial reasons, to support informal care.[20]

The present functioning of eligibility criteria is problematic in the extreme. It shows the naked need of major funding reforms. It arose because governments saw a huge and uncontrollable rise in public expenditure as increasing numbers of elderly people entered residential and nursing homes. Their solution was to transfer responsibility to local authority social service departments. The cash-limited grant to fund care and the requirement for social workers to assess people was also intended to encourage alternatives.

The means test has been an important axis. We should, of course, recognise the necessity of the means test, otherwise the taxpayer would have to fund everyone. This is beyond the capacity of already high current tax levels. However, the way in which local councils have operated the criteria has created a lottery in care. This helps highlight the need for fundamental reforms. Many elderly people do not qualify for local authority help according to some councils, but they would be helped in other districts. The 'Fair Access to Care Services' (Facs) policy is very inconsistent in its application and results. In the lottery, some win. But those who do manage to get a ticket do not always get good care. There are large numbers now struggling at home, with inadequate savings and no local authority help. Those who have no ticket, and who have no savings to fund their care, are in serious trouble. They are described by the Henwood and Hudson report as 'lost to the system'. The cohort is growing as councils raise the height of the hurdle.

The present local government 'Facs framework' permits councils to meet 'needs' in categories: low, moderate, substantial, and critical. CSCI shows a trend of tighter rationing as demand grows. Henwood and Hudson reported that two-thirds of councils were expected to set their entry level for funding at 'substantial' in 2007–08. Some already recognise only 'critical' needs as their core responsibility. Councils, of course, have little choice. Demographic pressures are irresistible, technological change continues at breakneck speed, but money is very tight. Scene-shifting or diversionary tactics also come into play, as applicants are referred elsewhere by hard-pressed councils, often into care cul-de-sacs where there is no funding. These manoeuvres undermine individuals and increase dependency. By contrast, a recent study published in *The Lancet* (based on research conducted at the University of Bristol) suggested that elderly people are 20% less likely to go into a nursing home if they get proper medical and social care in their own home. However, if services are withdrawn save from those whose situation is 'critical', home visits, community-based care and other support will be insufficient.[21]

The apparent experience of many self-funders suggests that we need much more advice and support for decision making so that people who have saved are not faced with limited choices. Some vulnerable and isolated people are not equipped with the range of information which would enable them to choose between residential or home care. The PGCA – the mutual organisation to which they could take their funds – would, however, offer advice in making life-changing decisions, and offer independent and ongoing support. They would, too, be aware of the funding that the elderly individual has, and where this was proving to be insufficient they would liaise with the appropriate local state safety-net council to ensure that there was continuity of care. Innovators may also offer new approaches to funding. This would be a proper relationship between the PGCA and the member, and not merely a handing out of leaflets. The relationship would support self-assessment, individual self-determination and choice.

Personal budgets: revolutionary impacts

As I have argued throughout this book, personal budgets in social care are truly revolutionary. Much more so than seems to have been realised. The personal budget in social care – and potentially, in all aspects of the NHS, too – is thus the most important of all the initiatives concerning choice, provided that it does what it says on the tin. It will enable many elderly people to stay in their own homes, buying the necessary support. And it is difficult to see how personal budgets can for very long be restricted to particular areas of health and social care. It is the most radical social reform we have seen. Its wider implications and likely demonstration-effects for the NHS are literally revolutionary. If the elderly, the chronically ill and the disabled can control the money – and they may have been foolishly thought by some to be among those less likely to be able to cope – then why not all of us, and for all services? By preference in a lifelong personal health savings account (supported by tax incentives), or by voluntary insurance, or from tax-transfers to the poor.

Personal budgets are already encouraging competing private provision, and much more independent thought by service-users in social care. They are freeing from mystification both prices and individual possible choices. People want to know what they can get for their budget, and how costs are constructed. Consumer preferences are changing the shape of services, and the identity of who provides these, too. People are rebelling against the poor services previously published by cash-strapped and paternalist local authorities. They are using their budgets to get services tailored to their wishes. Free prices reveal consumer preferences. We could ensure that everyone always had these freedoms if we revised the NHS system so that we each held and thus owned a health savings account.

The well-known Rand Corporation study showed as long ago as 1986 that when cash comes into the picture significant changes in behaviour in public services occur.[22] The introduction of direct incentives is educative in itself. Incentives ensure that resources flow to the organisations that do the best job, in terms of quality, access, cost and consumer satisfaction. They bring new provision into the market. They empower consumer choice. They motivate purchasers, providers and insurers. For each of these must earn their incomes by satisfying customers, rather than by relying on money that falls from above in big bundles. Purchasers then buy selectively, rather than by bulk contracts. These changes, too, increase the flow of information, advice and advocacy – as they have done in direct payments from such valuable organisations as the National Centre for Independent Living.[23]

History, and consequences

The evolution of such an approach was signalled by the government's *Commissioning Framework for Health and Well Being*, published in March 2007.[24] That document asked for practice-based purchasing 'using individual budgets wherever possible, to give people more control of their own care and support arrangements'. Announcing the framework, the then Health Secretary Ms Patricia Hewitt said: 'Giving people more choice and more control over their lives – creating a truly personalised service – is the first goal of commissioning for health and well-being'. Practice-based commissioning is intended to devolve some of the commissioning work to GPs. But it has not offered the direct instruments of patient control. However, personalised services have been a continued emphasis by Alan Johnson as Secretary of State for Health. On 2 March 2008 he told Labour's spring conference in Birmingham that the key was 'a personalised NHS'.[25] He has pressed ahead with personal budgets, which can set in place the real levers of consumer control.

The evidence to support the idea of personal budgets was emphasised by Vidhya Alakeson (Harkness Fellow in Healthcare Policy at the Social Market Foundation). In *Putting Patients in Control* Ms Alakeson cited evidence from consumer-directed programmes in the USA which improved health outcomes and customer satisfaction as well as value for money. Capacity constraints were eased and individuals hired support from outside the official systems and at a cheaper cost. Coordination of services improved. Customers tended to underspend rather than overspend their budgets, too.[26]

The new Prime Minister has a reputation as an instinctive micro-managing centraliser who has tried to spend his way to security. Yet he and his new Secretary of State for Health, Alan Johnson, have broken the battle-line by pushing on more swiftly than expected with the next stage of the project to extend personal budgets. Tax funds will thus pass into the hands of more service-users and their families from April 2008. This has significantly shifted the agenda. At the same time it has opened up for debate liberal economic ideas. Perhaps among the most surprising dogs that have not barked in the past decade on behalf of individual freedom is that the Conservative Party has not responded to such calls to take personal budgets seriously, despite the clear tendency for British political parties to become increasingly similar. On these issues, indeed, all the dynamism has come from New Labour. New Liberal Democrat leader Mr Nick Clegg has also proposed that direct payments and individual budgets be extended to people with chronic long-term conditions, for mental health services and support for those with learning disabilities. But he wants taxes to rise to pay for it all. My PGCA would act effectively for those with no voice, such as those with learning disabilities.[27]

The dynamic decision by the new Gordon Brown government in *Putting People First* (December 2007) to put £520 million behind a three-year initial programme to transform social services for older and disabled people is an underestimated projectile which will make huge ripples in the largest of ponds, the NHS itself. Health Secretary Alan Johnson launched the *Putting People First* initiative to spread personal budgets – already held by the disabled – to those in social care at home. They will now define their wants, and negotiate these. This is tax-based money. But to fulfil all likely demand we will need to move to a savings-based structure. Otherwise, an expanding programme will require new taxes.[28]

Gordon Brown told health professionals gathered at King's College that 100,000 people with long-term conditions should now be given the ability to manage their care themselves, and 15 million patients with chronic or long-term conditions should have access to care at home. He said that,

> During 2008 we will bring forward a patient's prospectus that sets out how we will extend to all 15 million patients with a chronic or long-term condition access to a choice. Real control and power for patients, supported by clinicians and carers. And where it is appropriate, just as with personal care budgets for the 1.5 million social care users, it could include the offer of a personal health budget.[29]

If this occurs, it will be an enormous advance.

The entire proposal for extending personal budgets thus offers us the biggest opportunity yet to achieve clarity about purposes, funding and individual financial empowerment in *every* area of health and social provision. It does so not only for elderly care, or for children's services – on which a start was made with the *Children's Plan* issued in December 2007 – but in acute and chronic care in every respect, too.[30] Children's services are structured by the government's own outcomes framework – for example, in day care, children's centres, extended schools and training. These services, like all others including those for mental healthcare, should be the subject of personal budgets. However, although initially this may have to be funded by taxation, we should move towards a generational change whereby everyone invests in a health savings account, which they own, which it is in their interests to keep in good repair by adding to, and – when they have to use it – to spend prudently.

The concordat signed by central and local government and other partners – *Putting People First* – effectively delivers a version of the patient fund-holding which I have been calling for since the early 1990s, although not yet across the entire spread of health and social care. It will put personal budgets into the hands of large numbers of social care users so that they can define and choose their own services. This budget may be taken either in cash or it can be administered by a local authority on behalf of an individual and with their agreement. The individual may spend the money on any reasonable means of enhancing their own well-being. No doubt there will be a debate about 'reasonable', but the intention is to offer autonomy. Individuals may, for example, pay their family to support them or to employ people who have previously been excluded under the direct payments scheme which was initially introduced for the disabled.

Putting People First follows the 13 pilot schemes involving some 3000 people in personal budgets. These emphasised a new direction for social services, building on the success of direct payments made to the disabled. They have promoted personalised services, independence, choice, and user-defined quality of life. The funding issue was fudged here, however, as the pilots were enabled to tap into several additional funding streams, including the Supporting People housing subsidy. The wider scheme requires urgent attention to funding, to enable consumers to fully benefit from the concept and from more information services, support networks, advocacy and user support which the scheme is prompting.

Andrew Cozens (Strategic Adviser for Children, Adults and Health at Idea), summarised the challenges: 'How do you turn a cash-strapped service, dependent on means-testing and needs assessment, into a service for all based on entitlement and choice?' And: 'The big step is to reorient the planning for adult social care: from individual need [*sic*] to the whole population; from need to entitlement; and from packages of support to a more dynamic recognition of changing individual need.'[31]

We should ask how? We should remark, too, on the use of the word 'need'. The important distinction, which the reforms underline, is between 'need', which experts decide for us, and 'wants', which are our specific individual preferences. It is 'wants' which will drive the personalisation of service and the shift from inputs to user-defined outputs which is at the heart of these issues and of this proposed transformation.

These changes offer an opportunity for an open discussion about the whole role of social services, which began with the idea of collective responsibility and the objective to relieve poverty. It challenges, too, the existing widely varying degrees of mean or adequate provision, eligibility criteria and assessment systems. It takes us from what was initially a rigid destitution approach, to a wider concept of a national minimum standard, then to a modern approach where the individual defines services. It is the most powerfully explicit statement of the approach of liberal economics to public services ever made by government. Indeed, it goes much further than the Thatcher governments of the 1980s, which hardly touched the demand side in reforms.

But won't people make the 'wrong' choices?

Current (spring 2008) discussion of this development is itself both informative and revealing. On the one hand, there is talk of taking services away from the remaining Poor Law heritage.[32] On the other, there remains a suspicion among providers and in local government that people will make 'the wrong choices'. Of course, in choice the individual does not need to be the *technical* expert, but there are points to be made here. First, we are all in many senses the expert on ourselves – on our values, preferences, history and hopes. We know which values we most prize, and which trade-offs we might or might not be prepared to make. When we make purchases in our ordinary lives, too, we rely on the market. That is, on the data and guidance that markets supply with reputation, advertising and other information we gather from several sources such as word of mouth, recommendations from friends and from consumer organisations (e.g. *Which?*), and on the advice of a trusted agent. The agent may well seek to guide us to make 'good choices'. But it is (or should be) our money, our life and ultimately our own choice. Thus the folklore quip: 'You pays your money and you takes your choice!' When Andrew Cozens of Idea, for example, writes of funding services so that people can make good choices and of a system which will get 'the right services to the right people at just the right time' we must hope that he means this fundamental notion, and not an echo of experts making 'the right choices' for us.

New Labour initiatives on these budgets, however, are starting to get us to the actual workings of instrumental measures which actually attach personal control over funds to individual healthcare and social care provision. This is starting to get us beneath the surface simplicities of rhetoric and 'policy' and beyond general statements about 'community', 'involvement', a 'say' (even a 'greater say'), more consultation and decentralised 'democracy'.

Learning from the pilots

We can make further progress when we have the full publication of the learning from the 13 government pilots on personal budgets.[33] We need analyses of the experiences of individuals, of the impact of the changes on providers, and what they have meant in terms of staffing, organisation, financial management and other cost issues. We need to understand the impact on residential and care homes as well as on domiciliary care. We need to be informed, too, of the impact on different individuals – for example, on how successfully those with learning and other disabilities have been enabled to move from residential care back into the community. Competition, too, has both expected and unexpected consequences and we need to assess these. For example, Des Kelly, executive director of the National Care Forum (representing not-for-profit care homes) pointed out that the larger corporate providers may do better, with all the benefits of economies of scale, but it is important that smaller facilities survive to widen choice. And that there is also spare capacity to permit choice. However, in residential care high occupancy rates are essential to the survival of facilities, and these commonly run at 90%, so spare capacity is not easily to hand.[34]

We are getting some of this information about the shifts in facilities due to new market pressures, as well as on the successful experiences of some service-users. This has been published by newspapers, notably, in the Social Care supplement in *The Guardian* in February 2008 which gave very informative details of individual experiences with personal budgets. It is important to be careful, however, not to let those in social services and in some providers who necessarily feel the impact to try to derail the policy by going hunting for market failures. These are self-correcting, whereas government failure is not. Indeed, it is government failure – national, and local – which is now being but partially addressed by the introduction of personal budgets and markets, but as yet with insufficient encouragement of personal savings for long-term care.[35]

The experiences of service-users already speak volumes. Christopher Bott, aged 26, from Newport Shropshire, has complex physical and mental disabilities, and is unable to speak or move unaided. In June 2007 his family secured an individual budget for him. He had been going to a day centre for 15 hours a week and they were very unhappy with the arrangement. He seemed to spend a lot of time sitting in his wheelchair. His family can now offer the quiet, personal attention thanks to the budget. 'Christopher now has a structured day, has undivided attention from a personal assistant, is spending less time in the wheelchair and is becoming more mobile. After a lot of difficult years with health and social services, it's good to be able to endorse an arrangement wholeheartedly,' his mother told *The Guardian*. Others have been asked what is important to them, and helped to secure this support by using a personal budget. Sean Dunn, 20, of Clitheroe in West Lancashire, has learning disabilities. He said, 'I set goals with my supporter workers and I work towards them. I'm learning new skills and my confidence has grown enormously. I can see a future now.' These individuals, their families and others like them have found that the budget arrangements need not be complicated and difficult to oversee. They have successfully handled the arrangements for payments, national insurance contributions, personal liability insurance, PAYE etc. Already in February 2008 there were an estimated 70,000 people working as personal assistants – often, they were family members or close friends – to support holders of personal budgets.[36]

There are many other examples of an imaginative approach to social care, notably enabling people to move out from the roles allocated to them – such as 'disabled', or 'elderly', or 'mental health patient' or 'service-user'. There is a whole range of things which affect people's well-being that are now being addressed by a new emphasis on personal self-organisation rather than administrative control or 'being cared for'. In one example, the elderly social care client, usually looked after by her husband, chose to go on holiday for a week with a carer rather than go into respite care. Her husband had a break and she had great benefit from the holiday at no greater cost than formal respite. In another example, a man who was isolated and seriously overweight said that rather than going to exercise classes and a day centre, having a dog would help him. He was provided with SID, which stands for Social Inclusion Dog. This sounds amusing, but it is very serious. It opened up his life, both beyond the narrow confines of an isolated existence and enabling him to go beyond the category to which he was assigned. SID helped an isolated, dependent person to have loving and loyal companionship, including that of other dog-owners whom he met when he went out for short walks every day and he got the necessary exercise. It gave meaning – including a time-frame – to every day. It showed that services could be imaginatively restructured, and could go beyond basic home care, necessary as that was. It showed a local authority responding to specific individual concerns, and genuinely changed experiences of individuals because of personal budgets. For the individual it is infinitely better than popping a pill or going to the surgery. Novelist Clare Allan, a mental health patient, reported a similar experience in her own life.[37]

Similarly, a Pakistani mental health patient purchased a personal trainer's time rather than a day service. A man with learning disabilities employed his neighbours to offer respite care instead of using local council facilities. One personal budget holder reported that 36 people used to visit him for assessment and service activities. Now it is five. Not only is this about improving lives by people improving them for themselves, it is also about encouraging workforce development, and greater staff satisfactions in achieving personal and customer fulfilment. This, too, is contributing to the shaping of the market, changing quality standards and shifting purchasing to help maintain an individual's independence over time. Tangible and quantifiable new efficiencies are resulting. For example, redirected funding here includes reducing inappropriate hospital admission, or admissions to residential care, and facilitating timely discharge from hospital.[38]

However, there are at present many different assessment and charging policies in different local authorities. There remain inequalities in how different sources of personal income are treated in different assessments. There are, too, some unhelpful assumptions being made about the capacities of people in residential care. Co-payments are viewed differently in the control of overall local budgets. We do, of course, want local variation and imaginative approaches. But the failing structure of funding remains the most urgent local and national issue. Here, a former local authority treasurer and chief executive of Bolton Council, David Collinge, has drawn attention to some of these major issues which need to be resolved in favour of emphasising individual empowerment and appropriate funding.[39]

Clear principles on which to base changes are evident, and these need to be reaffirmed. First, empowerment and not cost-cutting is the chief purpose of personal budgets. And, of course, if informed purchasing reduces costs, clearly the savings should be used to improve benefits. Second, funding must be sufficient so that the system does not fail. If it is allowed to fail then unsympathetic officials will be enabled to blame service-users for being unable to manage their own affairs. Third, we should not rely on the existing system of eligibility judgements being made by local authorities. Indeed, there should be a lifelong, incentives-based structure to secure sufficient funding. At present, local authority average-banded assessments take away from the individual those precision-based service responses to individual preferences which individuals clearly want. They also leave councils free to trim payments or to raise the ceilings on eligibility. They can do so without reference to a national decision in principle of how to set the means-test ceiling to encourage the most savings by individuals. Of course, if there were individual health savings accounts the owners would negotiate for the services they want.

Meanwhile, a national contract which specifies what will be offered by state-funded services is necessary to clarify what you can get, and what else you may wish to provide for yourself by savings. The state-funded services should be at a higher moral minimum than present social care services, and with a less stringent means test. This would deter the disposal of personal assets by individuals so as to 'beat' the means test. And it would be much better than the present requirement for councils to offer only 'reasonable' budgets. But what is 'reasonable'? It is at present defined as 'the amount of money needed to purchase a service that your local authority deems to be no worse than services already available to other local people with the same kinds of need'. This is clearly very unsatisfactory. David Collinge pointed out, too, that it does not square with the principles of the government's own *Valuing People* programme for learning disability.[40] There needs to be much more transparency, and firmer national guidance on charging and assessment. In addition, those in receipt of personal budgets should cooperate in purchasing, so that cooperative (and competing) local purchasing bodies could emerge which would negotiate with potential providers and on behalf of otherwise isolated individuals. They would encourage, too, adequate support for informed choices among a varied clientele.

Both in social care and in all aspects of NHS care the way to do so best could be to encourage each of us to save throughout our lives. I am not an expert on insurance, and we need those who are to do more work on how this could best work in this new model to facilitate best care. My expectation is that the individual would join a mutual, cooperative patient guaranteed care association, which would also be the insurer, and which would buy the care on their behalf. These PGCAs would be competitive, which would discipline them and the market. The poor would have tax transfers. The funds would be individual and guaranteed, under the control of individuals and not under the control of central or local authorities. These funds would then be taken to a preferred insurer. The funds would cover all necessary care. There could be an inducement (the negotiated but voluntary 'excess') to encourage consumers to consider their demands, and the costs, and to pay the first small sums, thus allowing the HSA to be saved and to grow. The best inducement is price, and differently priced offers of care. This accepts a principle of insurance: the voluntary variation of premiums with risk.

Voices from Brussels

More change may come from Brussels. The Commission is taking a serious interest in consumer issues and empowerment. These enquiries – and possible interventions – are likely to be very wide-ranging, although not yet much noticed in the UK. If the European Commission extends the right to British patients who face an 'undue delay' for treatment to travel anywhere in the EU for an operation – with the NHS paying for this – an effective 'voucher' would be introduced. This proposal was expected to be announced as a draft plan early in 2008.[41] It would inevitably impact both on NHS and on social care. I have previously forecast that the EU would extend the single market into the public sector, and that this could have the most profound effects on healthcare delivery. For example, in France the majority of citizens pay '*complimentaire*' assurance to top up the French government's 75–80% contribution to medical costs, which amounts to £75 per month for a couple. Delays are virtually non-existent, and outcomes are good. It seems likely that the EU will encourage the British government to introduce a system of 'top-up' insurance premiums if it seeks to unify health systems throughout the EU. Top-ups will clearly influence social care. In acute care, if people do travel to the continent for care, arrangements for dealing with later complications and follow-up care will be necessary. However, the same free movement for care, using such a voucher, could be extended for all care in the UK, too.

Personal budgets have been widely welcomed. They give service-users control and choice over what care they receive and prefer. They encourage innovative and imaginative solutions. They change workforce practices. There is also some evidence that they may be cheaper. However, as I have said, the key issue is individual financial empowerment, at suitable funding levels and in empowering financial packages. The aim is to build independence. To facilitate choice. To encourage voluntarism. To seek yields from lifelong savings, in a contributory scheme. To focus on helping people to live their own lives. To benefit from a framework of incentives, freedom and thrift. This includes those commonly labelled as 'the disabled'. We should not automatically assume that users of services who are seriously disabled or in difficulties with dementia (for example) are unable to do anything for themselves. Those who say that they need help to control a personal budget must be able to get it. We can improve arrangements for families, friends, or an available independent advocate to help them to do as much as possible for themselves.[42]

All of these challenges should not be a local authority responsibility, subject to local cost-cutting in a restricted budget. They are national responsibilities. This is best discharged by encouraging a stronger financial structure – and one which emphasises a gradual move to the savings of the individual not the taxes of the collective. One where local variations in services are not only permitted but endorsed, too, so that we can all achieve access to a variety of services, and above the level of a high moral minimum.[43] In these important respects, we begin, I think, to see the statue in the marble.

However, Dr Nicholas Misoulis has given us fair warning that in the economy at present 'the trend is for saving, investment and economic growth to decline, for the population to age, and for the provision of adequate income during retirement to become more and more difficult'.

The policy problems are deeply problematic. However, 'In a changing environment, "business as usual" is never a good option.'[44]

Notes

1 I am particularly indebted to my colleague at the IEA Professor Philip Booth for our discussions and for his invaluable comments on an earlier draft of this chapter. There is an excellent summary of current views being expressed by those representing major provider and charitable interests, and by the DoH, in Judy Hirst, 'An agenda on ageing', *publicfinance.co.uk* (internet magazine), 9 November 2007, accessed 3 March 2008.

2 Not 'free', of course, but paid for by compulsory central government taxation.

3 Philip Booth, 'The young held to ransom – a public choice analysis of the UK state pension scheme', *Economic Affairs*, 28(1), March 2008, pp. 4–10. See also E.K. Browning, 'Why the social insurance budget is too large in a democracy', *Economic Inquiry*, 1975, 13, pp. 373–88.

4 Nick Clegg, speech 'Nick Clegg sets out his vision for a people's health service', 22 January 2008.

5 Oskari Juurikkala, 'Punishing the poor: a critique of means-tested retirement benefits', *Economic Affairs*, 28(1), March 2008, pp. 11–16.

6 Philip Booth and Nick Silver, 'Editorial: New perspectives on the economics and politics of ageing', *Economic Affairs*, 28(1), March 2008, pp. 2–3.

7 Ibid., p. 2.

8 Nicholas Misoulis, 'Demographic effects on economic growth and consequences for the provision of pensions', *Economic Affairs*, 28(1), March 2008, pp. 29–34.

9 James Lloyd, *A National Care Fund for Long-Term Care* (London, International Longevity Centre, 28 February 2008). See www.ilcuk.org.uk.

10 Oskari Juurikkala, 'Punishing the poor', op. cit., pp. 11–16; Nicholas Misoulis, 'Demographic effects', op. cit., p. 33.

11 See note 24, Chapter 1, 'Vignettes and Visions', above.

12 Melanie Henwood and Bob Hudson, *Lost to the System? The Impact of Fair Access to Care* (London, Commission for Social Care Inspection, 2008); also, article by these authors, 'Checking the Facs', *The Guardian*, Society section, 13 February 2008, p. 6.

13 JP Newhouse and the Insurance Experiment Group (1993), *Free For All? Lessons from the RAND Health Insurance Experiment* (Cambridge, MA., Harvard University Press, 1993); Kathleen N Lohr, Robert H Brook, Caren Camberg *et al.*, *Use of Medical Care in the Rand Health Insurance Experiment. Diagnosis – and Service – Specific Analyses in a Randomised Controlled Trial* (Santa Monica, Calif., RAND Corporation), originally published in *Medical Care*, 24(9), September 198, pp. S1–87.

14 See Care and Support debate, House of Commons, *Hansard*, 5 June 2008, cols. 963–1028; John Carvel, 'Johnson admits to £6bn black hole in funding of care for older people', *The Guardian*, 12 May 2008, p. 2.

15 Gordon Brown, 'Speech at the social care event', King's Fund, 12 May 2008, transcript at www.number-10.gov.uk/output/Page15496.asp.

16 See www.careandsupport.direct.gov.uk. Also, Rosemary Bennett, 'Insurance could free the people from fears on old-age', says Brown', *The Times*, 13 May 2008, p. 8; Alice Miles, 'Spare a few quid for the rich old folk?', *The Times*, 14 May 2008, p. 17; John Carvel, 'Ministers look at social care insurance as costs rise', *The Guardian*, 13 May 2008, p. 10; Polly Toynbee, 'Despite the baby boomers ageing, we can afford the care', *The Guardian*, 13 May 2008, p. 31; Philip Webb, 'A return to Blairism as Brown looks back to save his future', *The Times*, 1 May 2008, pp. 6–7; first leader, 'Old Age Tension', *The Times*, 13 May 2008, p. 18.

17 On working models for insurance see Chapter 21, 'Getting it done 1', in my *Patients, Power and Responsibility*, op. cit.

18 CSCI Third Annual Report to Parliament, *The State of Social Care in England, 2006–07* (London, CSCI, 28 January 2008). There are, inevitably, many existing anomalies. On 29 January 2008 the Care Services minister Ivan Lewis MP ordered an urgent review of adult care eligibility criteria following publication of the CSCI Third Annual Report; '£80m to keep older people together in homes of their own', DoH press release 4 March 2008. Other anomalies include the case of a woman who broke her hip but who then needed nursing care due to a hospital-acquired infection. She was then cared for in a nursing home. Her fees there were more than £840 a week, but the state contribution to medical care for someone who can do nothing for herself was just over £100. Letter, Christine Anderson, *Daily Telegraph*, 14 May 2008, p. 21.

19 Philip Booth, *Caring for the Long Term: financing provision for the elderly* (London, Politiea, 2000), p. 1. He warns that this estimate should be treated with caution. See also House of Commons Committee of Public Accounts, *Improving Services and Support for People with Dementia, sixth report of the session 2007–08* (London, House of Commons, 14 January 2008).

20 Chris Philipson, 'Growing old in the 21st century', in Alessandra Buonfino and Geoff Mulgan (ed.), *Porcupines in Winter: the pleasures and pains of living together in modern Britain* (London, The Young Foundation, 2006). See also the classic study of family and informal support in early years, Michael Young and Peter Wilmott, *Family and Kinship in East London* (London, Routledge, 1957). Philipson (Professor of Applied Social Studies and Social Gerontology at Keele University) provides a valuable brief survey of some of the key issues, but does not mention encouraging savings.

21 Andrew D Beswick, Karen Rees, Paul Dieppe *et al.*, 'Complex interventions to improve physical function and maintain independent living in elderly people a systematic review and meta-analysis', *The Lancet*, 31(96114), 1–7 March 2008, pp. 699–700.

22 JP Newhouse *et al.*, *Free For All?*, op. cit.; Kathleen N Lohr *et al.*, *Use of Medical Care in the Rand Health Insurance Experiment*, op. cit.
23 There has been a stream of valuable analyses and commentary by the National Centre for Independent Living, the Care Services Improvement Partnership, the Commission for Social Care Inspection, the Independent Living Institute, the Social Care Institute of Excellence, the UK Home Care Association, the Scottish Office and others. See major evaluations directed by Martin Perkins at the Personal Social Services Research Unit at the London School of Economics, including V Davey *et al.*, *Direct Payments: a national survey of direct payments policy and practice* (London, PSSRU, LSE, May 2007). This contains a very useful note on references. See also especially DoH, *Direct Payments for People with Mental Health Problems: a guide to action.* (London, Care Services Improvement Partnership, 2006), and Green Paper. *Independence, Well-Being and Choice: our vision for adult social care in England*, Cmd. 6499 (London, Stationery Office, 2005).
24 Department of Health, *Commissioning Framework for Health and Well Being* (London, DoH, 2007); Patricia Hewitt, speech announcing the new Commissioning Framework, 8 March 2007.
25 Speech, Paul Johnson, Secretary of State for Health to Labour Party spring conference, Birmingham, 2 March 2008; Deborah Summers, 'Johnson promises personalised NHS', *The Guardian*, 3 March 2008. Johnson also announced reforms to enable married couples to stay together in residential care homes. Rosa Prince, 'Elderly couples to stay together under care reforms', *Daily Telegraph*, 3 March 2008, p. 14.
26 Vidhya Alakeson, *Putting Patients in Control: the case for extending self-direction into the NHS* (London, Social Market Foundation, 2007); Victoria Vaughan, 'US evidence backs individual budgets', *Health Service Journal*, 15 March 2007, p. 10.
27 Nick Clegg, speech, 'Nick Clegg sets out his vision for a people's health service', 22 January 2008.
28 Paul Johnson, speech, '*Putting People First: launch of new social care concordat*', 10 December 2007. The policy may contradict much of Mr Brown's micro-management but it accords with his 17th Arnold Goodman Lecture, *Civic Society in Modern Britain*, given in London on 20 July 2000 and published by the Smith Institute, London, in 2001.
29 Gordon Brown, speech on the Future of the NHS, King's College, London, 7 January 2008.
30 Department of Children, Schools and Families, *The Children's Plan: building brighter futures* (London, Stationery Office, 11 December 2007). A Child's Health Strategy was to be published in Spring 2008.
31 Andrew Cozens, 'Poor law care due for an upgrade', in Social Care supplement on 'Personal budgets and beyond', *The Guardian*, 6 February 2008, pp. 1–2.
32 Ibid.
33 The Local Government Association, too, is to lead a consortium to help share experiences, with the Association of Directors of Adult Social Services and the Improvement and Development Agency for Local Government (Idea).
34 Des Kelly cited in Andrew Cole, 'Will care become a commodity?', Social Care Supplement, *The Guardian*, 6 February 2008, p. 3.
35 Social Care Supplement, *The Guardian*, 6 February 2008, op. cit., pp. 2–3.
36 See Linda Jackson, 'A new breed for care worker', in Social Care supplement, op. cit. Helga Pile, National Office for Social Care Workers at the trade union Unison, has pointed to some of the risks in changes in employment arrangements. Helga Pile, 'This scheme is unfair to both sides', Social Care supplement, p. 4.
37 Clare Allan, 'Out of the ward, and out of the control of others', *The Guardian*, Society section, 5 March 2008, p. 6.
38 Private information, January 2008. See also T Stainton and S Boyce, 'I have got my life back': users' experience of direct payments', *Disability and Society*, 19(5), 2004, pp. 443–54; Mark Gould, 'Liberation theory', *The Guardian*, Society section, 30 January 2008, p. 5 – interview with Simon Duffy, Chief Executive of In Control.
39 See Alakeson, op. cit., and Andrew Cole, 'Will care become a commodity?', and David Brindle, 'We must be wary of cost-cutting', *The Guardian*, Social Care section, op. cit., pp. 3, 5.
40 Department of Health, *Valuing People: a new strategy for learning disability for the 21st century* (London, DoH, July 2006). See also White Paper of same title, published by the Stationery Office, London, 20 March 2001. Also, consultation paper, *Valuing People Now: from progress to transformation* (London, DoH, 4 December 2007).
41 Editorial, 'Health care and the BBC need the competition', *Daily Telegraph*, 20 December 2007, p. 21. Jeremy Laurance, 'NHS will be put to the test by EU plan to open healthcare borders', and Peter Popham, 'Thinking of travelling to Italy for treatment? I would think again', *The Independent*, 20 December 2007, pp. 2–3; John Carvel, 'EU delays move allowing patients to travel for care', *The Guardian*, 20 December 2007. See also 'Patient mobility' at www.euractiv.com.
42 See Mary O'Hara, 'Bridging the gap', *The Guardian*, Society section, 6 February 2008, p. 1 for action by dementia patients in Scotland in the campaigning group Scottish Dementia Working Group for examples of people well able to do much for themselves.
43 Cabinet Office Minister Ed Miliband MP has recognised the point. Speech to fifth annual Guardian Public Services Summit, 7 February 2008. Patrick Wintour, 'Miliband: no turning back on reform of public services', *The Guardian*, 7 February 2008, p. 19.
44 Nicholas Misoulis, 'Demographic effects on economic growth and consequences for the provision of pensions', *Economic Affairs*, 28(1), March 2008, pp. 29–34.

18

To see the statue in the marble

'No matter who you vote for, the Government gets in.'

– FOLKLORE

'The fog lifts, the world sees us as we are, and worse still we see ourselves as we are.'

– EVELYN WAUGH

We will not get to the right answers until we get to the right questions. We will not get to the right questions unless we understand what counts as an answer and what counts as a fudge. To properly phrase the questions and to discover some answers the first step is to go right back to first principles – to their explanations and implications.

As the previous chapter showed, the advent of personal budgets in social care has revealed the perennial dilemmas concerning funding, provision and choice to which we need to find secure and clear answers. The necessity of moving to a genuinely funded approach is once again highlighted by what we have learned about the state of elderly social care. We should now institute an urgent major study of the British possibilities for a health savings account to cover both NHS and social care. This should be part of the current review of eligibility criteria for state funding of social care, which care Minister Ivan Lewis instituted in early 2008. If all care funding was integrated into a health savings account for every individual then other major disparities could be addressed, too. For example, where a patient suffering from alcohol-related liver damage is now automatically treated by the NHS but a person with dementia is not.

Our present funding arrangements for long-term care significantly depend on transfers of income from those currently in the labour force to those who are retired. Yet these transfers by taxation from the employed to the no longer employed seem very unlikely to be able to sustain the system in the near future. The tax burdens, too, undermine economic success, which further weakens the structure. We need to find dynamic alternatives. Under existing arrangements we are already staring at enormous and unfunded costs. And the gaps are widening.

Notably, this is due to the tensions revealed by current problems of funding provision and by the lottery of local government decision making. These perennial issues have been exposed once again, like the beams of ancient shipwrecks uncovered by the changing tide. Personal budgets in social care – and their present limitations – show, too, that solutions need to be such that they do not resolve one problem by exacerbating others. Incentives cut both ways. We need relatively simple solutions – at least, which can be understood in headlines – although in practice these will inevitably be characterised by complexities given how difficult the problems have become. There will also inevitably continue to be push and shove by vested interests demanding increases in state spending.

The answers to funding elderly care are among the most pressing to discover. These turn on three words, 'choice', 'tax' and 'save'. The key principle which can take us forward successfully is to believe in choice and to use tax allowances to promote voluntary savings. Then those who make the choice of more careful consumption and suitable long-term provision will be rewarded by the yields from using savings accounts and by further investing in extra insurance cover and in other savings such as equity in housing. They will then be independent of future state funding, and their care requirements will to that extent be more inexpensively funded, too. We need to encourage as many people as possible not to resort to the state as last resort. And, instead, to reduce this demand as we reduce the role of the state. The encouragement to save would counter the present discouragement to make private provision. But to achieve this, there must be more disposable income to dispose. Lower tax levels and incentives can do much to enhance this. However, a tax allowance system would automatically shift disposable income from the Treasury to the individual, and at the same time would ensure some reduction in the role of the state. This would genuinely return funds for savings to the individual taxpayer. There would be less for vested interests to fight about, and provision would be taken into a structure of community without politics.[1] There are thus fundamental choices to be faced, notably concerning how to strengthen the funding position while at the same time substituting private action for collective compulsion.

As we have seen, a major issue is who will pay for the rising and costly demand for long-term elderly care. It is now a pay-as-you-go government system which has no call on capital to support it. There is no secure and invested government funding, except from current taxes. Nor is the financial commitment sufficiently covered by individual savings. What central funding there is comes from a current budget, distributed through local government. This cost is being charged to a diminishing proportion of the population. But changes in fertility patterns have introduced a new source of financial instability. This is shifting what is known as the 'dependency ratio' unfavourably. The cumulative disadvantageous funding impact is likely to be stupendous. Professor Philip Booth (the actuary and economist) has said that,

> Long-term care costs are a particular aspect of this general problem. Consider the ratio of those in need of care to the working population. This dependency ratio is projected to increase from 1.6% to 3.7% between 1991 and 2031 for those in need of continuous care. The total cost per adult of working age (including the cost of informal care) was projected by Nuttall et al. (1994) to increase from £1345 in 1991 to £2014 in 2031 at constant prices, assuming that costs grow at the same rate as GNP.[2]

This was written in 1996. But 12 years later we still try to 'pay-as-we-go', with no savings fund invested forwards.

In addition, what long-term care the state does provide is means tested. Many people discover this to their surprise when it is too late to start to save. A similar shock arises when there is a call on the sale of a middle-class family home to fund care. This also challenges popular ideas of equity, since those who have saved nothing have nothing to sell. But they get similar care 'free' from the taxpayer via the local authority budget. The anguish caused by being unable to transfer a property asset to the next generation has been considerable, especially since people regard healthcare and elderly care as no different in kind. These disincentives and distortions were avoidable. If we had introduced a proper savings system in the 1940s this would now be funding long-term care. Meanwhile, we persist with serious disincentives to earn and to save. And this despite our understanding that savings are a social and economic mechanism which are positive, effective, equitable, sustainable and which keep people clear of making demands on the taxpayer.

It is a fair question in such a crisis to ask whether the state will, can and should always fund and provide for all of us? Or is this not only immoral but also inefficient, unnecessarily costly and unaffordable? If we are to move towards a more diverse and fertile structure of savings, which are the possible economic instruments? We have mentioned health savings accounts, insurance and self-payment. How can such financial approaches be best structured? The generally fit are insurable for most of their lives. They can save. We could use tax reductions to create a health savings account for all, and then also encourage people to add to this and also to their pension fund with additional long-term care savings. Such funds would have to be additional, rather than just permitting part of an existing pension to be drawn down for care funds. Otherwise, an often insufficient pension fund would be even more thinly spread. Tax breaks would be less expensive to the state than otherwise providing a more extensive elderly-care safety net. An insurance scheme, too, would allow individuals to make choices about the level of benefits they want in the future, and to face what these will cost. Our years as elderly people are, after all, *our* years. They are not some unexpected and surprise add-on which are someone else's responsibility. In addition, a pre-funded system would have a much wider economic impact. It would increase the savings ratio and investment and generate economic growth which would help fund the increasingly costly safety net. This has been the insight of private pensions reform. We should learn this lesson with our eyes on the crisis of elderly care. We should emphasise it, too, as a counter-balance to the voting power of the elderly which (as a special kind of special interest) may itself encourage demands for much increased taxation to pay for care.

Signposts to cul-de-sacs

We should be alert, too, to properly read those signposts which would take us all in the wrong direction. One recent bell-weather article is that by Professor Chris Ham and Dr John Glasby, of the Health Services Management Centre at the University of Birmingham.[3] This article and ideas like these should not, however, count as an answer. These writers proposed a shift in the funding of social care, but in ways which would compound existing errors. They do not offer the necessary revolution in thinking. Instead, they underline prevailing ideas of state intervention and state control. We should, indeed, be cautious about such approaches which – in Flora Thompson's phrase in *From Lark Rise to Candleford* – would be like 'putting a poultice on a wooden leg'.[4]

Professor Ham and Dr Glasby would increase taxpayer support by bringing NHS and social care together into one budget. This is right. But they then call for an end to means testing and the creation of a statutory right of entitlement for elderly care. This is not right. These are inappropriate and certainly unaffordable ideas. As they fail, as they would if attempted, they would be followed by further demands for more taxation to fund more payments. Which would worsen the problems, and offer no solutions. However, to confuse the picture further, they place their own call in jeopardy by adding that 'People with a certain level of need would automatically be eligible for services and support at an agreed level.' Who would decide on the 'needs'? And on the levels? Ham and Glasby propose to fund social care from extra taxation, and from the surpluses which the NHS 'efficiency-drive' has generated. This is not an economically sophisticated argument, even if the surpluses were reliable. But they are not. The robust evidence shows that these NHS surpluses are temporary. They are due in the main to a combination of recent funding increases and a pause in centrally prescribed cost increases, which are already building up again. The future costs of hospital construction have also been significantly underestimated. To look to such a short-term surplus for a long-term solution is a delusion. In addition, under Treasury rules any surplus stays with the NHS. These temporary cost savings were made by squeezing emergency care, reducing prices paid to hospitals for care and cutting staff by 8500 – the first fall for a number of years. Staff numbers are, however, increasing again, and cost-of-living increases will also be expected to grow. It is an illusion that the NHS has suddenly become more efficient. Indeed, as Nigel Hawkes of *The Times* said, 'It has jammed on the brakes, squeezed its staff and denied some patients the care they would take for granted in other countries. As a result it is in surplus. But it won't last.'[5]

Ham and Glasby propose a widespread extension of individual budgets, drawn from taxes, and 'a partnership approach in which additional public funding is combined with increased private spending may be the way forward'. This last point is very vaguely stated. But there is no mention of incentives or of savings. And so this tax-funded plan seems to be another twitch of the tail (or tale) of the state-running-the-show. It *is* a response to a crisis, but only within the intellectual framework which has itself produced the crisis. Instead, direct incentives for individual savings and a properly pre-funded system must be the objective. Is such savings provision to be voluntary, or compulsory – which effectively means increasing taxation? If compulsory, what kind of society is that?[6] If voluntary, which incentives work best, and which models do we already know work well? It is time we learned from places like Singapore, on health savings accounts, and from insurance models such as those of Switzerland or Holland and other nearby European countries – as well as those of more distant lands like Australia. Oz has an excellent system if we decide that health savings accounts or insurance is the preferred model. Sweden, too, has shown what the voucher can do to improve educational provision. Professor Ham has made other important contributions. But on this occasion he is wide of the mark.

The role of charity

In addition, what creative and supportive roles can charity and voluntary bodies add to the picture, for example, in fund-raising for community projects and in extending informal support for the elderly? In February 2008 Age Concern, in a new report titled *Out of Sight, Out of Mind*, said that one in five of over 80s suffer from social exclusion and are largely neglected by the state. People say they are lonely, and that there is insufficient help from public services. However, such reports are in part an integral element in the bidding process of 'the iron triangle' – of vested interests, politicians and the bureaucracy – for more taxes to pay for more services. So, too, is the warning by Age Concern in February that local councils face a £1 billion shortfall in funding within three years as a result of the rising cost of elderly care. Before we can move to a savings model we shall certainly have to find significant new money to fund services. In January Liberal Democrat leader Nick Clegg called for a care guarantee of £2 billion for personal care payments for all elderly people requiring care 'based on need and not on ability to pay'. This call, however, does not deal with how to pay for this.[7]

The commitment that very many people make to voluntary and charitable bodies shows that we should not automatically look to the state, but to ourselves. Malcolm Dean, founder and editor of *The Guardian* Society section for nearly 25 years, shows that in the last decade the numbers of charities has increased from 98,000 to 170,000. There are an estimated further 400,000 community associations, neighbourhood groups and small charities that are not required to register. The number of employees in this sector has risen to 1.5 million, backed by 6 million volunteers. Just under 20 million people regularly volunteer in their communities on a monthly basis – an increase from 18.4 million in 2001. There are estimated to be some 865,000 'civil society' organisations in the UK, with an annual income of over £109 billion. In addition, 26 'social enterprise' ventures have been backed by £1.4 million from the Department of Health as 'pathfinder projects'. In March 2008 Ivan Lewis announced a further £27 million for the sector. There is also £100 million allocated to create a social enterprise fund for health and social care.[8]

This tale tells us an important story about the possible alternatives to the centralising state. For very large numbers are giving their time and money to private charitable, cultural and educational societies organised on a non-profit basis through strictly voluntary arrangements. And, unlike governments, these organisations are spending their own money – or, at least, the money of their supporters, given to them without coercion and with some tax incentive in 'gift-aid'. The role of charitable endeavour and of subsidy and support for elderly people can be a much larger part of the whole. These organisations, too, are – at least in theory – accountable to their members, although some are so large as to be very difficult to make accountable by annual meetings or elections to their councils. For example, The National Trust. However, there are a number of very successful mutual organisations such as cooperative and friendly societies offering members health services or cash benefits for these. Many of these serve large numbers of trade unionists under employment benefit schemes. They include the Benenden Hospital, which is one of the largest independent facilities; BUPA; the Civil Service Healthcare Society; Medicash; the national charitable network of the 40 Nuffield Hospitals; Shepherds Friendly Society and a number of others of significant size and membership. They show a willingness to spend private individual funds on healthcare.

In the wider voluntary and charitable sector the present picture of engagement is, however, evidently very mixed. A few very large charities dominate in terms of income. There are, predictably, more active charities in affluent than in poor areas. Nevertheless, about 40% of personal social care – childcare, support for the elderly, care of disabled people – is now provided by the independent sector, both voluntary and private. But Norwich Union recently reported that a generation of adults faces the triple pressure of having to support their parents and their own children while themselves having made no provision to safeguard their own futures. Three in five over 50s admitted that their pensions and savings are unlikely to see them through retirement. One in four adult children were, however, ready to cash in their savings and investments to fund their parents' retirement. But this is hardly a reliable commitment, and it merely transfers the challenge for a generation. The 'savings gap' is thus an enormous and urgent challenge. In March 2008 the Skipton Building Society said that more than half of under 35s contribute nothing to a pension, and a quarter of those who do so save £50 or less a year. Some 58% said they knew they should save but said they simply could not afford to do so. Two-fifths were struggling financially already. Almost half had less than £1000 saved, and 22% had no savings whatsoever. The Centre for Economics and Business Research also reported in March 2008 that average household disposable income had fallen during 2007.[9]

However, neither compulsory private insurance nor an extension of compulsory national insurance is the most positive way to make progress. It does not seem sensible or politically feasible or morally right to demand that more taxation is raised to pay for long-term care costs in this way. In addition, any attempt to return to compulsory and universal benefits would clearly hinder our ability to help the poor, the weak and the disadvantaged. Professor Booth has said that an attempt by the state to finance care for all on a non-means-tested basis would have damaging effects, besides being very expensive. It would reduce choice. It would erode the informal sector. It would have serious effects on future long-term care costs. Indeed, he has suggested that the means test be less severe, to help remove negative disincentives which prompt individuals to get rid of assets to 'beat' the means test. This would help make private solutions affordable. There will always be members of the public determined to 'game' the system. Any easing of the means test may discourage 'gaming', but it increases the unfunded costs to government and thus to the taxpayer. At present the structure discriminates against those who save, own their own house, live in close and mutually supportive family groups, and who make direct or indirect provision for long-term care. At the same time, tax discrimination in favour of informal care and saving should be strengthened. Just as UK tax encouragement to pension funds since the 1920s has provided choice, independence, security and economic stability, so too we could achieve these gains in long-term care funding by the individual and the family.[10]

Savings are crucial. But compulsion is very problematic, even if unavoidable. Voluntary actions engage ownership. Being told that you must do something deters individual willingness, not least to save voluntarily. But if medical savings or insurance is voluntary what do we do when people who have not volunteered, who have failed to provide find themselves in difficulty later in life? How can we do more, too, to use the financing system to encourage those who do most to help themselves or to help their own families? Is the state or the private sector best equipped to offer a pluralist range of funding solutions in diverse financial instruments, to try to meet individual wishes? We need to consider these issues in terms of the specific situations of a variety of individuals.

Ms Careful-Foresight, Mr Sid Spendthrift *et al.*

Let us look at some specifics, and some representative if fictional individuals.

At the risk of being too specific, some examples can point up the contrasts between individuals, and show the difficulties of devising positive policies. Those who make no effort to save – whether earning little or much – have little prospect of anything but dependency unless they have the capital of a property. But many of those in better-paid work and who do save also face difficulties. The modern economy has been characterised by rising incomes, new supplies and falling prices. We have, however, become used to spending in an unprecedented way on many new opportunities. Yet even those in steady work at reasonable income levels need to save significant sums, to fund 'ordinary' pensions and long-term care, although if they buy a home via a mortgage they can look to that capital value to help them when they are old. Let us introduce some specifics.

Ms Careful-Foresight of Bristol has insured and saved from income by deferring gratifications and investing in a long-term care plan. But Mr Sid Spendthrift of Tooting Bec and his associates have consumed, smoked, drunk, used illegal drugs, holidayed abroad, driven fast cars and gambled. Why should he and they expect to pass the social care bills to Ms Careful-Foresight, the taxpayer and saver? What is to be done to encourage *both* to save sensibly, and also to give incentives to their families to informally help, too? What does a moral society do about Mr Spendthrift, who will be there in old age demanding services, however powerful the incentives to save?

Mr and Mrs Solidcitizen of Bedford did their best to save. But they were a low-income family. They are now among the impecunious elderly who have made an effort to save but who underestimated costs and also underestimated their longevity. They now need tax transfers into a personal budget for social care.

Their daughter is Ms Try-my-best Solidcitizen. She is an NVQ-qualified care assistant working at a residential home in North Yorkshire. She is 29. She is diligent, and forward-looking. She is also thrifty. She is, however, an example of someone who works really hard, does the best they can, but who life – in the American phrase – 'doesn't give a fair shake'. She only earns £7.25 an hour. She is, too, one of the many who suffer from our continuing pay discrimination by gender. She is also one of many families dependent on a woman's wages. By dint of self-denial she has saved several hundred pounds over five years. Unfortunately, like many young women, she chose an unsuitable father for her child. She is not married. Her partner, Mr 'Dunno' Dave Dreadnought, is on income support. He left school at the first possible moment. He was a determined truant before that. His mother did her best for him, but his father was virtually an alcoholic. Dave is long-term unemployed. He has no marketable skills. He has held no job for more than a few weeks. He has attempted training several times but never stuck at it. And even when he goes for a shelf-stacking job at the supermarket he is in a line of hundreds of similar unqualified applicants. They have a young son, two years old. They are unlikely ever to own their own home, or to be able to accumulate any serious savings. Their rent is paid by the grants system, and he is on income support. They pay no tax, so tax incentives have no bite. They have grown up in a generation which expects little of themselves but much of 'the state'. All the more urgent then for us to have a pre-funded savings system which generates extra wealth from investment to help pay for what they will expect when they are in elderly care. For they, like many, will inevitably survive in old age on state subsidies, as they are doing now. However, Dave's best friend Tony is seriously obese, already has heart trouble and is at risk of Type 2 diabetes. He may die before his parents.

Ms 'Sparkly' Champagne is a successful young woman. She is a highly paid account executive in the City of London. Like many young people, however, she lives for now. Even with a large annual bonus she has not deliberately provided for the future. However, she will be fortunate as she was encouraged by her father (who paid the deposit) to invest seven years ago in a house behind the Chelsea & Westminster Hospital in Chelsea. This is now worth £2.5 million. This will give her long-term capital growth, to help her pay elderly care bills. This was not, however, her intention in buying the property.

Her colleague Mr 'Prester' Johnny lives in a stylish but rented minimalist flat in Pimlico. He owns no property. He spends his money on foreign holidays, dining out, a new and sporty car every year, designer clothes and as many weekends away as he can manage. He was surprised to learn how much it costs to replace even half let alone two-thirds of final salary, and let alone long-term care costs. For example, that a pension pot of £500,000 would buy an income of just over £35,000 per annum at present. His response: 'I couldn't live on *that!*' But a very large number of ordinary workers would struggle to achieve even a pot of £100,000, for £7000 per annum on retirement.

As the figures demonstrate, the longer you leave it, the harder it gets. At age 30, on an income of £25,000 (and projected earnings at age 65 of £146,029 assuming 4% per annum earnings growth) it costs £414 (or 19.9% of current earnings) to fund two-thirds of final salary on retirement at 65. At age 40 the monthly contribution is £599 (28.8% of current earnings). These figures depend on technical details such as the pension fund being assumed to grow at 7% per annum. To finance a pension and long-term care is clearly very difficult indeed. It takes great willpower and self-denial. New tax breaks could be directly linked to elderly-care investments, on the same tax-gain basis as ISAs are at present. Meanwhile, it is perhaps unsurprising that more than half under the age of 34 in the UK have saved nothing. Few will be as fortunate as those civil servants – nearly 4000 in 2007 – who retired with pension pots of more than £1 million. Most received a tax-free lump sum of three times the initial pension. Ninety per cent of the 5.8 million public sector workers receive final salary pensions, compared with just 16% in the private sector. This may well not continue.[11]

There are other complexities. Women live longer than men on average. Many take career breaks to have children, and leave gaps in cash contributions. 'Final salary deal' company pension schemes are not likely to be offered anew for much longer. Even if you have a 'money-purchase scheme', the value will depend on how much your employer puts into the fund. Investment performance and annuity rates are unpredictable – the so-called longevity risk of saving. Rates may become more expensive in the time between investment and retirement. Lump-sum tax relief on retirement may change, too. The strain on pensions and on company finances is growing due to longer life. In February 2008 Mr Tony Hobman, the Pensions Regulator, warned company schemes that their liabilities would very significantly increase. A new report by Nick Hillman, published by Policy Exchange, shows that only one in four of Britain's 26.2 million employees has a private pension in addition to the basic state pension. This is a sharp fall since 1991–92 when 39% of people were setting funds aside for the future. The government's proposed Personal Account System, due to be introduced in 2012, has been claimed as the answer, with contributions to be matched by employers and by tax relief. This will divert 4% of employees' earnings in their pension fund, topped up by a further 3% from the employer and 1% in tax relief from government. This may be too small a shift, and means testing will reduce credit entitlements.[12]

Work and savings in context

All this places Ms Try-my-best Solidcitizen and her partner Mr Dreadnought and the challenge of funding care in context. At least she has a job, although as a young single earner on low wages she expected to be hit by the abolition of the 10p tax band which had been planned to come into effect on 1 April 2008.[13] Even as an employed person and a small saver she has no hope of accumulating a pension pot of any consequence, nor any long-term care investment. She cannot work more than part-time as she only has some informal child-care help. She cannot rely on her partner. She lives on benefits and various state credits, which pay for her rented maisonette. She accumulates no capital, and started with none. At least she is trying as best she can to support herself and her young son. Unfortunately, the incentives within the benefit structure deter many like her from doing more for themselves, even if she was in a reliable relationship of mutual support, even if she earned more than £7.25 an hour.

It is often more profitable to be on benefits than in work. This is in part because wages for those with few qualifications or skills are so low, in part because some benefits are major disincentives to try harder oneself. Even those in work but on low pay are caught much too soon in the tax net. This reaches too far down the ladder. As Michael Fallon MP has pointed out, a single man on the minimum wage in the UK earns about £11,482 a year, but he pays £1722 in tax and National Insurance, or almost 16% of gross earnings. He receives just £2 a week in working tax credit. If he lived in Ireland, he would have to earn twice as much before he paid the same amount of tax.

In addition, council taxpayers on low or fixed incomes are increasingly unable to meet their bills. Mr Fallon reported that recent work by the Low Incomes Tax Reform Group – which is an initiative of the Chartered Institute of Taxation – has shown that the current rules make it virtually worthless to work between four and 16 hours a week because of the interaction of income support, working tax credit and child tax credit. In addition, there are some 1.4 million agency-employed temporary workers who can make little or no forward provision. Ten per cent of this group were claiming out-of-work benefits in 2007, although the Department for Work and Pensions said that since 1997 youth unemployment was down by almost 40%. That there were 2.9 million more people in work. And that there were 1 million fewer on out-of-work benefits. There are also said to be an estimated 2 million 16 to 24 year olds living below the present poverty line. Ten per cent of nearly one in 10 unemployed are officially classed as not in education, employment or training. Youth unemployment early in 2008 was also rising.[14]

One result is that in 2008 more than 2.2 million British children – *one in five* – now live in such households, dependent on state benefits. In areas of Manchester, Liverpool, London and Glasgow *almost half of children* are growing up in entirely benefit-funded homes. Britain now has Europe's highest proportion of children in workless households – in part itself due to the consequences of the 'benefits culture' and its negative incentives. Sixty areas of Britain are now so dependent on state handouts that more than half of all adults are unemployed or on benefits, new figures showed in March 2008. The benefits system for workless British households now costs more than £12 billion a year. How will those in this situation, and their children, ever fund savings? In addition, for those too late to provide for themselves, a basic single pension of £87.30 a week or £139.60 for a couple – when measured, too, against the official poverty level of £134 a week – offers no room for extra payments for care once an individual depends on a state pension alone.[15] Even if we can introduce incentives to much strengthen the savings effort for taxpayers there will seemingly be many people like the prodigal Mr Spendthrift, or the unfortunate Mr and Mrs Solidcitizen, their thrifty daughter Ms Try-my-best Solidcitizen, and her partner the idle Mr Dreadnought.

In addition, due to 'the credit crunch' in February 2008 it was reported, too, that there were record numbers of bankruptcies in England and Wales, the figure having doubled in the past four years. Even taking into account the regular builder's dodge of closing up on Friday and re-opening anew on Monday, these are alarming figures. The number of pensioners living below the poverty line has risen by 2.5 million in 2006–07. Average mortgage debt of the over-seventies has also worsened in the last 12 months. Mortgage payments now account for a record £1 in every £4 of take-home pay. Income distribution figures published by the Office of National Statistics on 13 June 2008 showed, too, that middle England median earnings were at c. £23,700. Disposable incomes had hardly risen between 2001–02 and 2006–07. There had been a rise of only 1% a year. The bottom third, which includes skilled manual workers, saw their incomes fall between 2004–05 and 2006–07. The ability to save is clearly very weak among some earners, and either tax transfers or tax incentives are necessary if we are to encourage this.[16]

Clearly, it will remain essential to fund and target benefits where they are most necessary. But we also need to so structure incentives for the future to reduce as much as possible the numbers who need the safety net. This is a very considerable public policy challenge. Here, we can make an important argument that charity and voluntary bodies could offer much, too, encouraged by tax changes.

Principles and solutions

These are all very serious issues as we consider the case for making individual funds available to every individual. We know that when people do hold such funds this can genuinely empower choice, prompt more competition and increase diversity. This can also raise standards in provision, or at least change these to standards which consumers determine – which is in principle the same thing. Such evolution would certainly encourage a more active role for service-users. We should make no mistake about this: personal budgets are a major step towards reducing the power of the state and its bureaucratic machinery over our lives while at the same time assuring people of the greater potentials of competition, reliable access, equity and safety. But we need to highlight the true lesson that a system which guarantees such funds to all is the next essential step, just as we need to evolve the necessary financial instruments. It is, indeed, a large 'narrative'. Yet this is no abstraction. It is a potential reality which can be much more effective in individual lives than philosophical discussion of increased local accountability, a 'new localism', or an NHS 'constitution', and other quasi-market substitutes. If we ask, too, whether people would and could accept similar responsibilities for decisions about acute care as for social care then I believe the answer must be 'yes', in collaborative discussions with purchasers of care such as my proposed patient guaranteed care associations. Mr Spendthrift may still say when offered choices, 'Don't ask me! You're the bloody doctor. You tell me!' Even so, this 'random shopper' will and despite himself benefit from the decision others make in the market, and the improvement this creates. And many others – as the experience of personal budgets in social care already suggests – are likely to take a dynamist view. Perhaps it depends on how you ask the questions. If you ask 'Are you in favour of privatising the NHS?' many say 'No', misunderstanding the question. If you ask 'Were you helped by tax breaks to actually hold a lifelong savings fund and thus be given actual cash to spend on the treatment, the doctor, and the hospital you prefer, would you support this?' many more would assent.[17]

All of this asks us to rethink solutions to the crisis in provision and funding of social and elderly care (as of the NHS itself). This book urges dynamist solutions to both funding and provision. Meanwhile, both seem increasingly uncertain, unpredictable and capricious. Yet as more people become accustomed to independent decision making about their social care we cannot take a static approach to a situation which is already one of great dynamic change. It is time to go back to first principles, and to think about what these represent. To find practical, real-world solutions we can see some clear principles which stand true despite the technical complexities of funding and provision. These principles should frame the fundamental aims of public policy. They emphasise humanity to all, liberty for all, and choice for all. To make these ideas effective we need an approach which gives more help to those in greatest difficulty, choice to those able to use it, and secure funds by which the individual can buy care, both out of a personal savings account and from tax transfers to the poor.

Critically, the chief purpose is to nurture and hasten individual independence, and to make as much voluntary provision as possible without the state. Personal budgets take us back to discussion about first principles. They highlight, too, key practical points.

First, that personal budgets should be available to all, in every nook and cranny of health and social care, if we wish to make a reality of choice and of self-responsibility.[18]

Second, that we need fundamental debate about how personal budgets are to be paid for, and by whom. How are sufficient assets to be accumulated in individual hands so that everyone has the buying power in the market? The best way forward seems to be to deploy tax discrimination in favour of dynamic public policies to encourage both savings and choice. Tax reductions which are used to set up health savings accounts in the first place, and then further tax-based incentives for the individual to grow and nurture these personal accounts are likely to be very fruitful.

Equality and esteem

The overriding purpose is to enable everyone to live without state assistance, and to do everything we can to nurture independence. Where this proves not to be possible we need to approach the problem by putting in place as few disincentives as possible. Where people are already in grave difficulties – the fragile and unfunded elderly, the mentally ill, and so on – we should make sure they have both formal and informal support if possible. And the funds to buy good services. Indeed, the most essential step – and the only effective way to create a social parity of equality and esteem – is to ensure that purchasing power is in everyone's hands, by giving purchasing power to the poor selectively and by offering powerful incentives to everyone else to save for grey rainy days. This is very different from state-engineered attempts at 'equality', in a nation where we are all unequal in our inherited DNA, parental inheritance, abilities and experience. It offers market opportunities to express our individuality, to take risks, and to decide what we prefer.

We should do as much as possible to encourage voluntary saving long term as the instruments of thoughtful provision in advance. We should make the assumption, too, that when costs do arise they will primarily fall on the individual who will receive the personal private benefits of care. This may sound harsh, but it is a moral and proper view. It is also workable under the health savings account approach. However, we need then to consider what we do as society when there are several groups who do not save, or cannot do so. We fear the stigma of the older ideas of the deserving and the undeserving poor, but somehow we must encourage everyone to make provision if they can, and yet have in place a safety net for those who do not do so. As I have mentioned, charity has a role, too. In addition, there are now many who are too late to join such a plan, and who already suffer from pre-existing and disabling conditions. Immigrant groups may have very varied attitudes to savings, too. Some immigrants arrive in the UK in adult life, and often bring no savings with them. Some become destitute and homeless. A study of older people living in inner cities recorded very high levels of poverty among certain minority ethnic groups, notably Somalis and Pakistanis, despite the entrepreneurship for which the latter are noted.[19]

The short-term question is how to pay for services now. The long-term question is how to encourage everyone to equip themselves financially, so that when those days come they have the individual financial power to access good services. The choices would be clarified if we stopped sustaining the myth that services are somehow 'free' and re-introduced prices for separable personal benefits while doing all we can to offer powerful incentives to enable everyone to be able to pay them. When we use tax-based transfers to help we should focus, too, on offering selective and not universal benefits. It makes no sense to give benefits to those who do not need this help, and who can pay themselves. This undermines the help we should give to the poor and disadvantaged.

Selectivity in benefits does most to assist the weak by concentrating scarce resources on those who most need help, while doing nothing to undermine the capacity of the strong to provide for themselves.

Our objectives should include increasing choice and competitive provision, increasing genuine welfare while reducing taxation, and targeting welfare to those who need it most rather than setting up a state-funded compulsory mechanism to pay unnecessarily for universal services. Here, it makes no sense to tax those to pay for the costs of services for which they then benefit most. It would be better to leave the taxes in their pockets, offer incentives to save, and to use tax-based funds to help those who are poor. The administrative savings would go into that pot, too. As Arthur Seldon wrote, 'equal treatment of people in unequal circumstances is not equality'.[20]

Seldon, too, emphasised again that one of the keys to answers is to reinforce the family, and what family members can do for one another. Tax changes are also crucial here. Seldon again on equality and the opportunity costs of wrong approaches:

> The change from universal to selective benefits is impeded by a variant of the equality principle that ranges from a wholesome rebellion against privilege to a little-minded indulgence in envy. It ordains that no one shall have anything -- better schooling, nursing, housing – unless and until everyone can have it. It is as potent a precept as any for postponing the day when all can have it. What is at stake is more than the blunting of incentives to individuals to earn more for their families, or indeed the role of the family in social life. It is even more than the logical dilemma of the egalitarian who is prepared to allow some inequality in income after taxation but no inequality in expenditure on education, medical care, even housing, and is content to see vast sums go to everyday consumption. The dilemma of the Egalitarian is that insistence on equality is insistence on *less than that possible for all.*[21]

We should recognise, too, that choices themselves support a dynamic system, which itself encourages effort and increases tax revenues while reducing costs. We should draw attention to the fact that charges are a better way to finance services, too, since they clarify the connections between services and payments. And that charges husband resources and minimise waste. In addition, we should regulate the market by setting out minimum standards. Here, we should focus on the benefits that arise from experiment, from trial and error and from adaptable change. Thus, we should make sure that everyone can be an effective purchaser in the market with a health savings account – and also from equity release, house sale, re-mortgage, other loans, annuities, self-insurance, or cash in hand. Tax reductions are essential initially to create an HSA, and enhanced tax relief should also encourage further investment. And, for the poor, government subsidies as vouchers.

The role of government is thus to work out the funding mechanisms and offer leadership in communicating the benefits. To regulate minimum standards, to protect competition, and to help the weak by doing all it can to promote positive incentives to save and to discourage perverse incentives. This includes ensuring that those who have not provided for themselves, or cannot, or who have tried but have done so ineffectively are not left in the gutter. How we try to avoid that happening in the first place is a large and complex question itself entwined with the demotivating 'benefit culture'.

Provision will necessarily change. The market, as we see in social care, will replace much state provision. We can hope to rely, too, on the continued rise in real incomes which raise expectations and increasingly enhance the ability of many people to provide for themselves by paying for private benefits in open markets. The entire corpus of social care provision, for example, could thus be placed in the realm of private decision making and private purchasing, supported by an HSA, by individual savings, by the deployment of personal capital assets, and by tax transfers to the poor. These principles rest on the idea that private provision is inherently superior since it empowers the individual, always provided that purchasing power can be placed in the hands of the poor. Thus, monopoly and tax-funded public services will be replaced by more self-funded purchasing of services provided in an open market. If the answers were easy, there would be no debate. However, there *are* some clear answers which we would do well to take very seriously as we consider the reform of the funding and provision of NHS care and of elderly long-term social care. We need, too, to find a system which is relatively simple to understand, visibly practical and viable – and which will appeal to the young who have to make the longest-term investments and who face the gravest future burdens.

Emphasis

There are some straightforward points to repeat.

First, to pick up again on the chief theme with which the book began, we must try to ensure genuine fairness, access and equality in a pluralist system. This is not the same as an imposed universal 'solution' for all.

Second, to urge that the problems of funding and providing both NHS and long-term elderly social care are complex, but that they are most usefully structured by flexible instruments, which are responsive to diverse wishes and offer individual approaches. Health savings accounts could cover all services. Meanwhile in social care dynamist approaches could include different annuity patterns in savings, and the individual being able to add long-term care benefits to pension plans. These could radically increase the money available for the provision of social care, chiefly by incentives to save signalled in the tax system. If additional insurance were purchased this would also pool risks, enable the premiums to be invested in economic growth, reduce costs and add compound benefits to policies. However, 'free' social care – which, as we have seen is itself not reliably available even when promised – increases costs by eroding formal and informal private sector provision, as the Report of the Royal Commission on Long-term Care for the Elderly said in 1999.[22]

Third, to argue that we can and should use exchequer transfers to help those too late to join a new savings scheme, or who have never earned enough to finance an insurance plan.

Fourth, to show that at the same time we should try to reduce disincentives to save or to self-provide out of assets.

Fifth, to outline how we can each be empowered to access good social care, whatever our financial situation.

Sixth, to consider the impact of personal budgets in social care now and to suggest that these can and should be extended to every NHS service.

Seventh, to encourage diverse solutions in an adaptive, trial-and-error market in order to meet unpredictable, changing and necessarily diverse wants which are best served by responsive markets which can meet the wishes of different people in differing circumstances.

Eighth, to recognise that funding long-term care through the state system is most unlikely to be cheaper than through the private sector. Indeed, experience suggests that the opposite must be true. As Professor Booth has said, 'If private long-term insurance were deemed unsuitable because of the costs incurred throughout working life, implicit insurance provided by the state through more taxpayer funding would only be cheaper if, for a given level of service, the state can provide finance more efficiently.' Indeed, levels of service seem more favourable in countries with different degrees of private and state health finance, both in social care and in healthcare.[23]

Ninth, to suggest that pressure on costs will continue to increase as demand for higher standards of care will continue to increase.

Tenth, imagination counts. The economists Richard Thaler and Shlomo Benartzi showed that in a scheme they called 'Save More Tomorrow', corporate employees agreed to boost their pensions by earmarking a proportion of future pay rises to go into their pensions funds. This idea has nearly quadrupled USA retirement savings.[24]

We need not forever be caught between a hard rock and the hope of an elderly care fund which we each own and control. It is savings which 'save'. And we need to re-think hard about them.

Notes

1 Philip Booth discusses many of these complexities – for example, concerning the qualifying rules for possible changes in financing in long-term care policies – and he finds many detailed solutions. See Philip Booth, *The Long-Term View: financing care for the elderly* (London, Politiea, 1996), and *Caring for the Long Term: financing provision for the elderly* (London, Politiea, 2000).

2 Booth, *Caring*, ibid., p. 5.

3 Chris Ham and John Glasby, 'Lifelong commitment', *The Guardian*, Society section, 30 January 2008, p. 6.

4 Flora Thompson, *From Lark Rise to Candleford* (1939; London, Penguin Books edition 2008), p. 49.

5 Bosanquet *et al.*, *NHS Reform*, op. cit., p. 7, pp. 23–9. DoH Head of Finance David Flory predicted an NHS underspend of £1.8 billion based on the first nine months results for the year ending 31 March 2008. John Carvel, 'Unions urge better pay as NHS in England predicts £1.8bn surplus', *The Guardian*, 4 March 2008, p. 7; Nigel Hawkes and David Rose, '£1.8bn surplus forecast for NHS after cutbacks in patient care', and Nigel Hawkes, 'Hitting the brakes created illusion of efficiency', *The Times*, 4 March 2008, p. 4. The NHS overspend of £800 million had become a surplus of £515 million by April 2008. However, one in five NHS bodies was still in the red, owing a total of £917 million. Savings had been made by cutting training, and halting some healthcare, with doctors warning that patient care may be suffering. House of Commons, Public Accounts Committee, *Report on the NHS Summarised Accounts 2006–07. Achieving Financial Balance*. 23rd Report, HC 267 (London, Stationery Office, 5 June 2008). There are also calls for carers to hold their own individual budgets. More taxation? See Sophie Moulin, *Just Care? A Fresh Approach to Adult Services* (London, IPPR, 2008).

6 On compulsion and its problems see also Andrew Cooper and Rick Nye, *The Future of Long-Term Care* (London, Social Market Foundation, Social Market Foundation Memorandum, 1995).

7 Age Concern, *The Age Agenda 2008: public policy and older people* (London, Age Concern, 26 February 2008); Rosa Prince, 'Councils need extra £1bn to care for elderly, says report', *Daily Telegraph*, 26 February 2008, p. 10. See also Stephen Burke, Caroline Bernard and Marie Morris, *Delivering a Sure Start to Later Life: exploring new models of neighbourhood services for older people. Project report.* (London, Counsel and Care, 27 February 2008); Richard Gray, '1.2 million older people "left lonely and isolated"', *Sunday Telegraph*, 24 February 2008, p. 10. Nick Clegg, speech, 'Nick Clegg sets out his vision for a people's health service', 22 January 2008; www.libdems.org.uk.

8 Panayotes Demarkakos, *Out of Sight, Out of Mind* (London, Age Concern, 15 February 2008); Rosa Prince, 'A million elderly people "ignored by authorities"', *Daily Telegraph*, 15 February 2008, p. 6; Malcolm Dean, 'The Voluntary Sector: roots, current health, future growth', in Alessandra Buonfino and Geoff Mulgan (eds.), *Porcupines in Winter: the pleasures and pains of living together in modern Britain* (London, The Young Foundation, 2006), p. 127. State-charitable/voluntary relations is a very lively area of policy debate. In May 2006 an Office for the Third Sector was created in the Cabinet Office. Dean reports that a third of hospice income is now from government and the government is now the largest funder of voluntary organisations, accounting for 37% of their funds. In his final Arnold Goodman lecture in 2001 Lord Dahrendorf expressed the concern that many charities working on government programmes 'to all intents and purpose had been nationalised'. It is important that the sector is not swallowed by government, either by grant-dependency or by unsuitable 'provider' relations. See *Stand and Deliver: the future for charities providing public services* (London, Charity Commission, 2000); Association of Chief Executives of Voluntary Organisations, *Replacing the State: the case for third sector public services delivery* (London, Acevo, 2003); *The Future Role of the Third Sector in Social and Economic Regeneration: an interim report* (London, HM Treasury and Cabinet Office, 2006); *Partnership in Public Services: an action plan for third sector involvement* (London, Cabinet Office, Office for the Third Sector 2006); *Public Funding of Large National Charities* (London, National Audit Office, 2007); *Hearts and Minds: commissioning from the voluntary sector* (London, Audit Commission, 2007); *Local Area Agreements and the Third Sector: public service delivery*

(London, National Audit Office, 2007). Other useful guidance is at The Serco Institute, www.serco.com and University Network of Social Enterprise at www.universitynetwork.org. See also Patrick Butler, 'Spreading the glue', *The Guardian*, Society section, 6 February 2008, p. 3, and National Council for Voluntary Organisations, *NCVO Civil Society Almanac* (London, NCVO, 8th edition, 2008) – previously the *UK Voluntary Sector Almanac*. In February 2008 evidence was reported that the 'third sector' is not being trusted to deliver services in large-scale public sector contracts. Sarah Wood [Programme Director, Third Sector Commissioning Programme], *Evaluation of the National Programme for Third Sector Commissioning* (London, National Improvement and Development Agency, 2008); 'Ivan Lewis announces £27m extra for social enterprise', DoH press release, 27 February 2008; Ivan Lewis, 'Social enterprise – a world class solution', Patrick Butler, 'Fresh thoughts on public tender', and Tash Shifrin, 'Social pioneers feel their way', *The Guardian*, Society section, 5 March 2008, p. 15.

9 Sarah Womack, 'One in 3 fears supporting children and parents', *Daily Telegraph*, 12 February 2008, p. 11; Sarah Womack, '"Tiswas generation" faces work until 76', *Daily Telegraph*, 7 March 2008, p. 13, and www.aviva.com. See also Daily Telegraph reporter, 'Soaring living costs leave families worse off than a year ago', *Daily Telegraph*, 4 March 2008, p. 12.

10 Booth, *Caring*, op. cit., p. 1. He warns that this estimate should be treated with caution.

11 Taxpayer's Alliance, *£1 million NHS Pensions*, Research Note 26 (London Taxpayer's Alliance, 25 January 2008); Andrew Porter, '£1 trillion cost of public pensions', *Daily Telegraph*, 25 February 2008, p. 1; John Greenwood, 'Diagnosis: NHS staff must top up their pension', *Sunday Telegraph*, 9 March 2008, p. M26.

12 See Paul Farrow, 'Live fast, die in poverty', *Sunday Telegraph*, Money and Jobs section, 24 January 2008, p. 24 for a helpful summary of these issues, and for more illustrative data provided by Standard Life. On 18 February 2008 the UK Pensions Regulator Mr Tony Hobman published a draft statement on the regulation of fixed benefit pension schemes that set out a new approach to mortality assumptions due to new evidence of mortality trends. See also Nick Hillman, *Quelling the Pensions Storm: lessons from the past* (London, Policy Exchange, 2008); Jonathan Wynne-Jones, 'Private pensions take-up drops to only one in four', *Sunday Telegraph*, 2 March 2008, p. 2. Also www.thepensionsregulator.gov.uk.

13 In fact, she escaped. See the policy change at House of Commons, *Hansard*, statement by Chancellor of Exchequer, Mr Alastair Darling, and debate 13 May 2008, cols. 1201–4; and debate, 5 June 2008, cols. 907–111.

14 Michael Fallon, 'Tories must champion fairer, lower taxes', *Daily Telegraph*, 13 February 2008, p. 21. See www.litrg.org.uk. Also, Polly Toynbee, 'MPs must fill Labour's pledge to low-paid and temporary workers', *The Guardian*, 22 February 2008, p. 33; Rosa Prince, 'Tories reveal "lost generation" of jobless youngsters', *Daily Telegraph*, 18 February 2008, p. 6.

15 Robert Winnett, 'Two million children growing up without a parent at work', *Daily Telegraph*, 13 February 2008, p. 1. See figures deposited in House of Common Library February 2008; Steven Swinford and Dean Nelson, 'Over half of adults on benefits in 60 neighbourhoods of Britain', *Sunday Times*, 16 March 2008.

16 Ministry of Justice company winding up and bankruptcy petition statistics – third quarter 2007. Published 15 February 2008. See www.justice.gov.uk. Christopher Hope, 'Record numbers seek bankruptcy', *Daily Telegraph*, 16 February 2008, p. 6. The figures are for actual court findings only. Department of Work and Pensions, *The Pensioners' Income Series, 2006–07* (London, DWP, 10 June 2008); *British Life-styles 2008: winners and losers in changing economic times*, research report published by market research firm Mintel; Kathryn Hopkins, 'Thousands fall prey to surge in cost of living'; Ashley Seager, 'Ministers risk missing key labour target', *The Guardian*, 11 June 2008, pp. 6–7; Stephen Adams, 'Mortgages take record quarter of incomes', *Daily Telegraph*, 16 April 2008, p. 4; Office of National Statistics, London, *Economic and Labour Market Review*, 2 (6), 13 June 2008.

17 See the detailed surveys of public opinion undertaken by the IEA, reprinted in Seldon, volume 6, *Collected Works*, op. cit.

18 Cabinet Office Minister Ed Miliband spoke of 'possibly using individual budgets' for people with chronic conditions. Speech to 5th annual Guardian Public Services Summit, 7 February 2008. Patrick Wintour, 'Miliband: no turning back on reform of public services', *The Guardian*, 7 February 2008, p. 19.

19 T Scharf, C Philipson, A Smith and P Kingston, *Growing Older in Socially Deprived Areas* (London, Help the Aged, 2002). I owe the reference to Philipson in Buonfino and Mulgan (eds.), *Porcupines*, op. cit., p. 88; Alexandra Topping, 'Nothing like the promised land', *The Guardian*, Society section, 20 February 2008, p. 4.

20 Arthur Seldon, *The Future of the Welfare State*, originally published in *Encounter*; reprinted in Robert Schuettinger (ed.), *The Conservative Tradition in European Thought*, 1970; then reprinted in Seldon, volume 6, *Collected Works*, op. cit. See p. 59.

21 Seldon, volume 6, *Collected Works*, op. cit., p. 61. Seldon's italics.

22 *Report of the Royal Commission on Long-term care for the Elderly with Respect to Old Age: long term care – rights and responsibilities* (London, Stationery Office, 1999), Cmd. 4192–1.

23 Booth, *The Long-Term View*, op. cit., pp. 6–7.

24 Thaler and Benartzi, 'Save more tomorrow: using behavioural economics to increase employee saving', *Journal of Political Economy*, 112(1), February 2004, pp. 164–87, part 2. gsbwww.Chicago.edu/fac/richard.thaler/research/SMarTJPEE.pdf. See Harford, *The Logic of Life*, op. cit., p. 63.

19

The picture in the frame

'Never speak loudly unless the house is on fire.'

– HW THOMPSON

'We have no guarantee that the after-life will be any less exasperating than this one, have we?'

– NOEL COWARD

Key questions

What do first principles tell us about the picture in the frame? What is 'the framing effect'? They help us to ask the right questions, to take a view of what might count as answers, and to look for these among the following interlinked questions:

How are personal budgets to be funded?

We have already seen that health savings accounts can be funded from reduced taxation. If individual budgets are to work well for all there must be a sufficient, secure, predictable and appropriate financial structure so that people can support their independence and not be constrained by local-government funding problems.

The most viable and secure approach to long-term elderly care is by long-term savings accounts (or through insurance) and other financial instruments, including house ownership. Savings accounts would be specific to every individual, held for life and be used to pay for all care services in a market. This is a creative and viable approach. Personal budgets funded by tax reductions, supplemented by long-term savings, insurance or other personal asset accumulation would be a more secure model than the present fragile local government funding model. This is unreliable. It is already seen to be at inadequate levels. It would be more secure than a collectivist but better-funded tax-based local government model. For there the individual has no future security or ownership. And future budgetary constraints may well further squeeze services. A health savings account offers us the chance to free the individual from the risks of the collapse of state tax-based funding.

As Professor Peter Beresford (Professor of Social Policy at Brunel University) has rightly said,

> The government is driving hard on its personalisation agenda, setting an ambition that all service-users have control over the support they need. But the good intentions of a

policy that currently is just a coating of values without the commitment of cash gives way, when scratched, to hidden rationing and restrictions, with choice and opportunity being overwhelmed by a declining quality of life and more stress.[1]

The solution is not to increase taxes. It is instead to ensure that every individual holds a lifelong health and social care fund – a health savings account – on which they can call. Professor Philip Booth has separately suggested advances could be achieved by insurance, or by other financial instruments such as paying when the need arises, if people can do so.[2] Indeed, these alternatives may be more rational for some. But many young people already struggle to rent let alone buy a home, and many may never achieve ownership of such a capital asset.

Meanwhile, with no health savings account in place yet – and for those too old to join a separate insurance scheme – we still need to sort out those who need help from those who do not. We do not now have a universalist scheme in social care, nor should we seek this. To help the weak and the disadvantaged we still need to concentrate on these, rather than to offer benefits indiscriminately. This makes a means test unavoidable, although we should simplify the cumbersome and costly bureaucratic structure of eligibility criteria and assessments in the system of allocating resources to individuals by a funding band. One purpose in doing so should include raising the means-test level to discourage the disposal of personal assets specifically to 'beat' the means test. Clearly, the existing banding approach is too crude. It undermines the individual assessment. It replaces this personalised assessment by the allocation of an individual to an average-banded assessment. It also implies a cap to the budget, which may mean that some in great difficulty are not helped.[3]

How could purchasing be strengthened?

Clearly, by encouraging everyone to hold a health savings fund. And then to bring people together to more effectively spend their money. Under present arrangements it is worth considering how the existing social care assessments work, and how purchasing functions. The present personal budget approach in social care is implemented in a series of local steps. Ideally, a care manager meets the individual and, hopefully, their carers. The individual completes a self-assessment questionnaire, with the help of their carers. The local authority makes an assessment in terms of its *own* eligibility criteria. The decision, if favourable, then produces an offer of a budget. A support plan can then be developed. The package is then reviewed by the care manager in the local authority. All this is usually very new to the service-user, and to their carers. It is an important learning process, and that itself can be empowering. However, there is also the greater potential for budget holders to share experiences, and perhaps to come together in mutual organisation. For example, following these negotiations services could be jointly purchased by a cooperative purchasing organisation. This would be member-owned and act on the behalf of members to secure that good care which the user defines.

Such an evolution of member-owned purchasing bodies could be an integral part of the social structure of a coherent society of solidarity and equity. They would enable willing individuals together acting cooperatively to deploy the power and resources of the nation to ensure appropriate and timely access to personal services which users define. They would do so irrespective of class or patronage or individual cultural clout. This would reinforce community identity while reducing bureaucracy, and curb and deter both centralised and localised uniformity. Such initiatives would be interwoven with the recovery of self-organising, cooperative but non-collectivist traditions of Britain. These offer both natural and personal liberty and individual self-responsibility. Collective action, without collective*ism*. Such an innovation within social care and the NHS would finally place the individual in the pivotal position. It would enable member-owned purchasing bodies to make the market. They would be part of a new and clearer structure of plural competing provision and purchasing. They would drive new models of services, and challenge existing risk-averse models of purchasing, provision and governance.

Such a purchaser structure defines preferences and good outcomes as the necessary currency of change. It makes the mobility of individual health savings funds the guardian of the market. It asks for permission for people to help it happen. Providers would have to deal with individuals, perhaps individually, perhaps via their mutually owned commissioner. And be capable of delivering a highly personalised and individual response. Clinical evidence, too, shows that the genuine involvement of service-users and patients in decisions improves outcomes, encourages 'compliance' with treatment, and helps reduce health inequalities.[4]

This is an as yet unexplored avenue of cooperative purchasing using personal budgets. If people holding their own personal budgets could join together in voluntary, member-owned bodies these, too, could encourage more imaginative provision and support. They would also give every individual a real democratic stake in the organisation of health and social care. They would encourage a local sense of belonging, and a genuine sense of mutuality. They would be independent bodies. Each member would meet on equal terms. The PGCA would be open, effective institutions of liberal democracy – as were the self-organising working-class institutions in the former world of mutual cooperation which we have lost.

Can we evolve a national framework, but one where the financial empowerment of the individual prompts as much local variation in the range of services as people are prepared to pay for?

Clearly, the 'yes' answer is directly illustrated by proposals to enable every individual to hold financial power. This will endorse local variations which prove useful. Here, too, we return to the issue of giving local providers and service-users permission to evolve local variations. They will do so in response to financially empowered purchasers.

Are people to be genuinely trusted to make their own decisions, including 'wrong' choices?

This is the perennial problem of knowledge. Again, a proper market will take us away from the idea that 'experts' can know our interests better than we know them ourselves. And that they can reasonably forbid us to make perfectly legal choices because they would not necessarily make these for themselves. There needs to be a positive attitude towards giving permission for change, as I have argued, and an acceptance of risk – both by the state, by purchasers and by providers. Service-users and those who assist them within social care should follow new directions, and be supported in being allowed to take and accept the consequences of their own decisions.

How will specific, individual, labour-intensive personal services be maintained, including those expensive services where some users are seriously handicapped and where flexible and intensive personal assistance is essential?

For example, the blind and deaf, those with advanced Parkinson's disease or with Alzheimer's, those who do not communicate verbally or for whom English is not their first language, and indeed who may not speak it at all. Here, the answer surely is that sufficient buying power would be gained and sufficient provision encouraged if these service-users held long-term funds, and if they also came together in member-owned cooperatives. Such mutual purchasing organisations would offer sufficient cash-flow to providers to encourage appropriate provision. Smaller voluntary and user-led organisations and ethnic organisations would play a vital role, too, together with larger providers.

How successfully are personal budgets now prompting new competition among existing care agencies and new providers, and what can we learn from these experiences?

Here we need new studies based on the actual experiences of individuals. There is now a great deal of knowledge scattered around the country. We can learn from one another. Informally, one hears that government is pleased with the results of the 13 pilots (in West Sussex, Bath, NE Somerset, Lancashire etc.), which is why they have pressed forward with personal budgets. However, we need the detailed information to be published.

Are we to seek individual financial empowerment, or cost savings?

Well, both! It is vital to continue to emphasise empowerment. But there can be significant cost-savings, too. James Bartlett, Niamh Gallagher and Charles Leadbeater, in their recent Demos pamphlet *Making it Personal*, suggested that significant savings averaging 10% on care packages have already resulted from the introduction of personal budgets, together with improvements in consumer satisfactions. These are the expected and normal effects of markets. We should welcome lower costs, and the successful provider will know to ensure that these gains are invested in better services and lower prices. Competition with private and voluntary providers will inevitably cut the administrative costs of wasteful local government and NHS bureaucracies.[5]

How can we do more to support and encourage care by family members or friends on an informal as well as a formal basis?

The informal (and 'uncommodified') sector carries a huge part of the burden of social care and much of its costs. This is morally positive. Here, we could do more by expanding income tax deductions to reinforce this help. But we have to be cautious, as voluntary work has a special moral value. Of course, the employment of family and friends through personal budgets is already aiding many, and large numbers do help with no thought of payment. Yet personal budgets used to pay family or friends puts an otherwise elusive financial value on this care, too, as there is now a market transaction, although earnings are not the only or for most the chief motive of family or friends. Nevertheless, the elderly are often helped by people not a lot younger than them and the extra income is clearly helpful. These carers are now partly in the informal sector, partly in the formal. We need to carefully consider positive incentives to sustain informal and loving help, and do nothing to undermine this help.

The 'economics of second best'

Funding, incentives and the social results are all one. This is not likely ever to be an area of interest free from the long shadow of government. Presently, however, as Professor Booth has said, government intervenes significantly by paying for care on a means-tested basis.

By doing so, it provides a strong incentive for people not to finance care themselves, not to save, not to take out insurance and not to use informal care. If the government is to continue to provide good quality care for those who do not have sufficient income or assets, as it has done since the 1983 reforms, this problem will remain. We are therefore in the realms of 'the economics of second best'. In these circumstances it is perfectly reasonable for the government to give favourable tax treatment to long-term care insurance or savings, or to help informal carers, thereby correcting the bias against self-reliance which currently exists within the system. Tax concessions might, indeed, reduce costs to the state of providing long-term care (it is worth noting that since tax relief for private medical insurance was abolished for pensioners over one million people have moved from the private to the state sector).[6]

Government *should* use incentives to encourage people to build up funds by which they can pay for this care and also make sure that the poor have financial clout in the marketplace, too. As Professor Booth makes clear, every individual, of course, has a variety of possible approaches to providing long-term elderly care for themselves. Each may be rational, depending on individual circumstances. They can pay taxes, and assume that government will deliver. They can do nothing extra, and rely on the same assumption. They can depend on informal care in the family. They can build up savings – in cash, equities, a house and the like or in a private pension and annuity, or earn interest and growth on capital. They can invest in one of a variety of long-term care insurance policies. There they can select specific cover; for example, domiciliary care costs but not nursing home care. Or both. They can decide instead to pay for immediate needs from current cash. They can decide to depend on equity release schemes. A free society should resist compulsion. It should be for the free individual to decide. It would be rational, too, for the Exchequer to offer incentives which relieve the state of high long-term costs. There are many lenses, too, by which we can try to consider the provision of services which are necessarily sensitive and often expensive. They should be particularly focused on individual wishes and preferences. An HSA is the most persuasive answer.

Learning to choose

My concern in considering funding and provision is with Hayek's perspective of the self-responsible and financially empowered adult. One who is learning to choose in an adaptive, incremental, trial-and-error market. A market where we each make every effort to provide the necessary funds for ourselves and our families out of our own incomes and savings (with taxes reduced) or investments in insurance and other products. It should be our own choice, just as the consequences of our behaviour and decisions should very broadly be our own. We should also want to live in a society in which social provision is made for those who do not or cannot provide, while doing all we can to supply incentives for the individual to look forward and to make financial provision for themselves. Here, too, we can make many gains by the influence of example and the demonstration effects of good reforms.

In discussing these questions I have not gone into great detail about the global figures of spending on elderly care, or social care or pensions, or health savings accounts. Nor into the complexities of such proposals as 'partnership schemes' in long-term elderly care (for asset protection), which are one means to promote investment in annuities and long-term insurance. But, as Professor Booth shows, like all else in this field, they bring gains and losses. And with 'partnership schemes' evidently more losses than gains. I do not examine the impact – for example – on mean testing, nor the locally varied approaches to means testing itself. The Commission on Social Care did this recently.[7] There are already excellent studies by Professor Booth, Joel Joffe and David Lipsey and others which expertly marshal these detailed numbers to support the arguments for reform. They examine, too, some of the possible economic instruments – such as a voucher to pay for long-term care insurance – and possible tax incentives. There is, as Professor Booth says, the possibility of a wider tax allowance which could be used to buy any number and any combination of 'social insurances' through the private sector – including pension provision, unemployment insurance, health insurance and long-term care, to promote choice and reduce the burden on the state, as proposed by Booth and Dickinson.[8]

The hazards of the state

The competing philosophical choices in the fundamental economic and social framework are clear enough. So, too, is the fact that the unpredictable costs of long-term care are growing and are unfunded, either by the state or by every individual at hazard. These hazards are not only due to health status. Increased state funding is a hazard, too. It involves higher costs, the unreliable promise of services which are unfunded, the future reduction of choice, and 'policy-induced risk' or the possibility that government will cut provision because under its state-financed model it becomes unaffordable. The Royal Commission Minority Report suggested that the cost of formal care could rise in the medium term to five or six times what it was in 1999. If services were universalised this would transfer at least £1.1 billion, rising to £6 billion by 2051, to be paid for from tax-based funds. Without increasing actual spending at all on services. This hardly seems credible politically. In addition, the Institute for Public Policy Research estimated that people who will need continuous care will require 97 billion hours of care in 2023, which is a 47% increase over 1995. *Someone* will have to meet the spending obligations, *somehow*. However, as the pay-as-you-go (PAYGO) pension system is increasingly unsustainable, will we make the same mistake with elderly care?[9]

We need much more creative thinking about the sources of income and wealth, and the incentives, which can make these costs affordable. At the time of writing (early March 2008) we are promised a government 'Green Paper' on social care. It is said that this may lead to a radically new funding system that would be 'easy to understand, accessible and properly funded'. Perhaps. It is widely believed that the work, based on 'progressive universalist principles', will be rooted in a guarantee of minimum standards of care with some co-payments to be made by the individual. Alexandra Norrish, in charge of the social care green paper team at the Department of Health – reporting to David Behan, Director General for Social Care, Local Government and Care Partnerships – has said that three principles will guide the work: independence, well-being and choice. However, trade-offs are unavoidable. Lord Sutherland, who is reviewing Scotland's services in social care – addressing a seminar convened by the online journal *Public Finance* and Deloitte's – has said that a new settlement should be based on needs as defined by professional judgement, equal treatment of frailties causing care needs, and a consistent application of services and guidance across local authority boundaries. As I argue, this is most likely to be achieved if holders of personal care budgets and those who are self-funding come together in mutual purchasing organisations. Then their wishes can be negotiated on their behalf by expert advisors, who would compete for their business.[10]

Meanwhile, the government and local authority rationing officials remain in difficulties, not least because of the cost-saving shunting between the NHS and the social care system. Here, the NHS has now paid out £180 million in compensation to people who remained in continuing care but who were moved into the means-tested care system, the rules being misinterpreted.[11] There would be much greater clarity if we decided what we would pay for individually from our health savings account, or from supplementary insurance or other personal assets.

The demographic balance

In terms of long-term elderly care we know that the demographic balance is against us financially, even though many of us are living longer and more fulfilled lives. The balance of life expectancy and of costs has shifted markedly in the past half century, and it will continue to change. The number of elderly people calling upon social and healthcare is constantly growing. People over 65 are responsible for 35.9% of all finished consultant episodes, although they are only 16% of the population. Those over 60 accounted for 39.7% of all attendances at NHS hospitals in 2005–06, although they make up only 21% of the population.[12]

However, the numbers able to offer informal care and support are decreasing. This matters greatly as in 1996 the estimate of the value of informal care, if charged at market rates then, amounted to 77% of all care. More elderly people have elderly children, who need help themselves. More women are engaged in the formal labour market. Families are smaller, and many children distantly located. More people live alone. And increasingly those who previously would have died due to serious disabilities are surviving. Many have co-morbidities. In addition, long-term care will have to be weighted towards the more serious levels of disability, requiring costly and labour-intensive continuous care, with which informal care may not be able to cope. The proportion of old and very old people in the population continues to increase, as do care costs due to rising wages. On some estimates, long-term care costs were projected to double between 1994 and 2031. As a consequence three common diseases – coronary heart disease, heart failure, and atrial fibrillation, among others – will predictably show rises in incidence rates. This will impact on many budgets including the drugs bill.[13] We already spend nearly half of the NHS budget on those over 64, and nearly a third on those over 74. These proportions are rising. The 2001 census showed that for the first time the number of people in England and Wales aged 60 and over was greater than the number aged below 16. In 1951 there were just 270 centenarians in England and Wales. In 2001 there were over 6000. By 2030 there may be 45,000.[14]

This is not, however, a subject over which we should lament, although one commentator notes that it is frequently filled 'by a demography of despair, which portrays ageing not as a triumph of civilisation, but something closer to an apocalypse'.[15] Indeed, we should rejoice, for it is many of us who will live to enjoy it. However, it is imperative to do more than tinker in the margins financially if we are to keep elderly people out of the margins of life. And if older people are going to be enabled to enjoy these extra years – the opportunity of 'the third age' with involvement in education, travel, voluntary activities, leisure, as well as in providing care and support within the family and community.

Some 31% of adult life is, indeed, now spent in retirement, by contrast with 18% in 1950, according to the Pensions Commission. We are then spenders, not savers.[16] The demand for adequate long-term care and thus of greater funding will not cease to increase. Professor Booth and, separately, The Gleneagles Group estimated that the number of people over 85 would rise significantly. More recently, government actuary figures have projected the number of people aged 85 or over to rise from 896,000 in 1991 to 2,768,000 in 2051, and with significant increases in the numbers between 65 and 84. Professor Booth has developed a sophisticated model of the UK economy which shows the anticipated numbers in different age groups from 2004 to 2078. This work was based on the Government Actuary's Department projections, using 2004 as a base year.[17]

In 2004 the number of people of pensionable age was projected to increase by 65%, from 10.7 million in 2003 to a little over 17 million in 2060, while the number of people of working ages was projected 'to increase much more modestly'. Dr Gabriel Stein has recently reviewed demographic information and dependency ratios. The older Gleaneagles report said that the increase would be from 1 million to 2.8 million by 2040.[18] And, as the aptly named Simon Godsave (then Head of Strategy at NatWest Life) has said, 'These individuals are not other people. If we live to a ripe old age, then many of them could be us.'[19] It is not the case, of course, that everyone calls upon care of this kind for very long. But many of us will do so in the last 18 months of our lives, and then it may be very expensive care.

The policy challenge is to face the fact that without a funding model such as a health savings account or voluntary savings – and preferably both – we will neither endorse a free society nor fund elderly social care successfully in the medium and longer term. Meanwhile, we need practical short-term solutions, too. Unless we can achieve both objectives we will not evoke the responses that can fruitfully help extend the potential of old age and recognise the vulnerabilities and the support for a good life which should be there in our old age.

Effective policies must be both practical and affordable. They must also be compassionate and inclusive. Meanwhile, the sun is setting.

Notes

1 Peter Beresford with Ray Jones, 'Fair shares: personal budgets must avoid one size fits all', *The Guardian*, Society section, 23 January 2008.
2 Philip Booth, *Caring for the Long Term: financing provision for the elderly* (London, Politiea, 2000); Philip Booth, *The Long-Term View: financing care for the elderly* (London, Politiea, 1996). On framing effect see Amos Tversky and Daniel Kahneman, 'Refining decisions and the psychology of choice', *Science*, 1981, 211, pp. 453–58; Harford, *The Logic of Life*, op., cit., pp. 12–13, p. 61.
3 D Brindle, 'We must be wary of cost-cutting', *The Guardian*, Social Care Supplement, 6 February 2008, pp. 3, 5.
4 See RG Evans, ML Barer and R Marmot, *Why Are Some People Healthy and Others Not?* (New York, Aldine de Gruyter, 1994). Also, R Marmot *et al.*, 'Contribution of job control and other risk factors to social variations in coronary heart disease incidence', *The Lancet*, 350, 1997, pp. 235–9; Michael Marmot, *Status Syndrome* (London, Bloomsbury, 2004); Bruno S Frey and Alois Sutzer, 'Happiness, economy and institutions', *Economic Journal*, Royal Economic Society, 110(127), October 2000, pp. 128–38. I owe the last two references to Geoff Mulgan, *Good and Bad Power: the ideals and betrayals of good government* (London, Allen Lane, 2006; Penguin Books edition, 2007), p. 71.
5 James Bartlett, Niamh Gallagher and Charles Leadbeater, *Making it Personal* (London, Demos, 18 January 2008). See also, Charles Leadbeater, 'This time it's personal', *The Guardian*, Society section, 16 January 2008, p. 6.
6 Booth, *The Long-Term View*, op. cit., pp. 18–29.
7 CSCI 3rd Annual Report to Parliament, *The State of Social Care in England, 2006–07* (London, CSCI, 28 January 2008).
8 Booth, *Caring for the Long Term*, op. cit; Booth, *The Long-Term View*, op. cit.; Joel Joffe and David Lipsey, 'Minority Report', *Report of the Royal Commission on Long-term Care for the Elderly with Respect to Old Age: long term care – rights and responsibilities* (London, Stationery Office, 1999), Cmd. 4192–1. At the time Joffe was formerly Deputy Chairman and a founder of Allied Dunbar, and later chairman of Oxfam; Lipsey was public policy editor of *The Economist*. See also Seldon, *Re-privatising Welfare: after the lost century* (London, IEA, 1996), reprinted in volume 6, *Collected Works*, op. cit; P Booth and G Dickinson, *The Insurance Solution* (London, European Policy Forum, 1997).
9 D Dullaway and S Elliott, *Long-term Care Insurance: guide to product design and pricing*, paper presented to the

Staple Inn Actuarial Society, 1998; Osaki Juurikkala, 'Punishing the poor: a critique of means-tested retirement benefits', *Economic Affairs*, 28(1), March 2008, pp. 11–16.

10 Lord Sutherland and Alexandra Norrish both cited in Judy Hirst, 'An agenda on ageing', *publicfinance.co.uk* (internet magazine), 9 November 2007, accessed 3 March 2008.

11 Nicholas Timmins, 'Payouts for social care patients', *Financial Times*, 13 February 2008, p. 4.

12 Office of National Statistics, *Regional Trends 39* (London, ONS, 23 May 2006); *Hospital Episode Statistics* [HES], at www.hesonline.nhs.uk. Hospital Episode Statistics.

13 SR Nuttall *et al.*, 'Financing long-term care in Great Britain', *Journal of the Institute of Actuaries*, 121, part 1, 1994, cited in Booth, *The Long-Term View*, op. cit., 1996, p. 3; A Majeed and P Aylin, 'The Ageing population of the United Kingdom and cardiovascular disease', *British Medical Journal*, 10 December 2005, 331(7529), p. 1362.

14 Chris Philipson, 'Growing old in the 21st century', in Allesandra Buonfino and Geoff Mulgan (eds.), *Porcupines*, op. cit., p. 82; UK 2001 census at www.statistics.gov.uk.

15 Cited in Malcolm Dean, *Growing Old in the 21st Century* (Swindon, Wilts., Economic and Social Research Council, 2004). I owe the reference to Philipson, ibid., p. 83.

16 See discussion in Pensions Commission, *Pensions: challenges and choice: the first report of the Pensions Commission* (London, Stationery Office, January 2005).

17 This was done for his work on pensions policy. Booth, 'The Young held to ransom', op. cit., p. 5. See also www.gad.gov.uk.

18 Booth, *Caring for the Long Term*, op. cit., p. 2; Government actuary figures 28 July 2004; Gabriel Stein, 'The economics, political and financial implications of ageing populations', *Economic Affairs*, 28(1), March 2008, pp. 23–8; Gleneagles Group, *Report to Government on Pensions and Long-term Care* (London, The Gleneagles Group, 1999); *Update of the Government Actuary's Quinquennial Review of the National Insurance Fund as at April 2006*. See also Patrick John Ring, 'Security in pension provision: a critical analysis of UK government policy', *Journal of Social Policy*, July 2005, 34(3), pp. 343–63; Government Actuary Department, *Interim Life Tables, 2004–2006* (London, Office of National Statistics, 22 August 2007).

19 Simon Godsave, Foreword, in Booth, *The Long-Term View*, op. cit., p. v.

20

World-class commissioning? 'Thanks, but no thanks. I think I will go round the corner'

'It is unbelievable how many systems of morals and politics have been successively found, forgotten, rediscovered, forgotten again, to reappear a little later, always charming and surprising the world as if they were new, and bearing witness not to the fecundity of the human spirit but to the ignorance of men.'
— ALEXIS DE TOCQUEVILLE

'The problems [which social scientists] try to answer arise only in so far as the conscious action of many men produce undesigned results, in so far as regularities are observed which are not the result of anybody's design. If social phenomena showed no order except in so far as they were consciously designed, there would indeed be no room for theoretical sciences of society. . . . It is only in so far as some sort of order arises as a result of individual action but without being designed by any individual that a problem is raised which demands a theoretical explanation.'
— FRIEDRICH VON HAYEK

Money moves. There is nothing more powerful than a consumer saying, 'Thanks, but no thanks. I think I will go round the corner to the other provider.' Then money talks, and preference walks. We can then see the potentials of the 'triple whammy': of members, purchasing and power. Of savings, sensibilities, and shifting buying patterns. Of the mutual purchasing organisation, the competing patient guaranteed care associations, and individual choice. This would establish new structures and policies to address key priorities – those of fundamental moral ideas as well as the important objectives of individual autonomy and improved health and social care.

To turn the corner, the consumer must be able to go round the corner. The move to *competing* purchasers would be the clearest possible statement that *we mean it*. And that change is not an illusion. That it is not one step forward and two quick steps back. That the stone will be moved. That we will not allow it to roll back upon us. That time and money marches on.

The PGCAs would be an integral part, too, of the social structure of a coherent society of solidarity and equity, fairness and morality, and the proper release of subjectivity and individual authenticity. They would enable willing individuals together to deploy the power and resources of their own and of the nation to ensure appropriate and timely access to personal services. They would do so irrespective of class or patronage or individual cultural clout. They would reinforce community identity while reducing bureaucracy, and centralised uniformity. All this change would be interwoven with the recovery of self-organising, cooperative but non-collectivist traditions of Britain, offering both natural and personal liberty and individual self-responsibility. None of this will arise from monopoly PCTs.

There are thus key operational, moral, social, national and functional benefits to be had from financially empowered choice where the individual can take their fund to a preferred purchasing organisation. This innovation within health and social care would place the individual in the pivotal position. It would enable member-owned purchasing bodies to make the market. They would market and manage care and ensure choice. They would be part of a new and clearer structure of plural competing provision both of purchasers and of providers. They would drive new models of services, and challenge existing risk-averse models of purchasing, provision and governance. They would prevent monopoly, and where this is a problem (as in A&E) then managements must be contestable.

This purchaser structure defines preferences and good outcomes as the necessary currency of change. It makes the mobility of individual funds the guardian of the market. Providers will have to deal with individuals, via their commissioner, and be capable of delivering a highly personalised and individual response. Clinical evidence, too, shows that the genuine involvement of patients in decisions improves outcomes, encourages 'compliance' with treatment, and helps reduce health inequalities. We speak here, and throughout the book, of outcomes. We should keep in view a working definition of what we mean. Donabedin defined them thus: 'Outcomes record the effects of the care process on the health status of the population.' Good outcomes include many benefits, including those predicted by treatments. These are both clinically and personally defined. Bad outcomes include death, medication errors, post-operative loss of an organ, a limb, speech, sight, hearing or smell; or hospital-acquired infection. 'Quality is not how well or how frequently a medical service is given, but how closely the result approaches the fundamental objectives of prolonging life, relieving distress, restoring function, and preventing disability.'[1]

These voluntary, member-owned bodies would give every individual a real stake in the organisation. They would encourage a local sense of belonging, and a genuine sense of mutuality. They would be independent bodies, and each member would meet on equal terms. They would be open, effective institutions of liberal democracy – as were the self-organising working-class institutions in the former world of mutual cooperation which we have lost. As David Green has said,

> The friendly societies were not just benefit societies. They treated people as if they had a moral dimension to their character as well as a material one. They appealed to the best in people, and enabled them to face the challenges of leadership and self-organisation. When national insurance was introduced [in 1911] it attended only to the material dimension, and in separating the cash benefits from the moral and educational role of the societies destroyed their essence.[2]

The recovery of this salient spirit would be one of the several benefits of the system I have outlined.

In the face of genuine plurality of provision and a choice of a purchaser there would be the necessity for every competing PGCA and every potential provider to offer a genuine client-centred service. There would need to be different models of management from existing PCTs, and different partnerships as well as competition between providers. Providers would have to contract and cost services based on unit costs and outcome criteria set by purchasers and providers, and not by politicians. This means a massive cultural change, especially in the expectations of clients and staff. The role of commissioners would then be to manage by evolution, but to be fast and sure-footed. This structure would ensure that the consumer must remain at the centre of all thinking in the system. Purchasers will be the leaders in health improvement in their localities, working in collaborative partnerships with providers and with their own PGCA members. They would prompt and require new investments in services and drive continuous innovation. They would thus effectively deliver what Mark Britnell, Director General of Commissioning for the NHS, has called for – 'world class commissioning'.[3]

The Department of Health's consultation document *Commissioning Framework for Health and Well Being* of March 2007 challenged purchasers to commission for 'what outcomes people want for themselves and their communities'.[4] But, as we have seen, the NHS and social care still struggles to make sense of empowering the individual save in those areas where personal budgets have been permitted. To that extent it remains a freehold and not a leasehold business.

Individual control over funds would make purchasing and provision work better. My proposed membership bodies, the patient guaranteed care associations, would function in a system designed on the basis of individual choice, better outcomes, improved productivity and what Professor Michael E Porter and Dr Elizabeth Teisberg have called 'value-based competition'.[5] In addition, the allocation of public funds should be removed from the Department of Health. Instead, this, would become a Ministry responsible for preventive care information and for some strategic consultations. The oversight of health savings accounts should, too, be administered separately from the Treasury and the DoH, by a new independent body. This structure, too, would help curb the power of pressure groups.

The competing PGCA

In my Introduction, and in my discussion of the serious deficits of cancer care especially, I emphasised the importance of *coordinated care*. Crucially, the competing PGCA would exert all its management and leadership skills to achieve coordinated provision and care, since we know that many of the failures in British cancer care, for example, arise from the absence of just this coordination. In addition, the PGCA would exert great influence on many other issues, which PCTs are failing – inadvertently, or quite consciously – to do. Thus:

1 Strong, legally independent local purchasers

The competitive PGCA would make commissioners of services strong, legally independent and locally accountable. This would offer local legitimacy to local decisions. It would give purchasers teeth – which has been called for by Anthony Kealy, the Department of Health's Commissioning Policy head.[6] This is, indeed, a much more attractive means to independent operation than setting up an NHS board, which would remain on political strings. PGCAs, too, would be directed by managers and doctors fully aware that modern medicine is delivered by teams.

2 Impact on providers

General practice fund-holding in the 1990s reduced waiting times, reduced elective hospital admissions and cut prescribing costs. The project shook up hospital management and challenged consultant complacency, as did no other policy as I well remember from my time in the Chair of the Brighton Health Authority and then the Brighton Hospitals NHS Trust.[7]

One of the chief benefits of financially empowered choice would be the impact it would have on providers. It would make them sit up, reward the best providers and encourage other providers to enter the newly stimulated market. It would test traditional referral patterns. Individual choices would have a cumulative effect on services. This would improve services and build leadership capacity. It would also encourage the entry to the market of those entrepreneurs and innovators who understand how to give service to those with choices – as in the much more transparent financial services market and travel markets, for example.

In December 2007 the Government's Chief Medical Officer, Sir Liam Donaldson, set out a radical plan to fine hospitals if patients contracted superbug infections while in their care. But this would reduce patient care, without moving the money to a preferred provider which would be the case in my own purchasing proposals. Mr David Cameron has called for the funding of hospitals where patients are infected with MRSA or other hospital-acquired infections to be cut. But this would be best achieved in a market, not by central diktat. The PGCA would have this power over all suppliers, by negotiating this condition in contracts, by writing state-of-the-art infection control into the system, by insisting on cleanliness (including doctors and nurses washing their hands properly between seeing patients – which the NHS still fails to achieve despite patient deaths from hospital-acquired infections). In 2007 more than 8000 deaths were linked to two of the most serious hospital-acquired infections – MRSA and *Clostridium difficile*. The PGCA would move business elsewhere if necessary.[8]

In addition, if the PGCA were to offer employment on fixed-term contracts to GPs there would be a resolution of Alan Johnson's continuing struggles with them over their hours and services. Direct incentives would do the trick.

3 Impact on quality and on costs
Competition would drive up standards, and reduce costs by better management of the complex set of pathways and networks linking together the care elements, including individual preferences, quality and outcomes, access and costs. Purchasing contracts would also be as specific as possible about the data required on outcomes, from providers and in patient reports. In addition, gains in cost controls by purchasers would free funds to provide additional benefits for members. Thus, the successfully managed PGCA would be able to attract new members, including the next generation of recruits. Careful financial management, too, would safeguard member funds and the financial viability of the organisation. Good and regular external audit would be a condition of the structure.

4 Coordination of choice
The purchaser would have the responsibility to ensure that at all stages in the patient pathway they would be accountable for the quality and coordination of care and of choice. This would be a safeguard against the quality of care being a trade-off for choice, for example in the treatment of those with long-term conditions.

5 Improved end-of-life care
The PGCA would take very seriously the necessity to much improve end-of-life care. They would be transparent about services commissioned, their costs and details of such important aspects as support for choices of where to die when terminally ill,

and support for families. They could help patients have much more control over their death, which is itself one of the keys to a good life. They could significantly help end the indignities of death in hospital. This would be one of the major discussions they would have with members. They would discuss using the HSA for palliative care, including nursing, physician care, social services, counselling, inpatient and respite care, and bereavement services. They could thus much improve support for hospices and other relevant services specialising in palliative care and pain control, rather than these being sucked into the state sector by increasing central grants. Almost half of all complaints to the Healthcare Commission relate to end-of-life care. About 60% of people die in hospital, where less than 20% would choose to do so. The number of all complaints, too, is surely understated; many do not complain as they are so vulnerable.[9]

6 Make payment-by-results a reality
This flagship NHS policy continues to struggle. But the PGCA would make it a reality by negotiating appropriate local tariffs and costs. For example, as Sophie Christie, Chief Executive of Birmingham East and North PCT pointed out, 'Truly incentivising good chronic-disease management would differentiate between planned and unplanned admission. And with pay regardless of length of stay. If we really engaged to make hospitals pay attention to infection control, should a commissioner pay at all for a patient episode that results in iatrogenic disease or disability?'[10]

7 Membership genuine
By enabling willing people to select a purchasing body this would be genuine membership, by contrast with the failed attempt to make local people 'members' of foundation trusts, or by the supplicant status of being registered with the local, monopoly PCT.

8 Adverse selection/protection of 'the pool'
There would be no risk at all of exclusions and no 'moral hazard'. Every PGCA would be required to take all applicants. There would be no permitted shuffling of marginal applicants or those with poor health and pre-existing conditions. This would be a condition of any PGCA being registered and regulated.

9 Equal access and prevention of more inequality by protecting the disadvantaged
Unless every user of services has control of a health savings fund then improved choice, by itself, will favour the affluent and educated, who know how to exercise effective choice. The individual, acting via the agency of the PGCA, would have an equal chance.

10 Visibility of costs/spend
The public would see what their fund was buying for them. This would also encourage prudence among both purchasers and subscribers.

11 Specific measures to make sure the elderly, and those with poor literacy and language skills, benefit
Holding an individual health savings account would achieve this. It would be assisted by advocacy. But advocacy is no substitute for the power of money.

12 Individual involvement in treatment decisions

This is constantly called for, and the PGCA would contract on this basis. It would ensure that patients are well-informed about treatments, and help them make choices. It would ensure that appropriate information is available, and that treatment options were discussed with them by the PGCA and by those to whom they were then referred. It would make a reality of government hopes of putting patients 'at the centre of commissioning' (which is at present no more than a completely meaningless and incantatory phrase).

13 Ensure that choice within consultations becomes a reality

The PGCA would contract on this basis, and remove funds when it was not delivered. There could be no clinical slip-sliding here.

14 Focus on outcomes

As I have argued, provider (and doctor/nurse) incomes should be *directly* linked to outcomes over time. For example, why not pay providers on behalf of sufferers of long-term conditions on the basis of how well they have been kept this year?

15 Registration of purchasers and providers

As the economist Professor John Kay has shown, the distinction between state and market is in some senses an unreal one since all markets are embedded in social and cultural structures. There would thus be national regulation and registration. There would, too, have to be appropriate audit to secure the financial viability of each individual PGCA. A government audit could determine, too, how much of their income and assets would have to be held in contingency funds. These contingency funds should be administered centrally on behalf of members, as was the case with the Government Actuary under the original National Health Insurance scheme of 1911–48.[11] There could be one national financial regulator. Or there could be alternative regulators for other aspects of their work. I do not assume this must be with the Health Commission (to be replaced by Ofcare, The Office of Health and Adult Social Care, in 2009). Indeed, it should be a general principle that there should be competing regulators, and organisations should be able to choose how they are badged. The public could then take a view. Regulation can ensure standards and quality of care. But regulators can be captured by government, the DOH, and providers, too.

16 Focus on quality improvement

Regulation would nevertheless be necessary to ensure that both purchasers and providers focus on quality improvement, rather than only on cost-shifting. We need careful discussion about these aspects of the business model, once we agree that individual financial control is the key element in change for improvement.

17 The competing PGCA would meet the calls regularly reported as being made by users of services, where they are frustrated at not being heard

Thus, wanting information and involvement in decision making about their care; being treated as an individual; being offered choice; having alternatives and side-effects explained; given time to consider; assured of predictable and convenient access to services; guaranteed equitable treatment and access to preferred outcomes; being treated in a safe and protected environment.

18 Respond to the necessity to develop management skills

The deficits in management skills, in economic understanding and in an appreciation of how markets work to fulfil the wants of consumers must be put right. One example of failed management concerns the national policy of shifting services from hospitals into the community, where success has been patchy. An evaluation of projects chosen as the basis of the NHS Institute for Innovation and Improvement's 'Making the Shift programme' found only mixed success. Professor Chris Ham (the evaluation team leader and Professor of Health Policy and Management) at Birmingham University's Health Services Management Centre pointed to 'basic project management resources and skills which the NHS doesn't often have'.[12] This after the NHS spent £72 million on the failed NHS University, its own internal training and education body, scrapped in November 2004 after just two years in operation.[13]

19 The PGCA system would meet the key demands of the 2005 White Paper, 'Our Health, Our Care, Our Say'

By properly supporting people to understand and control their condition at an early stage, and to self-manage where possible both during and after treatment, resources would be well used, medication not wasted, and individual control of individual health much improved. The rhetoric of the 2005 Department of Health White Paper and the arguments of the subsequent 2006 publication *Choice matters: increasing choice improves patients' experiences* would thus be fulfilled.[14]

20 Preventive care

The PGCA would negotiate individual health improvement plans with members, to meet sensible health promotion objectives without being suffocated by nannying. It would expect to impact on lifestyle and disease prevention, occurrence, and management in discussion with individual members who became more aware of all the associated costs of behaviours including the impact on their HSA. For example, it could offer relevant incentives for the individual. If you are a supporter of The Arsenal, you are more likely to make an effort to meet an agreed health plan if the reward is a much-valued season ticket (much cheaper than years of treatment). I proposed such an approach in my book *Patients, Power and Responsibility* in 2003. In December 2007, Gavin Croft (aged 40) of Rochdale applied for cash to buy a season ticket under the scheme to help him improve his 'quality of life', the *Putting People First* initiative.[15] Mr Brown has introduced an 'MOT' for middle-aged men and other groups at risk from heart disease, strokes and diabetes. But without direct incentives – as in the Pruhealth example we considered earlier – and no direct rewards. Of course, if you listen, you live longer and avoid much chronic pain. But we need to have real rewards for doing so, especially to those who otherwise do not seem to value longer life or the avoidance of pain in their last decade, And who decide nevertheless to drink, smoke, eat junk food and take no exercise. We need financial bite with genuine individual incentives.[16]

21 Divide purchasing and provision

As the government's *Commissioning a Patient-led NHS* urged in July 2005, we should have professional, specialist purchasers, rather than the present situation where PCTs can be both purchasers and providers. The two tasks are different. In addition, there is clearly an implicit (and sometimes, a very explicit) conflict of interest. It is important that a wide variety of alternative providers are encouraged. 'In house' provision by purchasers dilutes this objective. Purchasers as PGCAs would use members' money to send patients to GPs whom they decide to commission, for example, and be able to exert pressures for improvement. PGCAs (and existing PCTs) should not be direct employers of GPs. They should sub-contract, and thus prompt alternative provision.[17] GPs, too, are going to have their hands very full as routine patients go to community hospitals and the more complex patients come to the tertiary centres with GPs much more closely involved with district general hospitals. The Australian 'Medicare' card is a good model here for the HSA. In Oz patients can pick and choose between any GP at any time, carrying the 'Medicare card' which entitles them to care. They have access to specialised practices for different kinds of problems.[18]

22 Prevent monopoly purchasing
Larger PCTs – or smaller ones if formed into commissioning clusters – representing a million people or more can and do rapidly become monopoly buyers, just as large acute trusts are often monopoly suppliers (which is why their managements must be contestable). It is important that competition is protected by regulation, and if markets tended towards monopoly in a structure of PGCAs this would have to be very directly and quickly addressed.

23 Voice less effective than choice
One working example: which is more likely to be effective in making choice real – a maternity service liaison committee or a mother with the ability to select where she will have her child? What works best, a block contract, or a single choice made by a parent who has control of the money? Which is most likely to enable an individual to secure a timely, personal, intimate and suitable service: holding a personal fund, or signing a petition? Which is more likely to secure the service: waiting in line, or being able to take your fund to an alternative independent purchaser? We have seen the contrast between real 'choice' and the possibility of 'voice', with all its cultural and practical limitations.

24 A real chance to deliver key policies
Competing PGCAs would negotiate with members about essentials: reliable access to preferred services; personal efforts to remain healthy, or to alter lifestyle; encouragements for early intervention; bringing services closer to home; offering integrated services; promoting independence and choice; dramatically influencing inequalities of access and care, by working with financially empowered members. It would also impact on inequalities of access, and thus of health status.

25 Transparency on affordability
I have previously proposed a legally enforceable system of patient guaranteed care, in my book *Patients, Power and Responsibility*. This discussed what the state should legally guarantee to deliver. This explicit approach would do much to help people manage their own expectations as well as offering opportunities for personal top-ups, including the purchase of effective drugs now denied to them by the NHS as it at present exists.

26 Save rather than consume
The contract between the willing subscribing member and the PGCA could offer incentives, such as money back for not consuming. This money could be saved into the long-term health savings account. Some 'frivolous' demand might be deterred, and self-care encouraged. This model would also contribute to improving the very weak funding model for elderly care, as we have seen. Here the incentives to save for long-term care are weak and need strengthening. Too few save, except for the wise and reflective who look ahead (and who can afford to do so). Similarly, such incentives

could work alongside educating people to avoid the chronic disabilities of old age wherever possible, as well as appreciating that if a care home is necessary one day then good ones can bring companionship, security, activities and good care.[19]

27 Transfers between PGCAs

Efficiency is the result of market systems, not of planning. A competitive allocative mechanism must be protected, with individuals free to move between organisations. The market depends in part on the freedom of the individual to move their business. It would be important to facilitate inexpensive transfers between PGCAs when a member wished to move. It may be necessary to have rules which limit such moves, perhaps only at the end of a year or two years. This would need to be an inexpensive and not a complicated and over-bureaucratic process. Electronic patient-held data would facilitate relatively inexpensive shifts. Some may say that a balance will have to be drawn between apparently 'frivolous' moves [but *who* decides what is 'frivolous'?] and the autonomy of the fund-holding individual. Here, I fear, we hear the tiny steps of yet another regulating quango.

28 Owning capital

The individual ownership of an NHS fund would strengthen democracy. The knowledge, particularly for the poor, of owning an asset would enhance personal status, self-worth, and thus the wider society. This individual capital fund would be universal, unlike the ill-fated, misconceived and transparently futile earlier Conservative proposal for 'patient passports' to offer an extra privilege to the middle classes. This was rightly rapidly abandoned by Mr Cameron.[20] For, as Mr Milburn has said:

> The most substantial inequity today is not simply between income groups, but between those who rely solely on wages and benefits. That is why I believe the biggest contribution to enhancing social mobility is to establish asset-owning democracies in the developed world. People rarely spend their way out of poverty. While income support fuels consumption and a 'live for today' mentality, building assets leads people to save, defer consumption, plan ahead, and work hard to turn what they have into bigger assets such as a home. Owning assets creates a buffer in times of crisis. People act differently if they own assets. It gives them a real stake in the future. It enables people to act independently and make their own choices. Ownership works. It enhances responsibility. After all nobody ever washed a rental car.[21]

29 The successes would be such that bringing PGCAs back into central political control would be impossible

Government's role is to enable the architecture of health and social care to evolve adaptively, with sufficient funding and with regulation over concepts that count such as the protection of competition. It should establish an independent body for the rapid publication of outcomes information on surgeons, physicians, clinical teams, and GPs, to assure safety and quality. Much stronger incentives at local level – institutional and personal – through payment by results to competing purchasers who work for willing members is what we have to ensure and then protect. Safety and good outcomes would be a key marketing tool, and not just waiting times or access or costs – all of which would necessarily improve, in any case, with more competition.

30 Integration of health and social care

The competing PGCAs could join the argument that health and social care must be integrated if there are to be properly coordinated and collaborative services, to prevent people from falling through the cracks. This has already been achieved in Northern Ireland. The health savings account would accomplish this change. Professor Paul Corrigan, a key adviser on healthcare to Tony Blair and Alan Milburn, later Director of Strategy and Commissioning for NHS London and a continuing key adviser to No. 10, told the King's Fund in June 2006 that the primary responsibility for delivering improvements depended on purchasing.[22] The real choice here is between the failures of government, which are very hard to correct, and the benefits to be achieved by competing purchasers who are the buyers for their members. As we saw with GP fund-holding, this shakes the tree. It did so even when GP's were – as they remain in many areas – local monopolists. Older providers awake. New providers emerge when disappointed providers find they have less money to spend because consumers cease to give it to them.

Why are we waiting?

Notes

1 An unnamed physician, quoted by Chilingerian, op. cit., p. 449. A Donabedian, 'The quality of care: how can it be assessed?', *Journal of the American Medical Association*, 23–30 September 1988, 260, pp. 1743–8. See also Vivienne Nathanson, 'Patients' big chance to call the shots', *Health Service Journal*, 15 February 2007, p. 8 discussed this.

2 David G Green, 'The Friendly Societies and Adam-Smith liberalism', in David Gladstone (ed.), *Before Beveridge: welfare before the welfare state* (London, IEA Health & Welfare Unit, 1999), p. 24.

3 Mark Britnell, 'The grand plan for the NHS to lead the world', *Health Service Journal*, 18 November 2007, pp. 18–19.

4 Department of Health, *Commissioning Framework for Health and Well Being* (London, DoH, 2007).

5 Michael E Porter and Elizabeth Olmsted Teisberg, *Redefining Health Care: creating value-based competition on results* (Cambridge, Mass., Harvard Business School Press, 2006).

6 Anthony Kealy, presentation, reported in Helen Mooney, 'NHS and councils could be placed under "single regime"', *Health Service Journal*, 25 January 2007, p. 5.

7 R Lewis, *Practice-led Commissioning: harnessing the power of the primary care frontline* (London, King's Fund, 2004); J Smith, N Mays, J Dixon et al., *A Review of the Effectiveness of Primary-led Commissioning and its Place in the NHS* (London, The Health Foundation, 2004); T Gosden and DJ Torgeson, 'The effect of fund holding on prescribing and referral costs: a review of the evidence', *Health Policy*, 1997, 40, pp. 103–14.

8 David Rose, 'Hospitals to pay for harming patients', *The Times*, 14 December 2007, p. 1. Tania Branigan and John Carvel, 'Cameron calls for funding cuts at super bug hospitals', *The Guardian*, 3 January 2008, p. 13. The same problem arises with the Office of Rail Regulation fining Network Rail £14 million in February 2008 for chaos caused by over-running engineering work on the west coats mainline. Fares just rise, investment is deferred or standards fall. On not washing hands, see Archie Clements et al., 'Overcrowding and understaffing in modern health-care systems: key determinants in meticillin-resistant *Straphylococcus aureus* transmission', *The Lancet Infections Diseases*, 8(7), July 2008; Kate Devlin, 'Overcrowding and overwork on the wards blamed for hospital superbugs', *Daily Telegraph*, 24 June 2008, p. 2.

9 See my *Who Owns Our Bodies? Making moral choices in health care* (Oxford, Radcliffe Medical Press, 1997); Richard Smith, Nancy Williams, and Keri Thomas, 'The American way of death', *Health Service Journal*, 24 May 2007, pp. 28–9. Vivienne Nathan son, 'Patients' big chance to call the shots'. Greater choice in end-of-life care was called for in response to the government's command paper *Building on the Best* in December 2003, but has made little progress. Helen Mooney, 'Government consults ahead of new choice framework', *Health Service Journal*, 24 August 2006, pp. 6–7. In 2005 the Healthcare Commission reported that 54% of all complaints about hospitals concerned end-of-life care. Healthcare Commission, *State of Health Care 2007: improvements and challenges in services in England and Wales* (London, Healthcare Commission, 2007).

10 Sophie Christie, 'On money and morality', *Health Service Journal*, 9 August 2007, p. 15. The article also discusses relevant ambiguities and problems of some incentives in some situations.

11 John Kay, *The Truth About Markets: why some nations are rich but most remain poor* (London, Allen Lane, 2003; London, Penguin Books edition, 2004). See also Noel Whiteside, 'Private provision and public welfare: health insurance between the wars', in Gladstone (ed.), *Before Beveridge*, op. cit.

12 Jo Stephenson, 'Pilots making little difference', *Health Service Journal*, 30 August 2007, p. 8.

13 Charlotte Santry, 'NHSU: "embarrassing" failure', *Health Service Journal*, 19 April 2007, p. 7.

14 DoH, *Our Health, Our Care, Our Say: a new direction for community services*, Cmd. 6737 (London, The Stationery

Office, 2006); DoH, *Choice Matters: increasing choice improves patients' experiences* (London, DoH, 2006). See also DoH, *Delivering 'Choosing Health': making healthier choices easier* (London, DoH, 2005).

15 Paul Waugh, 'Footie fan is bought season ticket on NHS', *London Lite*, 18 December 2007, p. 5.

16 Gordon Brown, speech on the Future of the NHS, King's College, London, 7 January 2008; Robert Winnett, 'Private style health MOT to be offered', *Daily Telegraph*, 7 January 2008, p. 4.

17 Liverpool PCT, for example, advertised in spring 2007 for 'willing providers' for community-based dermatology services in the south central area of the city. Two companies it accepted had links with GPs in the practice-based consortium. One company had several GPs from the area on its board. Alison Moore, 'PCTs grapple with grey areas of GP-led commissioning', *Health Service Journal*, 24 May 2007, pp. 14–15.

18 See Anna Donald, 'On lessons from Australia', *Health Service Journal*, 5 July 2007, p. 17. The BMA's proposed 'rational' single-system is contrary to sense and purpose. See BMA, *A Rational Way Forward for the NHS in England: a discussion paper* (London, BMA, 2007).

19 But see the important report and guidance from the Commission for Social Care Inspection, *See Me, Not Just the Dementia: understanding people's experience of living in a care home* (London, CSCI, 3 June 2008).

20 On passports, see Sean Williams, *Alternative Prescriptions: a survey of international healthcare systems* (London, Conservative Policy Unit, 2002). I was consulted in 2001–02. I strongly advised against this ill-conceived and misdirected policy in meetings with my good friend Mr Rick Nye, then Director of the Research Department, and with Sean Williams, who was in charge of developing the proposal.

21 Alan Milburn, 'Empowering citizens: the future politics', Speech to the Global Foundation, Sydney, 2 May 2006.

22 Professor Paul Corrigan, King's Fund, London breakfast seminar on *Effective Commissioning*, June 2006.

21

My body, but *your* decision? 'Concordat', and shared decision making

'Nothing lies like the truth.'
– NELSON DE MILLE

'We are discussing the end of the world – or how to delay it.'
– ARCHBISHOP STUART BLANCHE

'One by one, we were tapped on our shoulder by our maker.'
– LLOYD JONES

People *are* different. Every patient and user of services is an individual. Doctors are individuals, too. Each needs the certainty of respect.

The idea of shared decision making is that we each bring different kinds of knowledge to the discussion. Including those unstated thoughts, which are often only 'seen' or 'heard' in the silent spaces between words. There are anxieties we cannot necessarily even express to ourselves, but which affect the shape of the choices we may make. We need help in understanding who 'I am' and 'what might happen to me'. We need an honest engine on which we can rely. But in the final outcome it is *our* body. None of us wants to be nobody in an unfamiliar city, and we all seek the future. We would all like to remain utmost and securely ourselves, even when and perhaps especially when we are confronted by serious illness.

In this often frightening situation, doctors and patients should work side by side as peers. The issue is to improve lives, not just to delay death by whatever scientific means possible. Shared decision making is essential. Doctors, too, should achieve recognition not because of the white coat but from the satisfaction of those they help.

When we are ill, we want to see a doctor, not a manager. But it is not, however, the role of the doctor to make the patient do what the doctor wants them to do. The task is to set out clearly possible courses of action, for the patient to decide. This cannot sensibly preclude a recommendation when the patient asks, 'What would you do if you was me, doc?' – but the patient's values and preferences must come first. Faith in the doctor as someone who is doing their best to help you matters, too. This has therapeutic value, and it is fundamental to the relationship.

One great hope has been that many of deficits of communications in care would be made good by 'shared decision making' between doctors and patients. That this would generate active choices by patients, in consultation with their doctors. That this would improve the approach to 'informed consent', itself a grey area of practice. That an improved relationship would encourage greater personal responsibility, and better shared understandings. This meant talking with and not at patients. 'Listening best', not 'knowing best'. The decline in British educational standards does not, however, help doctors explain to patients technical matters, nor does it help patients to express their wishes. This is a society-wide problem.

This 'concordance', would, however, if it worked, be a very important relationship, as Dr David Misselbrook has well shown.[1] However, a review of the literature indicates that doctors, patients and their carers often seem to understand quite different things by it. Many GPs resist it. Unchanging assumptions made by medical professionals still shape much of the discourse. Clinical views often remain privileged, patients' choices marginalised. This is so, for example, with regard to getting into hospital, and with regard to discharge planning from acute hospital care. Care routines are still procedurally driven, with insufficient opportunity for patients to be actively engaged in decision making. Again, on the deep blue sea, no plain sailing. And you sail nowhere without a following wind.[2]

The doctor/patient relationship can, of course, be a pivot of many improvements. It is best when successfully based in mutual respect. It represents many facets of the diamond. There are, too, outstanding examples of best efforts to make shared decision making a reality by sharing information and understanding. Such as the books by the leading urological surgeons Professor Roger S Kirby and Professor Tony Mundy, including their *Succeeding as a Hospital Doctor: the experts share their secrets*.[3] Shared decision making is especially important for sufferers of long-term chronic conditions, and these are the core of the NHS business. People with complex needs consume most of the NHS resources. Here, as elsewhere, care necessarily has to be negotiated and constantly re-negotiated as conditions change.

There are some paradigm examples of successful consumer influence changing practice, too. Consumer concerns about the approach medicine took to breast cancer and to obstetrics led a new attitude to choice. 'Routine clinical treatments' were rightly challenged. The feminist movement 'talked back' to doctors. Gay activists became expert patients, too, in order to secure different attitudes, more research funding, and prompt and more effective treatments for AIDS – both at onset and as the condition evolved into a chronic one. The focus on the person as well as the condition changed many relationships with professionals. Activism paid many collaborative dividends. They showed that patients need good information, personal skills and mutual support in order to handle the experience of illness. And to adjust to the rigours of medical treatment.[4]

My argument is that a person needs *both* informed dialogue, in a good relationship, and the economic power to make their own decisions and their self-responsibility *effective*. Lay advocacy may also make a contribution. But it is not a substitute for choice, although it may be a helpful support for it. Dialogue and informed and financially empowered choice are not alternatives, either. They are integral, one to the other. We need to continue to invest in every potential, including providing better decision aids. We are already able to make some assessments of change here. The necessity to improve information has resulted in the increased production of decision aids. The flow of new research, however, offers a very mixed picture of what these are yet achieving. This is in part due to the inheritance of 60 years of disempowered patients. In addition, the King's Fund recently showed that many GPs still resist patient choice. Many remain reluctant to even offer choice of which hospital a patient can select – from an official list – of where people can have their operation. This contravenes official policy. Many patients only get this choice – which was promised in the 'Choose and Book' project – if they *actively* express such a preference for choice. Some of these difficulties are rooted in the internal status structure of medicine. This has for long been a theatre of rank, with status integral to the everyday life of medicine and its social dispensations. Rank in this community has been one of a ladder of social degree and membership of exclusive guilds. It is not easy for many to extend space to others, not least because many have become accustomed as consultants to giving orders and having them obeyed.[5]

Once again, the NHS functions as a class-based structure. The incentives are insufficient, for both professionals and for patients. These are cultural problems, concerning who thinks who should make decisions, and who thinks patients are unable to do so properly. The review literature shows once again, too, that in the NHS the lack of information in forms which the lay person can understand and consider is deliberate. It misunderstands or misplaces the wishes of the consumer. It clearly hinders the test of predictability. That is, of the user being able to find out about the likely effects of a service in advance. A review of recent literature on 'concordance' between doctors and patients, of shared decision making and of the use of decision aids, shows that there is still a structure of highly restrictive practices among healthcare professionals. Especially in the sharing of information and knowledge, including respect for the special knowledge which only patients can bring to the situation.

Competing for purchasing again

Conclusions from an oversight of much of this research on concordance – and on decision-making aids to support its development – suggest that a purchasing structure dominated by GPs will not make sufficient progress in empowering patients. We need instead to move to a competitive purchasing structure. And one in which a PGCA employs GPs as outside contractors rather than being dominated by them. One which then guides GPs and other doctors and specialists to meet the preferences set out by the representatives of patients in these mutual, cooperative organisations, some of whose managers will (of course) be medical practitioners working as or alongside purchasing managers. Once again, we find that individual financial empowerment is a necessary incentive to counter-balance negative influences, some of which are themselves the result of government targets and financial rewards leading away from the ideal, some deeply embedded culturally.

Too often discovering any information that the individual may believe to be necessary information has been a matter of chance. For example, consultations with people caring for an elderly or a disabled relative in Birmingham identified lack of information about what help might be available to them. This was pointed out as one of the most significant problems. Consumer ignorance, as we have already seen, is no accident. Indeed, it has been a prerequisite of the NHS – of its entirely artificial processes of rationing, deficit and denial, of deterring informed demand since the sources of funding have been so artificially limited by ideology. The larger and more concentrated the state, the less there will be informed consumers. That information is poor has been a requirement of a rationed system. Clearly, it hinders the test of predictability, of the user being able to find out about the likely effects of a service in advance.[6]

This matters even if we accept the distinction between 'search goods' (which can be tested before purchase, like cars) and 'experience goods' (such as holidays, or medical treatments, on which a judgement about satisfaction is necessarily retrospective). For we do want to know what happened to other patients 'like me'. And which doctors did best; who does the procedure most often; what do other patients say about their experiences and results? Here, fortunately, many user groups are expert patients who have gathered much valuable information on experiences, performance and outcomes, which helps those who otherwise would have had no previous opportunity or need to investigate possible alternatives, and these groups do much to help people develop skills in choosing. Participation in active decision making has been shown to improve outcomes.[7]

As Dr Marian Barnes and David Prior rightly say,

> Access to any service depends on knowing that it exists, that it is relevant, and that one is entitled to use it. Choice between services depends on having such information about different options, and on having additional information about significant differences between services in terms of their essential characteristics, and/or effectiveness of their performance.

As to available options, these are enlarged by competition, and by more effective purchasing. Similarly, alternatives which people feel will meet their case are also stimulated. As to experience in choosing, this is in part about learning to choose, in part about the evolution of assistance and advocacy. Barnes and Prior recognise this in 'the world confronted by impermanence, ambivalence and diversity'. As they say, individuals are faced with the need to choose all the time. And they do so successfully from a vast and increasingly varied series of offers in all others areas of their lives, where markets guarantee variety, quality and feedback.[8]

A very important area of the relationships between their members and their medical colleagues for the PGCA as a purchaser will thus concern shared decision making between physicians and consumers. The power that these purchasers will hold needs to be put to the most constructive use. For example, when customers feel engaged they tend to be more 'compliant'. When they are asked how they feel, what are their views, on what would they like to comment, what do they not fully understand, they are more likely to be collaborative.

Here, we need more research. What we now have suggests the benefits of changes in training and behaviour to enable consumers and doctors to gain more from consultation – for consumers to benefit from their preferences and doctors to fulfil them. Such choices may, of course, include reliance on the doctor's decision if the patient so wishes. That is itself a choice. And, as we have seen, even such a random choice is benefited by the decisions of others in markets. Good information is an essential, and all that I have already said on this topic is clearly apposite here.

Those doctors in management who will be among the leaders of the new, competing purchasing organisations – the PGCAs – will want to work with clinical colleagues to make these gains. We can learn much from professionals skilled in shared decision making and in the difficult territory of communicating and assessing risk.[9] Communications skills – no common or garden thing, in the wider society – are transparently especially valuable. Listening best, not knowing best, even when you think you *know* you know best.

Research is now attempting to discern what involvement patients want in clinical decision making. It seeks to discover the underlying factors influencing choices, and then to identify aids which will help. The barriers to increasing patient involvement in decision making are also becoming more apparent. One study suggested that the NHS maintains a paternalistic approach. Results, too, showed that 20% of patients chose an active role in decision making and 80% chose a collaborative or a passive role. Major constraints in successfully focusing on shared decision making were the lack of staff, lack of information, and poor continuity of care. This study, published in a *nursing* journal, showed that nursing staff made patients feel disempowered.[10]

Traditionally, doctors have claimed to speak for the patient in order to demand more resources from government. Now, the state is insisting on greater efficiency, and it is seeking shared decision making as one means to achieve this. There has been investment in decision aids (DAs) as one result, but there is little information on the extent to which these approaches contribute to improvements, and how important shared decision making is relative to the other attributes of a consultation.[11] We are only now starting to get some useful studies of these initiatives, and their impact. Similarly, there has been a major theoretical commitment to 'concordance' between doctors and patients in shared decision making. Studies are again now beginning to show us more about who makes decisions, how, and what contribution patients make.

There has been a good deal of conceptual and experimental work here, but there is no consensus on how to make shared decision making work well both for patients and for doctors.[12] In terms of personal decisions about preferences, too, there has been little concern with the importunate issue of whether or not people can accurately predict or mis-predict their future preferences and feelings.[13] Nor, indeed, how problematic this might be. Substantial inequities in the provision and use of NHS services are made more evident, including the knowledge that those in the lower socio-economic groups use services less. This situation embarrasses NHS claims of equity. It is attributed both to factors of supply and demand and to differences in health beliefs.[14]

Generational change again

There seems here to be generational distinctions, with younger patients wanting to have more involvement in what happens to them, and to be more directive. Here, intuition seems confirmed by research. In one study more than half of older patients in their mid-60s and over placed great reliance on the doctor's opinion in the context of invasive medical interventions.[15] Another recent study in primary care practice showed that patients had a strong preference to be involved in clinical decision making, and that this is associated with patient satisfaction. However, preferences vary.[16] Shared decision making in mental health also needs careful attention.[17]

With aids to decision making, the provision of paper-based tools particularly helped elderly patients in general practice care in Europe and in Israel, according to one study. Here the tools encouraged patients to ask questions, and to offer their own opinions. However, we know little of who listened in terms of effecting changes in treatments (or refusal of treatment) in response to patients wishes.[18]

Patients seem to value more time in a consultation, a doctor who listens, easily understood information, and shared treatment decisions. Doctors seem to do best when they have received shared decision making training.[19] But not every patient valued shared decision making most among other factors. Despite an apparent general preference in favour of shared decision making, and what is said to be a widely accepted ideal by doctors, studies suggest that informed and shared decision making in primary care only rarely occurs, even among motivated physicians. A major barrier to changing practice seems to be the need to change well-established patterns of communications with patients.[20] There is evidently but unsurprisingly a wide variation in the ability of doctors to meet patients' preferences for involvement.[21]

Clearly, this research needs to be fed back to initial doctor recruitment and training, and into the perspectives of purchasers of care. As it does, too, into the design and use of decision aids. These are intended to promote patient choice and shared decision making. They include the Cochrane Databases of DAs, electronic databases, consumer and government websites, leaflets, pamphlets, videos and tape-recordings. What we know of patient experiences – what actually happened to them in treatments – is surely central to their validity if they are to help guide new potential patients. Especially since we know from work led by Dr Adam Darkins for the King's Fund using interactive video aids that people make surprising choices, including those we might not make for ourselves.[22] However, research suggests that although shared decision making has enormous practical implications for improving healthcare, it depends on largely theoretical frameworks and is not yet widely implemented in general practice. There is still a 'non-alignment' between patient preferences and the actual mode of decision making.[23]

Choices are not always offered. In making choices, only a third of patients studied in two surveys remembered being offered one, and only a third were aware of the choice policy.[24] One study concluded that patients' involvement in shared decision making has increased but not in key respects. When consent to a treatment was observed, patients were less often asked for their understanding. GPs who gave more information did more to involve patients, especially younger patients. But 'it should be questioned whether they are willing or capable of being involved and if so, how they could be encouraged'.[25]

In addition, the producers of decision aids have tended to rely more heavily on medical 'experts' than on guidance from service-users. Content evaluations have showed that DAs frequently omit descriptions of the procedures involved in treatment options. Screening DAs, too, frequently focus on false positives but not false negatives. Some half of DAs studied in a recent systematic review reported probabilities with greater emphasis on potential benefits than harms. In addition, these DAs were more likely to provide false positive than false negative rates: 'The review led us to be concerned about completeness, balance and accuracy of information included in DAs.'[26]

Other contradictions

There are, perhaps inevitably, other contradictions in routine practice. Video-recordings of primary care consultations when three types of DAs were used showed a predictable imbalance between doctor and patient, although both parties were reciprocally engaged in consultation. GPs dominated the conversation, taking up between 58% and 55% of the time. In giving information, they used highly technical language and gave little time (just 7%) to conversation which was socio-emotional in content, although this is an area which may be thought to be of great concern to patients. GPs worked primarily as information *givers*. But in their present form (paper-based guidelines; and computer-based DAs) the conversations did not lead to sufficient sharing by patients in treatment decision making, which may take too long to negotiate in use in routine (and unvideod!) consultations. Another study showed that GPs were often much less than frank about information and its meanings.[27]

The implementation of clinical guidelines for the management of common chronic diseases encourages doctors not to offer information in discussion about the choices to be made by patients and doctors in concordance. Studies indicate, too, that patients are not adequately informed about the treatment. In addition, the intellectual basis of large-scale randomised trials and the complexities of the data place grave limits on effective communication with patients. Time, too, is too short in consultations. There are also perverse incentives for doctors to comply with clinical guidelines, for which they are rewarded if they meet central targets. A recent study suggested that it is simply not in the financial interest of doctors to disclose accurate information. A negative incentive indeed! There is also an issue about what risks patients will accept if they are told enough to consider them. Faced with absolute risk decisions many decline treatments even if they are promoted by guidelines. The information issue here is clear. In my proposed structure of PGCAs doing the purchasing on behalf of their members it would be emphasised. This is, as the study by James Penston suggests, that the patient should be told that most patients receiving long-term medication obtain no benefit in treatments where only marginal benefits can be expected in managing chronic but common diseases. They are not usually told, and yet they are exposed to adverse drug reactions. Few know enough to be aware of the questionable validity of clinical trials. If there were genuine 'concordance' many would reject the recommendations urged by guidelines. And doctors would encourage a more critical approach to clinical research, to guidelines and to 'concordance' itself. The PGCA framework would achieve these changes. In the NHS there is no incentive or reward to decline treatment. In an HSA the patient would be offered an inducement to consider much more carefully the benefits and cost of the possibilities. We need incentives to encourage people to consume responsibly.[28]

It is individual financial empowerment alone which will change the locks on all these doors. It will produce a new confidence in the minds and attitudes of service-users. It will change the expectations of all involved. It will also please forward-looking professionals, too. What research tells us will then be transformed into better results.

The biomedical model: what is locked in the attic

Meanwhile, much of the difficulty embedded in the deficits of shared decision making arises from the biomedical model. The biomedical model needs to be set into a more modest perspective. It has done much for many, but we do not want our lives medicalised to the extent that this undermines our self-reliance. The biomedical model does much to limit our lives, and it evades the full consideration of a good death. The model, too, over-emphasises the hospital context. It was developed in hospital medicine, but the majority of patients are seen in general practice, 'where a biomedical model is either insufficient or even inappropriate', according to Dr David Misselbrook. Here, the GP deals both with the presenting problem and often with the 'real' problem, which is often social and/or psychological. I refer the reader again to the superb discussion of these issues in Misselbrook's book *Thinking About Patients*. Here he shows that much gets left out by the biomedical model: 'humanity gets left out. Care gets left out. Biomedicine is great for fixing biological parts that go wrong. But I am not just the sum of my biological parts. If we believe that people matter then biomedicine is not enough.'[29]

Biomedicine has contributed very significantly to fixing many medical problems. But the doctors' gaze is too restricted. Of course, much that was not previously treatable can now be addressed, and there have been enormous advances, although the total burden of ill health – much of it self-imposed – remains huge. Yet major progress has been made with cancer, cardio-vascular disease, mental illness, drug abuse, AIDS and so on. However, there are increasingly widely recognised limits to the success of biomedicine. There are concerns that it improperly makes normality problematic. And there are proper anxieties about what the model omits. As Misselbrook says this is 'the dark side to biomedicine, which we [doctors] prefer to keep locked in the attic'. There are a number of issues:

- ❒ The limitations of the scientific foundations of medicine
- ❒ The limits of biomedicine's success
- ❒ The importance of the values that the patient brings to the conversation
- ❒ Iatrogenic problems
- ❒ What biomedicine leaves out
- ❒ Functional illness
- ❒ The problematisation of normality
- ❒ Biomedicine's vulnerability to hijack (by politicians).

Medical intervention does good and bad. It also changes people's perceptions of their own health. Outcomes – such as reduced disability – are subjective phenomena. We know from disability groups and from individuals that there is no simple relationship between the severity of disease and the degree of disability experienced by the patient. Look, too, at the career of Helen Keller, deaf and blind at 19 months, unable to communicate through language until seven, yet she became a famous crusader for the disabled. Or of the author Christy Brown, who wrote with his foot, and who retained a clear mind and wonderful literary gifts. Or of Milton, who went blind at 43, and whose *Paradise Lost* sprang from what to many would have been a personal catastrophe.[30]

In addition, what would be an intolerable burden to some is something to which another adjusts. My own mother's disability with her legs damaged at birth was an example, as was her brother Alfred's partial blindness due to measles when a year old. Both lived very full and active lives. Biomedicine is reductionist. It can shift the focus from the *whole person*, who matters. Each of us should be enabled to take charge of our own lives, assess risks and weigh benefits and costs. And be equipped to access good information by which we may make judicious assessments and private trade-offs for ourselves. We should be enabled to do so among the choices offered by biomedicine, and by other treatments, including non-treatment. Where this discussion is facilitated, where patients are enabled to consider *both* what doctors call 'evidence-based' information and what patient's own values count to them as 'evidence' – their own subjective feelings as well as information about treatment options, likely different outcomes, and self-care – they usually make rational choices that are often more conservative and involve fewer risks than their doctors would choose for them (if not for themselves?).[31] However, Isaiah Berlin would have been perhaps judiciously intrigued to notice that the activity of considering choices can itself make us feel less well. Treatment within a medical model can make us feel worse.[32]

Dickens, as always, helps us see the case; for example, on the limits of the biomedical approach. Mr Venus, speaking to Silas Wegg, in *Our Mutual Friend* (1864–65) says: 'Mr Wegg, if you was brought here loose in a bag to be articulated, I'd name your smallest bones blindfold equally with your largest, as fast as I could pick 'em out, and I'd sort 'em all, and sort your wertebrae, in a manner that would equally surprise and charm you.'

But we can endorse the girl who turned him down: 'I do not wish,' she said 'to regard myself, nor yet to be regarded, *in that bony light*.' Similarly, just as the boy Bitzer, in *Hard Times* (1854) described the horse without in any way capturing its essence, we exclude the patient's realities by subsuming all to biomedicine. The reader will recall Bitzer's view:

> 'Give me your definition of a horse,' demanded Mr Gragrind of Sissy Jupe. The girl being too alarmed to utter a word, then heard 'Girl number twenty unable to define a horse', proclaimed Mr Gradgrind to the assembled school. But the boy Bitzer at once

came up with a sharp definition: 'Quadruped. Graminivorous. Forty teeth, namely twenty-four grinders, four eye-teeth and twelve incisive. Sheds coat in the spring; in marshy countries sheds hoofs too. Hoofs hard, but requiring to be shod with iron. Age known by marks in mouth.' Mr Gradgrind was gratified. 'Now girl number twenty you know what a horse is.'

If we are to truly see a patient-centred healthcare system we must do better than the boy Bitzer.

Notes

1 David Misselbrook, *Thinking About Patients* (Newbury, Petroc Press, 2001). I do, of course, appreciate how awful, irresponsible, demanding, uninformed and bullying some patients can be in a crowded GP's surgery on a Monday morning or in A&E on a Friday night. However, the lack of incentives for self-responsible behaviour, and the failures of educational policy, have not helped at all. See my Chapter 2, 'Patients, culture and anarchy' in my *Patients, Power and Responsibility*, op. cit.

2 Guro Huby, Jenny Holt Brook and Andrew Thompson, 'Capturing the concealed: interprofessional practice and older patients' participation in decision making about discharge after acute hospitalization', *Journal of Interprofessional Care*, January 2007, 21(1), pp. 55–67.

3 Roger Kirby and Tony Mundy, *Succeeding as a Hospital Doctor: the experts share their secrets* (Abingdon, Oxon., Health Press, 2000; third edition, 2007); Roger S Kirby, *The Prostate: small gland big problem* (London, Prostate Research Campaign UK, 2000; third edition, 2006).

4 See M Gerteis, S Edgman-Levitan, J Daley, and TL Delbanco (eds.), *Through the Patient's Eyes: understanding and prompting patient-centered care* (San Francisco, Calif., Jossey-Bass, 1993), p. 96; Millenson, op. cit., pp. 556–7.

5 See note 2, in chapter above, 'The present reforms: "coherent and right?"'.

6 Older people in Fife, too, who were involved in a project to explore their experiences of growing older and using services intended to enable them to stay living at home also highlighted lack of information and efforts to access it and services and an 'uphill struggle', or 'a fight'. 'Having exhausted their energies simply trying to find out what is available, people may feel little inclination to seek information about alternatives, or to question solutions which are offered'. M Barnes and G Wistow, 'Consulting with carers: what do they think?', *Social Services Research, 1*, 1992, pp. 9–30. I owe the reference to Marian Barnes and David Prior, 'Spoilt for choice? How consumerism can disempower public service users', *Public Money and Management*, 15(3), July–September 1995, pp. 53–8.

7 See RG Evans, ML Barer and R Marmot, *Why Are Some People Healthy and Others Not?* (New York, Aldine de Gruyter, 1994). Also, R Marmot et al., 'Contribution of job control and other risk factors to social variations in coronary heart disease incidence, *The Lancet*, 350, 1997, pp. 235–9; Michael Marmot, *Status Syndrome* (London, Bloomsbury, 2004); Bruno S Frey and Alois Sutzer, 'Happiness, economy and institutions', *Economic Journal*, Royal Economic Society, 110(127), October, 2000, pp. 9128–38. I owe the last two references to Mulgan, *Good and Bad Power*, op. cit., p. 71.

8 Barnes and Prior, 'Spoilt for Choice?, op. cit.; Anthony Giddens, *Modernity and Self-Identity* (Cambridge, Polity Press, 1991), p. 81. The classic statement is, of course, Berlin, *Four Essays*, op. cit.

9 Adrian Edwards, Glyn Elwin and R. Gwyn, 'Shared decision-making and risk communication in practice: a qualitative study of GPs' experiences', *British Journal of General Practice*, 55(510), January 2005, pp. 6–13.

10 Carole Doherty and Warren Doherty, 'Patients' preferences for involvement in clinical decision making within secondary care and the factors that influenced their preferences', *Journal of Nursing Management*, 13(2), March 2005, pp. 119–27.

11 Mirella F Longo, David R Cohen, Kerenza Hood and Adrian Edwards, 'Involving patients in primary care consultations: assessing preferences using discrete choice experiments', *British Journal of General Practice*, 56(522), January 2006, pp. 35–42.

12 Siobhan O'Donnell, Ann Cranney et al., 'Understanding and overcoming the barriers of implementing patient decision aids in clinical practice', *Journal of Evaluation in Clinical Practice*, 12(2), April 2006, pp. 174–81.

13 Nick Sevdalis and Nigel Harvey, 'Predicting preferences: a neglected aspect of shared decision making', *Health Expectations*, 9(3), September 2006, pp. 245–521.

14 Anna Dixon and Julian Le Grand, 'Is greater patient choice consistent with equity? The case of the English NHS', *Journal of Health Services Research and Policy*, 11(3), July 2006, pp. 162–6.

15 Dennis Mazur, David H Hickam, Marcus D Mazur and Matthew D Mazur, 'The role of doctor's opinion in shared decision making: what does shared decision making really mean when considering invasive medical procedures?', *Health Expectations*, 8(2), June 2005, pp. 97–102. Some researchers, I think unpersuasively, suggest that the public is not very interested in accessing or using current sources of information. But to increase the use of performance information by the public it is necessary to move beyond provider-led information and professionally constructed approaches to providing information. Martin Marshall, Jenny Noble, Helen Davies, Heather Waterman and Kieran Walshe, 'Development of an information source for patients and the

public about general practice services: an action research study', *Health Expectations*, 9(3), September 2006, pp. 265–74.

16 Benedicte Carlsen and Arild Aakvik, 'Patient involvement in clinical decision making: the effect of GP attitude on patient satisfaction', *Health Expectations*, 9(2), June 2006, pp. 148–57.

17 Tony Colombo, 'Model behaviour', *OpenMind 2005*, No. 131, January/February 2005, pp. 10–11. See also Lesley Warner, *Choice in Mental Health Care* (London, Sainsbury Centre for Mental Health and King's Fund (2006), SMCH briefing: 31; Jennifer Rankin, *A Good Choice for Mental Health* (London, Institute of Public Policy Research, 2005).

18 Anja Klingenberg, Hilary Hearnshaw, Michel Wensing *et al.*, '"Older patients' involvement in their healthcare: can paper-based tools help?: a feasibility study in 11 European countries', *Quality in Primary Care*, 13(2), December 2005, pp. 233–40.

19 Mirella F. Longo *et al.*, op. cit.

20 Angela Towle, William Godolphin, Garry Grams, and Amanda LaMarre, 'Putting informed and shared decision making into practice', *Health Expectations*, 9(4), December 2006, pp. 321–32.

21 Sarah Ford, Theo Schofield and Tony Hope, 'Observing decision making in the general practice consultation: who makes which decisions?', *Health Expectations*, 9(2), June 2006, pp. 13–37.

22 Adam Darkins, 'Shared decision-making in health care systems', in *Proceedings from the Annual Research Conference 1994, Profession, Business or Trade: do the professions have a future?* (London, The Law Society Research and Policy Planning Unit, 1994); 'Introducing and evaluating an interactive video system designed to give patients detailed information about the likely outcomes of medical care they receive', *Abstract International Soc. Technol. Assess. Health Care Meeting*, 93(9), p. 61; J Spiers (ed.), *Dilemmas of Modern Health Care* (London, Social Market Foundation, 1998).

23 Adrian Edwards and Glyn Elwyn, 'Inside the black box of shared decision-making: distinguishing between the process of involvement and who makes the decision', *Health Expectations*, December 2006, 9(4), pp. 307–20.

24 John Appleby, 'Data briefing: patients' memory of choice', *Health Service Journal*, 117(6039), 21 January 2007, p. 21.

25 Atie van den Brink-Muinen, 'Sandra M. van Dulmen, CJM de Haes Hanneke, 'Has patient's involvement in the decision-making process changed over time?', *Health Expectations*, 9(4), December 2006, pp. 333–42.

26 Deb Feldman-Stewart, Sarah Brennenstuhl, Kathryn McIsaac *et al.*, 'A systematic review of information in decisions aids', *Health Expectations*, March 2007, 10(1), pp. 46–61.

27 Eileen Kamner, Ben Heaven, Tim Rapley *et al.*, 'Medical communication and technology: a video-based process study of the use of decision aids in primary care consultations', *BMC Medical Informatics and Decision making*, 10 January 2007, 7(2). Published online at www.biomedcentral.com/content/pdf/1472-6947-7-2.pdf.

28 James Penston, 'Patients' preferences shed light on the murky world of guideline-based medicine', *Journal of Evaluation in Clinical Practice*, February 2007, 13(1), pp. 154–9. I owe this and some other references to the very helpful reading list 'Patient decision-making – (including Patient Advice & Liaison Services [PALS] and the Patient Choice initiative', published by the King's Fund London, July 2007. See also, DoH, *Developing the Patient Advice & Liaison Service: key messengers for NHS organisations from the national evaluation of PALS* (London, DoH, 2006) and DoH, *Independence, choice and risk: a guide to best practice in supported decision making* (London, DoH, 2007).

29 Misselbrook, op. cit., p. 25.

30 Helen Keller, *The World I Live In* (London, Hodder, 1908); Christie Brown, *My Left Foot* (Cork, Mercier Press, 1964).

31 AM O'Connor, A Rostom, V Fiset *et al.*, 'Decision aids for patients facing health treatment or screening decisions: systematic review', *British Medical Journal*, 319, 1999, pp. 731–4; RB Haynes, PJ Devereaux, GH Guyatt, 'Physicians' and patients' choices in evidence based practice', *British Medical Journal*, 324, 2002, p. 1350.

32 Misselbrook, op. cit., pp. 21–2.

22

How many fingers make five? Culture, kultur, and permission to change

'It was a bright cold day in April, and the clocks were striking thirteen.'
— GEORGE ORWELL

'At eighteen our convictions are hills from which we look; at forty-five they are caves in which we hide.'
— F SCOTT FITZGERALD

'Culture is not life in its entirety, but just the moment of security, strength and clarity.'
— JOSE ORTEGA Y GASSET

'How do you describe a sunset to the blind? What is appealing about new possibilities for those who do not seek them?'
— LLOYD JONES

It is cultures which shape who we are. It is cultures which form how we give service. It is culture which exercises the most significant roles in structuring, sponsoring or obstructing long-term changes.

The broad cultural context here is set by controvertible questions both about the life of the imagination and about social organisation. What is ominous and what opportune, for the individual citizen? What can I live with, as a healthcare employee? What do I want as a service-user, and how can I be sure to get it? What are the wider cultural potentials? Are the likely changes in culture positive, or not? And was the NHS itself notably destructive of a separate, different, older, more promising if often regionalised working-class culture? What were the unfulfilled potentials, which were subjugated and submerged by the state? How can we recover these now? Can the individual – whether employee or service-user – cope with new and major change? Can we recapture the lost potential of a dynamist culture? How might this be recognised, represented and empowered? These are all vital moral and practical questions.

Cultural change asks people to adopt new practices. To share new understandings. To adjust to new relationships. To endorse new realities. To believe in them. To work with them. Or to deny them. To resist them. To decry them. The most necessary cultural change is to involve people *willingly* in new engagements. This is one of the hardest things to achieve. Cultures serve as repositories of memories and of assumptions. To take part in change people need a different sense of 'me' before they can fit into a new sense of 'them'. Just as an organisation's culture flows directly from its values and ethos – representing the guiding beliefs which define it – so a new identity must be found in a very new context when the older ideas no longer fit. These moral and practical conundrums may be elusive of solution, but they are unavoidable now. Particularly so as the values of the public sector are defined for it from outside, and the expectations of its patients/service-users/customers are themselves changing radically and rapidly. Particularly as the prop of proto-Marxist values has crumbled, too. Particularly as even the senior civil service is having to find ways to enunciate vision, to value imagination and to endorse innovation rather than run by the rule-book and rule by the cosy group cohesiveness of Sir Humphrey's 'mate-ocracy'.

All this points to one of the most difficult problems concerning how organisations learn. And how they manage the 'interim' territory of change. And what people can fail to imagine. How hard it is to push through a door into a different world. In the public sector, too, unlike with private firms, services cannot be shut down overnight. Very large numbers of staff have to be linked up to changes, and as work continues to flow.

It is a very difficult task to manage reluctance, or fear of being hit by a wave beam-on, or even bloody-minded resistance. And to introduce dynamism and the capacity to learn anew among those habituated to very different ways of doing things. How then to support belief that change can happen, and that it will be permitted? How to support a well-rewarded and well-motivated workforce with permission to change, in a responsive system of enterprise and innovation, pluralism and choice? These are a key part of the changed ethos we expect from providers and what consumers expect from them – and from themselves. Slowly, perhaps, but *surely*, change must come. Sean Connery, in the role of the reclusive novelist William Forester in the film *Finding Forester* (2000) says: 'Do you know what people are most afraid of? What they don't understand. When we don't understand we turn to our assumptions?' We need to open out these assumptions, and to discuss them. But they are often like very old folded linen maps, with deep creases.

As I said in the Introduction to this book, the choice between dynamism and statism is in effect a clash of civilisations. We are thus looking at the prospect of huge cultural changes. There remains a huge canyon to cross.

We need a bold big bang of reforms. I favour a big bang change, and hope for political courage among our leaders to achieve this by empowering the consumer. Certainly consumer control will require a transformation and some shock therapy. We do need to jolt a new system into gear. Equally, we do need to think carefully about how to manage this. Changes can, by their rapidity, generate some of the difficulties which their implementation is intended to defuse, including shaken staff morale. It can prompt more determined resistance. We need to show how the well-being of staff and patients is a joint objective. Both staff and patients have to live through the process. It is a quandary how to deliver a change which is sufficiently fast, economically efficient, effective in outcomes, and socially acceptable.

Even a 'big bang' approach or a 'clean break' must itself then prompt adaptive changes and re-combinations. Transience is permanent. WM Thackeray taught us about *vanitas*. All of our own experience underlines the elusiveness of general statements and the imminently transitory nature of life. We need always to take an adaptive, trial-and-error approach. The success of personal budgets here offers pointers for the success of any project which can combine the economic approach of free markets with the political ideas of democratic rule. Staff satisfactions appear to be growing here. As the market changes we will discover more of how the workforce and the work flows are being influenced. So, too, on staff selection, training, and the necessary literacy, communications skills, empathy and recruitment at better pay levels.

You cannot change a culture by a new law. Some change may be achieved by demonstrable benefits seen in pilot projects. Some by persuasion. Some by powerful employee incentives. Some by contestability of services, and the replacement of managements. Some by much fuller publication of information, including reports from consumers. In all this the staff are essential partners in change. We should not assume that providers know best. Equally, we should not think that the people running the present system are necessarily bad people. Many are very good people who do their best to give a good service, despite the often inadequate resources. The future picture is not necessarily bleak. Especially if we hold onto the concept of every person as an independent individual who is also a social being. And that social relations also change with changes in modes of production. We need to believe that there is a moral role in participation. And that people respond to incentives and rewards.[1]

The key to successful change is to take people with us. The cost-benefit principle suggests that individuals will indeed take actions when they perceive that the personal benefits exceed the personal costs. This is not only about money. In several different ways – notably including job satisfactions – the individual can reap many of the benefits as well as bear some of the costs associated with change. Here we see Adam Smith's invisible hand again, as individuals generate benefits and costs that accrue to themselves but also to others. We need to consider how convergence between individual and group or social interests can be demonstrated. It is essential that people do not think change is not really there in their own work, and that they are not quite part of it.

Conciliation, and reconciliation?

We have already started to see some of the very fruitful impacts of personal budgets on workforce development and on the working satisfactions of employees in changing social care. The challenge here is thus not the language of hyperbole or of imposition. It is one of negotiation, conciliation and reconciliation. Yet there seem likely to remain many who are not now and will never be prepared to make the moves. These will inevitably have to leave the stage. The key elements in improving or in preventing health and social care delivery concern cultural change, psychological understandings, and those economic instruments which enable responsive markets to evolve. As we try to deploy all possible levers and encouragements for cultural change we should certainly use economic incentives to enable consumers to control the two crucial areas of our lives, health (and education). And for us all to benefit from the incremental consequences – *including* the staff themselves – both at work and later when they are ill or old.

We can talk big from the centre about cultural change. But this needs to be expressed in local initiatives. It can be difficult for people to take local initiatives when there is so much central direction with targets and block contracts and so much inertia or just plain political objection to innovation and to entrepreneurship. These attitudes conflict with necessary local variation. If we expect to enable free choice we have to have permission for variety. This is what markets provide. Otherwise, it is problematic for people to give up power, especially when they have always been closely accountable to those above. They are now being asked to let go, and to let things happen for which they are not accountable. Not that is in the old ways, but in new ways in a market. Some suspect they will be rolling the ball up the hill when government suddenly pushes it down again. Yet if we expect cultural change we have to give people permission to allow local differences, individual preference, and free choices for service-users. And then to survive it.

This is a vital part of the argument for change, particularly in cultures and for the individual financial empowerment of the consumer. And, too, for the different but empowering conciliation of the provider. The permission to be different, in order to meet the wishes of real people living their lives, rather than 'services' defined in terms of volume, block contracts and preconceptions. This is an argument about the nature of genuine individual choice, what it is, why it's a good idea, and what the necessary conditions are for it to be genuine, if risky.

Cultural – and thus structural – change is of the essence to achieve the prevailing objectives of justice in access, and a new balance between the individual and the state. The cultural message of the health savings account is that we need to think differently about the relations between surface and substance, aesthetics and value, the patients' experience of services, and what they think of them. The HSA supplies the direct mechanisms which can reliably enable and support health providers *willingly* to respond to these messages. The result can be more flexibility at work, freedom from politicised supervision, and a stimulating and creative environment, as well as significant improvements in preventive care. It can include the immediate satisfaction of the customer's wishes, and the prestige which that will bring to the provider and the purchaser. The talents of creative, thoughtful, sensitive staff can, indeed, be the essential complements to the technical or engineering skills of specialists. We can give new value to feeling, emotion, perception and intuition. And to taste and aesthetics, too, as well by recognising and empowering economic and cultural realities.

These essentials have been made evident in the current struggles to encourage enterprise, innovation and entrepreneurship in the social care sector. The psychological barriers were, however, made explicit in the initiative by the Royal Society of Arts, the Social Care Leaders Learning Set and *The Guardian* to find projects to fund in encouraging enterprising change in the delivery of social care. Here people said they feared working outside their 'comfort zone'. One successful bidder, Rosie Callinan of Gloucestershire County Council, said, 'Yes, it's difficult to have the confidence to say, "Yes my idea is innovative, and yes it could actually work", because my experience is that good ideas often don't get past the drawing board because there isn't time, or the resources or the motivation, to think much out of the box.'[2] The task is to combine art and artifice. To integrate art and science. To value both emotion and cognition. To link science with sensibility. To hold onto rationality. And to recognise and respect the complete and often unavoidably emotive contexts of these fundamentals. Success requires teams of diverse talents, where medical and non-medical people talk to and not past each other. And where the priced satisfactions of the service-user are paramount.

To actually achieve these cultural changes the key is to try to show those who resist how, in Sidney Webb's words, 'Your arguments lead to my conclusions'. That is, that demand-led management, greater public information and choice (which people have shown that they want, and can use effectively) can achieve more for all – for patients and staff, for service-users and professionals, for the public and the private. But for everyone to be persuaded of this will require a key cultural shift. Each group will need to give up some of its conviction that its approach – and *only* its approach – is appropriate for solving certain problems. We need to integrate the knowledge and strengths of others, including the unique knowledge of themselves which only the service-user can have.

If the satisfaction of customers with good outcomes is the measure in a free market we shall have an independent source of legitimate value – and a morally superior measure, too. Then, goodbye to political measures by volume. Goodbye to politicised targets. Goodbye to politicised vote-buying as a manoeuvre to save St Hilda's on the Hill. Hello to genuine and individual financially empowered choice – and the consequent cultural change. This can be normal, natural and a cause of surprise to those who in the future notice that it was not always so. Choice, indeed, is no longer the frontier. The new forward boundary is the cultural change and the adaptive surprises which it can bring. We cannot know in detail what they will be in a creative, dynamist, evolutionary and adaptive environment. But as Virginia Postrel wrote,

> When we decide how next to spend our time, money, or creative effort, something else will top our priorities. Something else will disturb the familiar ways of business and culture. Something else will challenge our conventional notions of 'real' value. That something else may be radically new, the product of currently far-fetched technologies. It may be a major improvement in an existing good – a faster cleaner form of transportation, an instantaneous mode of manufacturing. It may be as ancient as story-telling or exploration.[3]

Porters and clinicians

Culture changes most indelibly locally – in the actions, attitudes and behaviours of individuals. It changes the switchboard. It changes the senior clinician and physician. It changes the porters. It changes the people in clinical records. It changes the approach of those who carry out social care assessments. It should change all health and social care work. Yet as we all know, it is not at all easy to achieve change. Fear is an issue. So is tradition. So is self-interest. So is anxiety about accountability. So is sheer bloody-minded selfish obstructiveness. So is vested interest proclaiming itself as 'the national interest'. In such a politicised structure as the NHS and social care it is especially difficult for people, too, to take local initiatives when there is so much central direction with targets and block contracts. And it is problematic for people to give up power. Especially when they have always been closely accountable to those above. They are now being asked to let go, to let things happen for which they are not accountable. That is, for service-users to make 'the wrong choices'. If, however, as I have suggested earlier, we expect cultural change we have to give people permission to allow it. And to survive it.

This is a key part of the discussion about how to achieve cultural change. It concerns enabling *both* individual financial empowerment of the consumer and the empowerment of staff in helping to achieve this. The *permission to be different* is essential if we are to meet the wishes of real people living their lives, rather than just to focus on 'services' defined in terms of volume, block contracts and politicised preconceptions. Many in public sector jobs still find choice confusing. One condition is that we need to recognise that many remain uncomfortable with the idea of choice, and of consumerism, in public services. Just as some do with a society of rising incomes, falling prices, and unexpected demand which can lead, they feel, to people making the 'wrong choices' about 'society'. Indeed, *The Guardian* 'Society section' is itself a weekly record of these anxieties. We need to address these concerns, too, if we are to encourage cultural change.

The necessity for the NHS is to move towards such a cultural recognition of the values and value of pluralist competition, choice, wider knowledge and independent validation, checks and exposures. This will require many changes in habits, attitude and beliefs, both in government and among purchasers and providers. This calls for a minute examination of every task and for the work of every staff member (including consultants – indeed, especially them) *by the staff themselves* to ensure that they all focus on customer care. And it requires that customer care is defined by customers, and by their purchasing representatives, their formal or informal carers, their family or friends. This involves careful and aware staff selection and training or retraining. Selecting and training people with appropriate qualities, those who know how to speak to another human being without condescension. We need the scientific skills, too. But very preferably combined with humanity. The challenge, too, involves properly maintaining the care environment – including faultless cleanliness. It remains a very considerable challenge, to link the values of patient safety and quality to reforms. For, as Professor Bob Sang has noted, 'Front-line staff – and especially clinicians – will resist further reform unless they can see the value.' And: 'there is growing evidence of clinical disengagement.'[4]

It is in the culture of the NHS and in social care that the greatest and most difficult challenges lie. Notably, with clinicians. We have seen, crucially, how the services cannot possibly solve 'the problem of knowledge' without putting market mechanisms in place. And that without understanding this, the services invest enormous sums of money and time trying to reorganise and manage [really, to administer] a 'new' but essentially unchanging structure. They invent, discuss, assess, consult, plan, counsel, forecast, confer, re-graph, re-consult, re-view, re-vise, audit, and seek to interest the uninterested public in strategic consultations, re-configurations, and those selective 'choices' set up by officials. As we have seen, this does not and cannot work. The knowledge necessary cannot be gathered save in dynamic markets. The individual cannot be empowered by these 'consultative' processes. The staff remain under unrelenting and unreasonable pressures. Not much of a deal at all.

Competence and capacity are, of course, relevant issues. But the most essential is culture and structure. The recent CSCI report *The State of Social Care in England, 2006–07* made this clear.[5] So, too, did the Cabinet Office 'capability review' of the NHS, published in June 2007. This pointed out that NHS staff did not feel ownership of NHS reforms and that they operate in silos. The categories of being asked to 'base choices on evidence' and to 'focus on outcomes' were both identified as areas for 'urgent development'. In addition, 'There is little evidence that the DoH has a systematic process for learning from past experience.'[6] Quite an indictment after 60 years of planning, but no surprise in a non-market structure.

Culture is, indeed, the realm of most resistance. Or, as two critics of choice put things: '. . . many people involved in the public sector, whether as policy-makers, managers or service deliverers, would reject competition and contracting-out as inimical to the public service values they hold . . .' These authors, sociologist Dr R Marian Barnes (then Senior Lecturer in Public Policy at Sheffield University), and David Prior (then Head of Policy Development at Birmingham City Council) openly stated that they believed that choice disempowered service-users. We have already seen earlier how unjustified were these arguments.[7]

Strikingly, too, almost all discussion within the NHS – as reflected on a weekly basis in the key publication, the *Health Service Journal* (or in such publications as the *International Journal in Public Services Leadership*) – takes the most limited view of choice and cultural change. And of the contribution of business and its creative disciplines. NHS Chief Executive David Nicholson has himself criticised managers for being too preoccupied with technical detail rather than with transforming services. Disappointingly, however, there is no evidence that he understands quite why the problems are so intractable. The polling organisation IPSOS MORI pointed to the necessity of cultural change. They found that 'One of the problems facing the NHS as a whole is that its staff overall, despite lots more money, are so negative about their leadership.'[8] In addition, key government targets such as expanding choice in childbirth to enable by 2009 all women to have a choice over where and how to have their baby and what pain relief they use look likely to be missed.[9] A careful regular reading of the *HSJ* shows that most who write there on choice still consider it paternalistically. And even when talking rhetorically of necessary improved 'patient involvement' or of ensuring that services are 'responsive to patients and local communities' they seem not to appreciate what this could mean, or to have thought through how to make it real.

This is not encouraging. Not, that is, if we want to see an entire change of the culture so that it becomes one of saying 'yes' to empowered and individual preferences – and *believing* in their legitimacy. We need a much more powerful structure of incentives and rewards. To enable health services to meet the requirements of today and tomorrow it is necessary for every spring lever and wheel, every member of every team to cooperate willingly, and to collaborate effectively. We need people to endorse in their daily round that choice is the *pulse* of change. And that any unnecessary friction, any cultural resistance to change, adds to disrepair. Every activity needs to proceed with as much ease as possible, with order and with successful outcomes. However, as Robert Owen noted, 'Opinions govern men'. And cultural resistance generates counteraction, confusion and dissatisfaction. This cannot fail to create poor outcomes and thus great human loss. If the self-adjusting powers of empowered choice are to help deliver better care these cultural trip-wires must go. Yet this is much easier said than done.

Permission to change is fundamental. And the reassurance that those staff who enable people to make their own choices will not be shot if the results are not what political or clinical 'experts' say they ought to be. Those users of services who make their own choices should be accountable for the consequences. This should not be the fault of those who willingly make the system work. Unless we make this change and shift in mindsets then large numbers will not be ready to change how they work. For the risk of empowering choice will seem like asking people to say that two and two equals five, as Winston Smith [6079 Smith W.] struggled to do in Orwell's *Nineteen-Eighty Four*.[10]

For many, financially empowered choice for the individual as customer will remain as difficult a concept as Winston Smith found when he tried to believe in opposites and when the requirement was not only the ability to believe that black is white, but to *know* that black is white. From this perspective, to ask many thousands of NHS and social care staff from another culture to believe in individual choice and to empower it come what may necessarily asks for what Orwell called 'doublethink'. It is risky and difficult. Even more so, too, for those many people who believe in an imposed 'equality' rather than in empowered individual access and in user-defined outcomes. Here, we should appreciate a fundamental core difficulty. Many of the staff struggle to hold two contradictory beliefs in their minds simultaneously. That is, that a state monopoly is the right one but that choice can be creative, too. We have to show that the cultural changes of dynamism and choice can achieve more than the old assumptions, and that the original values of equal access require different instruments to achieve these at last. In addition, the cost-benefit principle suggests that individuals will take actions when they perceive that personal benefits exceed personal costs. We need to show and prove that individual decision-makers can reap welcomed benefits as well as to bear the costs associated with cultural changes. Many benefits will inevitably accrue to others. But the change-makers must benefit, too. There needs to be a convergence between individual and social interests. We need to demonstrate that this is the only way to deliver the fairness and the reliable access by the poor to good, preferred and relevant services which many staff believe was the purpose which took them into the system in the first place. Pilots matter here, as we will see in a moment.

How reality is constituted

The archaeologist Lord Colin Renfrew has pointed out that 'Culture need not be seen as something that merely reflects the social reality; it is rather part of the process by which reality is constituted'.[11] In health and social care, culture particularly concerns how those employed by an organisation think and act as they do their work. How they perceive the guiding beliefs which guide the character of the inherited organisation, and the predominant role of the values and ethos which they hold up as a mirror when presented with potential change. These values and this culture are expressed in the folklore of beliefs, custom and practice: in 'our village', in 'why we are here', in 'what we stand for', in 'the kind of people we are' and in 'how we do things in this place'. These values are important as recruiters and motivators, but they can significantly obstruct necessary change if they are fossilised in outdated attitudes and working practices. Notably, they are mediated by 'public service' unions – for example, with an emphasis on redistribution – and also by the professional culture of medics, with an emphasis on self-regulation. These mediators can successfully protect failing organisations – and those inept clinicians among the good ones – within a highly politicised culture, especially when the failing St Hilda's on the Hill stands in a highly marginal parliamentary constituency.

In addition, many local people were born at St Hilda's, or became parents there, or saw relatives die there. Hospitals are a cultural, social and physical reality. They define 'community', as recent mass protests at hospital 'reconfiguration' demonstrate. They are resonant of personal memories, of self-recognition and of symbolism and 'tribal' loyalties – just as were the henges, stone circles and ritualistic monuments of our Neolithic ancestors. They are something tangible to hold onto in a world where many foundations seem unstable. These community commitments were formed by living together, with individual experiences as well as collective endeavours. They bear testimony to our individuality as well as to our collective memories. But this powerful combination of circumstances and memories can protect a culture that is no longer fully fit for purpose.

In addition, the NHS culture encapsulates non-financial incentives, whereas those seeking to alter the culture suggest that changes in financial incentives, costs and benefits can shift attitudes. Where people attach more importance to other values this is a difficulty, at least until the cumulative power of financial choices made by purchasers on behalf of willing members shakes the foundations and demonstrates that the original legitimacy of values is thus best delivered. Indeed, that they are delivered at last on behalf of the poor. Here we need to encourage experiment and an acceptance of the architecture of adaptive change while regulating the initial pace so that the roof does not immediately fall in. Thus, personal budgets are an important breach in the wall. They are incremental. And they teach by experience.

The 'Berlin wall', however, stands as firm as its defenders can manage. Here lies the disastrous disadvantage and the continuing damage to the huge potentials of creative change of statist ideas. For NHS and social care culture has not so far changed nearly enough. We have 'Foundation Hospitals'. But it is the *foundations* which need to change.

The many years of highly publicised deficits, denials, rationing and scandals have highlighted much avoidable individual suffering alongside the good work done. This shows something else that is important. That it is hard to *underestimate* the inability of people to adjust to *evidence* itself in terms of their own beliefs. And to truly believe that choice is the answer.

There is in the NHS a special mental atmosphere and – on many issues – a uniformity of opinion which reflects and endorses a hierarchical society. This is often unfortunately reinforced by some academic leaders. In the NHS many of these move in and out of a forest of governmental advisory roles, serve on many consultative committees (and on sub-committees of sub-committees), and share one statist mentality. They reflect a special and influential kind of provider capture. These 'experts', too, look to an outsider much like the coral captured in the paperweight that Winston Smith bought as a nostalgic survivor from 'the old days'. A crucial determining factor of resistance to cultural change is thus the mental attitude of the top levels of the NHS, of many academic commentators and local authority leaders. The structure of self-belief, habits, commitments, tastes, apparently instinctive rejections and emotions – Orwell's word was 'goodthinker' – which underpins the persistence of a certain controlling world-view and a way of life in a hierarchical structure. These attitudes are found at every level, from porters up. And as Lord Noel Annan said, '. . . those who have clear ideas on what life ought to be always have difficulty in reconciling themselves to what it is'.[12]

However, the locks on cultures can be changed by the locksmiths. The politics of the culture can be encouraged to move by politicians who can at least give a dynamist lead. Here, we have Hayek's guidance on the importance of ideas influencing the context within which politicians must function. Here, the drive for change and the empowerment of the individual have indeed been helped by some politicians, in the main from New Labour. Notably, from Mr Blair and Mr Milburn. And, latterly also from Mr Brown, Mr Johnson and Mr Lewis in extending personal budgets. The challenge they have posed concerns understanding, acceptance and learning. Surprisingly, the Conservatives have failed to take this lead. The drive for personal budgets implies other major consequential changes, too. More plurality of provision.[13] More investment in home-based care. For example, helping the frail elderly, those with diabetes, chronic heart disease, and chronic obstructive pulmonary disease. Payment by results. And the shift of hundreds of millions of pounds from the NHS to provide support for everyday help, a necessary shift emphasised by care services minister Ivan Lewis.

These fundamental questions especially ask us to think again about our insights into the culture of NHS organisation, the attitudes that underlie its processes, and the continuing relevance and compatibility of its values compared with the contemporary challenges of health and social care. As we consider how and why culture change occurs – and how to encourage this – it is what people think they are doing and what their motives are which are central to the landscape of reform. The objective here is to encourage people to adapt and adopt as they continue to re-express their own values in terms of best outcomes defined by service-users. As the creative commentator Perri 6 of the think-tank Demos has said, 'Solving problems is generally a matter of changing how people do things, or how they see the world.'[14]

The new 'information society'

The 'public service' (and the elite professional culture) is being challenged by the new information society, by interactive technologies, and by generational change and shifting expectations of many kinds from a more demanding but less deferential public. The question is how can we change cultures and services peacefully in a liberal democracy? One major challenge is to show how the legitimacy of the values – of 'fairness', equal access and the like – can best be expressed by new ways of working, in ever changing circumstances. However, this is much easier said than done, as Mr Tony Blair discovered.

Many contemporary individual and personal shifts in expectations – notably, in moves towards quality rather than quantity as a definition of successful outcomes – have been part of enormous global changes in technologies, and the consequent changes in institutions. Such driving ideas and concepts as fairness and equality are entangled with working cultural assumptions and practices, and with material engagement with work. Some of the change in this cultural framework has been managed by governments at the micro level, but much of it has been self-organised on the basis of opportunities presented by new technologies.

At the macro level in Britain Margaret Thatcher transformed much of the private sector, and she and Mr Blair changed parts of the public sector. Yet Mrs Thatcher hardly touched demand management in the NHS or in social care at all.[15] Here, Mr Blair made important changes, notably in direct budgets and in personal budgets that followed in long-term care. The re-inventors of government and the new public management pundits have had much influence, too. These approaches have included proposals for radically resizing government, its responsibilities and its take from GDP as well as improving its tools and capacities. This has sought to encourage economic dynamism within a system of social cohesion and public services. These initiatives have notably concerned contracting out, decentralisation, improving financial management, extending regulation while encouraging pluralist provision, enhanced financial incentives within the new purchaser/provider split, new pluralist partnerships with private sector providers and, latterly, if in contradiction, centralised targets, star-systems and league tables. Much of this was led by Osborne and Gaebler,[16] and, in the NHS, by Professor Alain C Enthoven from Stanford University.[17] The driving, dynamist idea was that society should so far as possible organise itself.

Pilots, and their value

An important point needs to be re-emphasised concerning pilots and their value. The imposition of change from above – and especially unpiloted change with no demonstrated virtues – solidifies opposition. It does not help to change cultures. It can easily be read as contrary to the values of many in the workforce. And be perceived as intended for cost-containment and more controls, rather than for patient-centred change. And so it is important that the incremental move to extend personal budgets was not offered as a Utopian policy, nor be imposed in one leap. It has, too, been presented as a means to add value, and to realise the preferences and self-knowledge of the users of services. Here, pilots have done a good deal to persuade reluctant culture-changers. It has been effectively the subject of many local trials, in specific areas of services. Clearly, when successes are shown these can be disseminated. And when difficulties arise we can learn from them. Thus, the policy meets the point made by Perri 6 about cultural change and cultural transmission – that this is most effective when it is at the micro level, is cumulative, and is on a slow burn. Greater trust together with mutual learning has been supported, both among users and providers.[18] We reach a point, however, when we must have the courage to take this new learning into a wider world. We must move to greater changes across the spectrum of all care. We have had the pilots. We now need to move into the wider ocean. For the task of the state is to encourage as much freedom as possible, to expand private decision making about the good life, to guarantee the order that makes such choices real, and to otherwise protect a legal structure which permits people to shape their own infinitely varied lives. Now that we have made some progress down this road government should protect and extend it to other services.[19]

Mr Alan Milburn is known to have taken the view that if you want to get it done you must mean it, and press ahead with a large change. Internet connectivity, too, is allowing new electronic transaction sets to facilitate much better management and an individual patient focus. Here a clear and big commitment is to be seen to *mean it*, combined with clinical leadership and market mechanisms. All are essentials.

Patricia (Pat) Natale, Chief Nursing Officer at Detroit Medical Center and a 'change leader' of very considerable experience, said to me in May 2008:

> 'What you say about change made me think how difficult this is. People in my experience do not do this willingly. Change is such a modest word for what is involved. What you are engaged in is transforming what we are doing, including clinical transformations from engagement to predictable excellence. It is very hard to achieve without actual lived experience. Without 'lived experience' we become anxious. Without lived experience we don't know what we don't know, and fear change. Without lived experience planning, too, is bound to be a mystery. Often, too, we discover that what was our best judgement often misleads us. Yet to achieve valuable change we do need to create a compelling vision for a healthcare system, a safe system with best outcomes. This is about leadership, tactics, speed, depth and excellence.
>
> 'My own view is that change has to happen in a Big Bang, and not in pilots. To do it incrementally does not work as people do not believe it is happening. In Detroit, in adopting new technologies and new electronic information systems, we were driven by the need for discriminating difference for the health system, in a very competitive environment. Implementation of change had to be rapid, thorough and deep. Never underestimate how difficult and stressful change will be. A successful approach has been that we have used the ethical imperatives of values and patient safety to enable clinicians to tolerate the churn of change and to create ownership. This is not a 'project' alone. It needs to be 'your pulse'. You need, too, to communicate at every step of the process. This takes leadership, insistence and training. This has to happen in the work flow, too, and not just in functionality and in outcomes. Clinical adoption and leadership is vital. In addition, you have to ask what do you educate for in terms of better practice and adoption. You should embrace patient safety and clinical outcomes, and be fully committed to the transition, always advocating for excellence. In hospital systems the move from a paper-based system to electronically generated records is revolutionary in term of quality and appraisal. It can now measure both adoption and change. It empowers staff. For example, a nurse can immediately see live information on the dispensing of drugs, and see if something important is going wrong. Improvements like this motivate. People like to work where care is good and where people talk about it. The effective rapprochement is between technology, safety and quality.'

It is experience which ultimately persuades. Meanwhile, we should recall the march of the weather-beaten and grizzled Old Guard in its retreat from Moscow and Borodino. Not to be underestimated. Not comfortable. Not creative. Not a pretty remembrance.

The Ministry of Truth had no windows. We cannot reinforce a failed system by bricking up our own windows against the light. As Virginia Postrel properly said,

'What was acceptable yesterday isn't today. Expectations increase, and tastes evolve.'[20] However, cultural change is much more likely if the people who have to make it possible can also be among the beneficiaries of its success. This is also more likely, too, if genuine incentives are in place, so that the jobs of those involved depend on success and not merely on securing extra funding from the Treasury. The system is human. It depends on people. We have to address incentives, rewards, satisfactions, comparative advantage, *and* dreams. We have to encourage, retrain and cultivate those who have to implement change, some of whom will be or feel hurt by these shifts. Those who join up, and who continue to think of smarter ways to do things and encourage efficient investment, should be rewarded properly for personal and service improvements. Bad ideas should be quickly abandoned. This is achieved by markets. Autonomy and choice should be supported for *both* patients and staff. This is all a necessity, while we attack the problems directly. The word that lights the magic lantern is usually 'price', for it generates information about costs and benefits and supplies the knowledge that planners cannot secure. So we return to the place we really started: is politics or economics to be the censoring force?

Finally, Dr Hunter 'Patch' Adams again. He met a man in the mental care facility to which he had admitted himself before he became a doctor. He was asked by him 'How many fingers?', as a hand was pushed into his face. From this man he learned to look beyond the question, beyond the problem, to imaginative and creative answers. He made a friend of the other patient, and when he founded his own special clinic on the revolutionary principles of seeing every individual *as an individual* this man provided the land and the funds. He made possible entirely new, revolutionary, much-copied initiatives.[21]

This all concerns a way of seeing arrangements, of setting in place the right incentives and combinations, of questioning why we thought a structure should be the way that it has been, and of directing thought and action by the guiding principles of patient safety and benefit.

The 'Frankfurt school' and Michel Foucault taught us to criticise power by philosophising from cultural phenomenon – especially of the modalities of everyday life. Foucault showed us that the flesh of our bodies is the site of both cultural inscription, political 'education' and individual resistance, as the Marxist philosopher Professor Buck-Morss stresses. She says that 'Dreamworlds are not merely illusions. In insisting on what is not all there is, they are assertions of the human spirit and invaluable politically. They make the most momentous claim that the world we have known since childhood is not the only one imaginable.'[22] Quite so. But we do not have to follow Professor Buck-Morss down the line she prefers, which rejects *both* Western capitalism and Soviet socialism for an unrealised communist alternative. We can still do our own imagining, without imposing a 'dreamworld' on others. We can, too, light upon the *practical* steps to take to improve all our lives, and in freedom and self-responsibility.

O'Brien of the totalitarian Inner Party asked Winston Smith how many fingers? Four? Five? Three? Winston had to *believe*. 'Sometimes, Winston. Sometimes they are five. Sometimes they are three. Sometimes they are all of them at once. You must try harder. It is not easy to become sane.'[23]

We should, however, very carefully, consciously and nimbly avoid such imposed statist 'sanity'. For we should now know that the real issue is *who decides who decides?*

Notes

1 As Emile Durkheim showed, the success of a political system depends on the extent to which it allows individual self-awareness to flourish. As anthropologist Mary Douglas put this, 'He tried to keep a delicate balance between reproaching utilitarianism for overlooking that humans are social beings and reproaching socialism for overlooking the demands of the individual.' Mary Douglas, 'Foreword: No free gifts', p. xi, in Marcel Mauss, *The Gift: the form and reason for exchange in archaic societies*, trans. WD Halls (New York W.W. Norton, 1990; reissued 2000).

2 Annie Kelly, 'All fired up', *The Guardian*, Society section, 5 March 2008, p. 5.

3 Virginia Postrel, *The Substance of Style: how the rise of aesthetic value is remaking commerce, culture, and consciousness* (New York, HarperCollins, 2003; Harper Perennial edition, 2004), p. 190.

4 Bob Sang, 'Don't let's forget, we're in it for the long-term', *British Journal of Healthcare Management*, 2007, 13(4), pp. 122–5 and 13(5), pp. 160–1. See also B Sang, 'Choice, participation and accountability: the potential impact of legislation promoting patient and public involvement in health in the UK', *Health Expectations*, 7(3), September 2004, pp. 187–90.

5 CSCI 3rd Annual Report to Parliament, *The State of Social Care in England, 2006–07* (London, CSCI, 28 January 2008). There are, inevitably, many existing anomalies. These embrace different assessment and charging policies in different local authorities; inequalities in how different sources of personal income are treated in assessments; unhelpful assumptions made about the capacities of people in residential care; how co-payments are viewed in the control of the overall budget. There needs to be much more transparency, and firmer national guidance on charging and assessment. In addition, those in receipt of personal budgets should cooperate, so that cooperative (and competing) local purchasing bodies could emerge which would negotiate with potential providers and on behalf of otherwise isolated individuals. They would ensure, too, adequate support for informed choices among a varied clientele.

6 Cabinet Office, *Department of Health Capability Review* (London, Cabinet Office, 2007) and the response, Department of Health, *Department of Health Development Plan: planning our future together: developing together: feeling the difference* (London, DoH, 2007); Richard Vize and Oliver Evans, 'Nicholson: let local managers drive health service reforms', *Health Service Journal*, 28 June 2007, p. 5.

7 Barnes and Prior, 'Spoilt for Choice? op. cit., pp. 53–8. They were discussing the relatively innocuous and very limited Patient's Charter, which fell from above.

8 Nick Edwards, 'Don't just focus on the technical details', *Health Service Journal*, 14 September 2006, p. 6. Ben Page and Jonathan Nichols, 'Progress is about perception as headlines and reality clash', *Health Service Journal*, 31 August 2006, pp. 16–17.

9 Belinda Phipps, 'How the push for local choice in childbirth is foundering', *Health Service Journal*, 20 July 2006, pp. 14–15. Helen Mooney, 'Warning over childbirth target', *Health Service Journal*, 24 August 2006, p. 7.

10 George Orwell, *Nineteen Eighty-Four* (1949; Harmondsworth, Penguin edition, 1961), p. 201.

11 Colin Renfrew, *Prehistory: the making of the human mind* (London, Weidenfeld & Nicolson, 2007), p. 155.

12 Noel Annan, *The Dons: mentors, eccentrics and geniuses* (1999; London, HarperCollins, 2000), p. 22.

13 I have much benefited from the invaluable and expert guidance to this literature and the bibliography by Jo Maybin, *Alternative Providers* (London, King's Fund, June 2007).

14 Perri 6, 'Governing by Cultures', in Geoff Mulgan (ed.), *Life After Politics: new thinking for the twenty-first century* (London, Fontana, 1997).

15 Indeed, towards the end of her time as Prime Minister she attended a lunch at a major London think-tank. She was pressed to tackle the demand side of the NHS. Her reply: 'Do you want me to *lose* the next election?' Private information.

16 D Osborne and T Gaebler, *Reinventing Government: how the entrepreneurial spirit is transforming the public sector* (New York, Plume [Penguin], 1991).

17 For his review of his own proposals see Alain C Enthoven, 'Introducing market forces into healthcare: a tale of two countries'. Paper delivered to 4th European Conference on Health Economics, Paris, 10 July 2002. See also A Enthoven and R Kronick, 'A Consumer Choice Health Plan for the 1990s', *New England Journal of Medicine*, 5 January 1989, 320, pp. 29–37.

18 Perri 6, op. cit., p. 279.

19 A succession of pilots followed by rolling out the successes takes account of the so-called 'Hawthorne effect', where people perform much better in pilots than they would if the system were the norm because they are given more resources and support. See E Mayo, *The Social Problems of an Industrial Civilisation* (London, Routledge & Kegan Paul, 1949).

20 Postrel, *Substance*, op. cit., p. 57.

21 Tom Shadyac film, *Patch Adams* (Universal Studios, 1998).

22 Buck-Morss, op. cit., p. 238.

23 Orwell, *Nineteen Eighty-Four*, op. cit., p. 201.

23

Postscript: Dazzled by Darzi?

'Repent, for the kingdom of Bevan is Nye.'

ELECTION SLOGAN, NORTHAMPTON, 1959

Should we be dazzled by Darzi? It would be easy to be so, for Lord Darzi of Denham is a very serious and prestigious figure who clearly emphasises patient care not politics. His Final Report of the NHS Next Stage Review, *High Quality Care for All* – published on 30 June 2008 – and its companion *Our Vision for Primary and Community Care* – published on 3 July 2008 – offer the prospects of fundamentally altering the picture so that the empowered customer is at last in charge.[1]

Lord Darzi, an eminent surgeon who in 2007 was ennobled and then appointed as a Parliamentary Under Secretary of State, has created an important report of the first rank which clearly focuses on many key aspects of care improvement. He has certainly significantly shifted the focus of concern to essentials. There is a new emphasis on quality, on accountability and on individual outcomes – including taking very seriously what patients say about their experiences. The focus on compassion, cleanliness, dignity and respect is vital, too – if still rather astonishingly necessary after 60 years of the NHS and after years of unprecedented investment.

The call for publishing more appropriate and more specific information is hugely welcome. There is a more direct discussion of individual choice and empowerment than has been conventional. However, there remain two significant concerns: how are further changes and improvements to be funded – given the narrow financial base of the NHS, despite much larger funding – and what are the economic incentives and economic instruments to effect indelible change? Including much improved self-care? In this book I have tried to address these questions. My hope is that what the book says can contribute to informing discussion on how to enable the changes which Lord Darzi proposes to become real.

In launching his inevitably celebratory report at Westminster Lord Darzi said that 'For the first time, patients' own assessments of the success of their treatment and the quality of their experiences will have a direct impact on the way hospitals are funded'. The report indicates areas in which patients should achieve more control. And it endorses some key economic principles, albeit on a limited basis. It introduces financial incentives for providers to respond. It says, too, that clinical incomes should be influenced by clinical activity and quality indicators. This is an enormous change, both of tone and content. There will also be new 'best practice tariffs', to encourage improvements. There is to be a new Commissioning for Quality and Innovation scheme 'to increase the influence that patients have over NHS resources.' What 'influence' will mean is at the core of the debate. There will be a new Quality Observatory in every NHS region to inform local improvement efforts. 'New funds and prizes' will be offered to innovators. Commissioners will also be expected to pay for improved outcomes. But these gains, I suggest, cannot be achieved by putting in place more complex structures and bureaucracies. We need markets which can demonstrably achieve these changes more directly, more simply, more surely and more adaptively.

In his Preface to *High Quality Care for All* the Prime Minister wrote that 'We need a more personalised NHS, responsive to each of us as individuals, focused on prevention, better equipped to keep us healthy and capable of giving us real control and real choices over our care and our lives.' These are important issues, and leadership here is very welcome. The question is how to achieve this control and these choices.

Here, we should rigorously apply the tests of consumer control, of competition, and of fully informed customers. Is the individual to be financially empowered to make choices? Are the medical professions to be empowered to respond in a new rapprochement in a market? We should assess in these terms what is being offered, whether it will work, and what still needs to be done. When the NHS publishes its new Operating Framework in October 2008 we should again interrogate it too in these terms.

The reader who has stayed with me thus far might ask:

1   Does the new vision pass individual financial empowerment to the individual?

No. It does not do so for all services. It proposes to extend personal budgets, but it still does not go far enough. The report says that 'The budget itself may well be held on the patient's behalf, but we will pilot direct payments where this makes most sense for particular patients in certain circumstances.' This is very tentative language. Who decides who decides?

Instead of the comprehensive adoption of direct payments based on existing pilots, we have another pilot. Here, 5000 individuals and families with long-term medical conditions such as diabetes, multiple sclerosis, motor neurone disease, and asthma will be given personal health budgets to give them greater control over the care they receive – 'with a view to a national roll-out'. In addition, all 15 million patients with long-term conditions will receive personal care plans – as NHS Yorkshire and Humberside urged in its *Healthier Ambitions* report in May 2008. But if the financial incentive principle is right, why not extend it into every nook and cranny of health and social care now? We have already seen the significant gains in social care from the pilots in personal budgets. The argument is not now about principles. It is about timing. Lord Darzi was reported as himself wanting a more immediate commitment to personal budgets for all chronic sufferers, but he was it seems curtailed by the Department of Health and No. 10. How long can such a line be held?[2]

2   Do the two reports create competing purchasing bodies?

Do purchasers have to seek the willing revenues from individual holders of health savings accounts? No. They do not. Notably, PCT monopolies – which are state created cartels – remain undisturbed, even if patients have the right to choose their GP. *Our Vision for Primary and Community Care* recognises that despite many positive experiences 'there is clear evidence that some services fall a long way short of the best' and that 'People want more control of their health and care.' But the necessary incentives for primary care practitioners to respond to customer power are not there yet.

3   Does Darzi introduce sufficiently powerful incentives for both purchasers and providers to be more effective by making local choices in response to financially-empowered customers?

No. It does not. Indeed, the report follows on nine regional reports – *Our Visions* – by Strategic Health Authorities which are incessantly prescriptive. The final Darzi report introduces some financial incentives, however. From 2010 onwards, NHS Trusts – with an average district general hospital now having an annual turnover of £250m – will be paid according to the outcomes of treatment they achieve, using indicators including surgeons' death rates. These have been already successfully pioneered by cardiac surgeons, as we saw earlier. There will also be surveys on how well patients feel after treatments. These are valuable gains. But we must hope for a much more extensive application of these incentives, and on a much larger scale. Initially, some £7m to £9m in bonuses will be paid to the best healthcare units and GP practices. This would be 3 to 4% of an average district general hospital budget. These are, however, relatively small sums. If the principle is right, why not enable the *entire* budgets of *all* units to be open to challenge? Why not pass the power to the consumer and to the consumer's representative in a mutual and competing patient guaranteed care association? The incremental financial impact – and its legitimacy – would then be a consequence of purchasers making decisions, on behalf of their members whose willing support they must seek.

4   Does Darzi tackle the problem of unexpected variations?

It begins to do so in a serious way. A list of 'never events' will be drawn up by the National Patient Safety Agency, which will include mistakes that were largely preventable. Hospitals will not be paid for botched operations and catastrophic medical errors. The financial impact needs to be on a scale that bites for the poor provider, for the inadequate purchaser, and for the GP who hospital staffs know often refers people too late, who is inconsistent in diagnostic skills and is inadequate in the use of appropriate treatments. The local purchaser should be empowered by their willing members to remove business on a larger scale. On clinical quality itself I continue to urge that Dr William Pickering's proposals concerning a medical inspectorate be re-visited. Meanwhile, what will happen to the surgeon to whom local doctors know they would not send their daughter? And will failing hospital services close? Or be involved in serious re-training and detailed review? Will the proposed incentives be sufficient to genuinely shift sufficient funding from the poor service and thus free up funding to reward the good? This seems unlikely, unless the sums involved are much much larger, and are the result of the cumulative decisions of individual, financially-empowered customers in a market.

5   Does Darzi achieve the full de-regulation of supply?

No. It does not. However, the private sector will be enabled to bid to manage 150 new polyclinics. Community nurses and others employed by PCTs will be encouraged to set up not-for-profit companies, under the social enterprise flag. But the full de-regulation of supply would only be the necessary consequence of fully empowered consumer decision making. For then the power to control such changes by politics would pass out of the hands of government. On 27 June 2008 Mr Gordon Brown said that he wanted to build on 'the success of the foundation trust model in the NHS' and create a 'growing role for independent public service providers, voluntary organisations and social enterprises' in the provision of public services. We still need strong incentives for this.[3]

6   Do the two reports introduce financial incentives to self-care –
     and thus directly impact on the crisis of chronic care and on the
     accumulating problems of obesity, alcoholism, drug addiction, mental
     healthcare and hazards to sexual health?

No. They do not. There are no tangible incentives to persuade people to re-consider their lifestyle, to do much more to avoid self-imposed disease and to invest in the prevention of ill health. Yet this is one of the most critical of all of the pivots for change, as the Darzi report emphasises. As long ago as 1889 the pioneering social investigator Charles Booth wrote of the dangers of people being 'divorced from the sense of responsibility which arises naturally from living in the reflected light of our past actions and pursued by their consequences.'[4] Lord Darzi's report is weaker than this famous comment. He reminds patients of their 'responsibilities' but with no incentives to do something more directly about these. Instead, there will be a new Coalition for Better Health to try to persuade you to eat more healthy food and take more exercise. From 2009, too, three million people a year aged between 40 to 74 will be invited to take a free blood test to check whether they are at risk from one of the big killers – heart diseases, stroke and diabetes. There will also be a 'Reduce Your Risk' campaign. These initiatives may have some impact. But past experience is not encouraging.

7   Does Darzi create a Disclosure and Information Commission, to
     publish audited information to guide consumer decisions?

No. It does not. It proposes a National Quality Board, to advise government and publish annual reports on standards of care in England. The Care Quality Commission will compare the performance of NHS units. This is a beginning, but the role of information gathering, audit and disclosure should be for an entirely independent body with no other governmental responsibilities. As to economic consequences, thus far Darzi does not propose issuing the detailed information on individual performance which we want and which will fully inform patients and influence individual incomes. There is no proposed link of new knowledge to individual financial clout. From April 2010 all NHS bodies will be required by law to publish 'Quality Accounts', which set out the quality of care they are providing. How specific will this be? How will people then be able to decide who decides? Information and economic power are necessarily intertwined. Thus far they remain separated.

8   Does an NHS constitution ensure that every user of services will be
     able to reliably access a personal, intimate, timely service?

No. It cannot. It will enshrine a patient's right to an approved treatment where they want to be treated. But it will not achieve the certainty of service which is necessary for the individual. Economic power will not be placed in individual hands to ensure the delivery of expectations. For this, we need genuine customer power and competing patient guaranteed care associations.

9   Does Darzi give patients the right to choose their surgeon and their
     GP, and then empower patients with economic instruments?

It does the first, but not the second. It offers 'a fairer funding system, ensuring better rewards for GPs who provide responsive, accessible and high quality outcomes.' But this funding will not be achieved by competing purchasers and by the incremental economic effects of individual financially-empowered decision making by the users of services. People will be guided by information on survival rates, length of stay in hospital, the frequency of re-admission, the incidence of hospital-acquired diseases, and patient satisfaction ratings. However, PCTs – in which most of the hope for change is invested by Darzi – will remain large local monopolies, directly funded by government. They will not need to compete for individual tax-based funds held by customers, who can then decide what they think about the information published and the competence of the purchaser. Nor is the contestability of large hospital Trust managements offered. The impact of information on the decisions made by individual patients and by PCTs on providers will very likely remain limited.

10   Does Darzi re-consider the funding of health and social care, with incentives to consume thoughtfully and to save for the personal future?

No. It does not. It summarises the changing nature of care, but it does not address the narrowness of the funding base. It speaks of rising expectations, demand driven by demographics, the continuing development of the 'information society', advances in treatment, and changing expectations. However, the budget for the NHS is effectively frozen until 2011. Meanwhile, cost pressures intensify, as do opportunities for improved care. As we have seen, there are many new drugs for cancer care, for example, which people will demand. The funding of social care remains the subject of a separate enquiry, and anxiety. Yet, as *The Times* pointed out in a first leader, 'Healthcare inflation, meanwhile, is likely to shadow the rate in the United States, where it is already double the underlying rate and projected to accelerate for at least a decade. Here as in the US, healthcare costs are driven by demographics and medical science.'[5] The right incentives are more than ever vital. As is the full reconsideration of the nature of the funding.

11   Does Lord Darzi's report solve 'the problem of knowledge'?

No. It cannot. It recognises the limitations of 'voice'. It speaks of 'those who for a variety of reasons find it harder to make themselves heard'. And of 'those people traditionally less likely to seek help or who find themselves discriminated against in some way.' But it offers no *economic* mechanisms by which purchasers and providers can discover what people want and are prepared to pay for, either by tax-based funds or by top-up co-payments and insurance. For this we need a properly functioning market.

12   Will the incentives be sufficient to persuade more than a million people employed in the NHS to change their ideas, attitudes, and behaviours?

It is a large ask. Lord Darzi has properly stressed that change requires 'the unlocking of the talents of frontline staff'. I have stressed, as he does, that effective change is led (or prevented) by local clinicians. I have carefully considered the necessary structural and cultural changes, including permission for change and the unrelenting incentives required. We have seen how far-reaching the changes must be if the ambitions of a modern, properly-funded, well provided service are to be achieved. The report asks for very considerable changes at work. But without sufficiently powerful economic incentives can it achieve these?

13   Does the report genuinely unleash the power of customers and of competition?

No. It does not. Lord Darzi recognises that those with least choices want more.[6] That empowered patients are more likely to take greater responsibility. And that 'Choice gives patients the power they need in the system, as NHS resources follow patients in the choices they make.' I have explored how to make this model really work. However, despite saying that 'choice should become a defining feature of the service', the report does not set in place the necessary economic instruments to achieve its ambitions. As its impact and its limitations unfold in practice then the case for these vital structural and cultural changes will become ever more insistent. It opens the door. But it does not step across the threshold.

14 What does Lord Darzi's report say or imply about the language of choice itself?

He has spoken of patients becoming customers. And that we should expect empowered choice. Lord Darzi properly emphasised the necessity of clear information on quality and on patients' experiences. In his own briefing when launching his final report Lord Darzi was reported as saying that 'wherever it is relevant, patients are able to make informed choices.' *Relevant?* When is it *not* relevant for a service user to make choices about what happens to them? Who decides who decides? We need to listen carefully, here. As Chief Inspector Montalbano observed in Andrea Camilleri's *The Patience of the Spider*: 'How did the Latin saying go? *Nec tecum nec sine te.* Neither with nor without you'. Yet there is no genuine half-way house.[7]

15 What does Lord Darzi say about end-of-life care?

On terminal care, it *is* an important new promise that the right to choose to die at home instead of in hospital should be for everyone. This is a significant change of emphasis. But very substantial and prompt investment in support staff in domiciliary care at home will now be required. Of course, a financially empowered customer could set aside part of their own health savings account with such a prospect ultimately in view.

16 Have politicians thus stood aside, to allow a market to function on behalf of the customers of care?

Not yet. But Lord Darzi has seen a new world through the key-hole. And the dynamist debate goes on.

Notes

1 Lord Darzi, *High Quality Care for All: NHS Next Stage Review final report* (London, Command Paper CM 7432, Presented to Parliament by the Secretary of State for Health, 30 June 2008) at www.ournhs.nhs.uk/ and Lord Darzi, speech, Royal Horticultural Hall, Westminster, 30 June 2008. Also, Roy Lilley, 'Darzi un-plugged, A stripped down briefing on the Darzi report', 30 June 2008, at roylilley@compuserve.com; Andrew Porter and Rebecca Smith, 'Patients given the right to choose GP as catchment areas ditched', *Daily Telegraph*, 1 July 2008, p. 4; John Carvel, 'Darzi plan offers patients more choice and more information', *The Guardian*, 1 July 2008, p. 6. Nigel Hawkes, 'Mind the gaps in promises', *The Times*, news section, 1 July 2008, p. 7; Profile, '"Robo Doc" scrubs up for radical surgery on ailing NHS', *Sunday Times*, comment section, 29 June 2008, p. 23. *NHS Next Stage Review: our vision for primary and community care* (London, Department of Health, 3 July 2008).
2 Rachel Sylvester, 'Gordon the snail finds it hard to be a whale', *The Times*, news section, 1 July 2008, p. 23.
3 Cabinet Office Strategy Unit, *Excellence and Fairness: Achieving world class public services* (London, Cabinet Office, 27 June 2008).
4 Charles Booth, *Life and Labour of The People of London. First Series: Poverty 1, East, Central and South London* (London, Williams & Norgate, 1889), p. 187.
5 First leader, 'World-Class Health Costs', *The Times*, 1 July 2008, p. 2.
6 John Appleby and Arturo Alvarez Rosete, 'The NHS: keeping up with public expectations?', in Alison Park *et al.* (eds.) *British Social Attitudes Survey 20th Report: continuity and change in two decades* (London, Sage, 2003); Julian Le Grand, *The Other Invisible Hand: delivering public services through competition and choice* (Princeton, NJ, Princeton University Press, 2007).
7 Andrea Camilleri, *The Patience of the Spider* (2004; London, Picador, 2008), translated by Stephen Sartarelli, p. 229.

Index